BIG SHOT

●

BIG SHOT

PASSION, POLITICS, AND
THE STRUGGLE FOR AN AIDS VACCINE

•

PATRICIA THOMAS

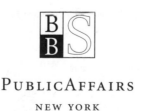

PublicAffairs
NEW YORK

BOOK DESIGN BY JENNY DOSSIN.

Library of Congress Cataloging-in-Publication data
Thomas, Patricia, journalist
Big shot: passion, politics, and the struggle for an AIDS vaccine / Patricia Thomas.
p. cm.
Includes bibliographical references and index
ISBN 1-891620-88-6
1. AIDS vaccines—Popular works. I. Title.
QR189.5.A33 T48 2001
616.97'92—dc21
2001031959

FIRST EDITION
1 3 5 7 9 10 8 6 4 2

CONTENTS

PREFACE

IN THE BEGINNING, the search for an AIDS vaccine was essentially a cottage industry. Individuals and small groups of scientists, with limited budgets and ambitious ideas, explored many different vaccine approaches in small labs dotted around the world. This was in the mid-1980s, when the human immunodeficiency virus had just been identified as the cause of this frightening and fatal new disease.

During those years, I was a young reporter living in Atlanta and writing about medicine for publications read mainly by doctors. Most of the news stories that I wrote about AIDS included a refrain that went something like this: "Because the disease is fatal and there is no treatment, a preventive vaccine is the only real hope against the epidemic." Nearly twenty years later, treatments are available—mostly for insured people in wealthy countries—but still no vaccine has proved that it can keep anyone in the world safe from AIDS.

Treatments moved faster than vaccines for a variety of scientific, social, and economic reasons. The AIDS virus was identified in early 1984, and within a year scientists had figured out how to determine whether a given chemical could kill it in a test tube. This opened the door to drug discovery by enabling major pharmaceutical companies to sort through their vast chemical libraries, pick out compounds that might have virus-killing potential, and test them in the lab. The most promising of these were rushed into clinical trials, and by the end of 1985, about a half dozen were being given to small numbers of volunteers.

Clinical testing expanded in response to top activists, who demanded that the government and industry go all out to help the soaring numbers of people who were dying terrible, highly publicized deaths from AIDS. Not only was AIDS a genuine public health emergency, but pharmaceutical companies could see that these treatments would be a very lucrative business. And because the disease itself was so frightening and lethal, they surmised that patients would tolerate toxic side effects if a medication helped keep them alive. AZT, the first antiviral drug against AIDS, was approved in 1987, even though it was only partly effective and was plagued by adverse effects. Other drugs followed, although not until 1996 did researchers show the superiority of a multidrug "cocktail" built around a new class of drugs called protease inhibitors. The hoopla surrounding this good news persuaded many people that AIDS has become just another chronic disease, as manageable as high blood pressure.

While it would be comforting to think that AIDS is a thing of the past, clearly this is not true. The World Health Organization (WHO) estimates that 36.1 million people are infected with HIV. Every day, nearly 15,000 previously healthy men, women, and children contract the virus—a figure that is soaring as the disease gathers momentum in China and India, the world's most populous nations. In South Africa, one in four adults already carries HIV. The spread of AIDS is fueled by poverty, inequality, and instability, both political and economic. Most of its victims are poor people who live in developing countries where HIV infection goes undetected until they come down with the terrible symptoms of AIDS—and by then they have inadvertently infected their loved ones. Once they do become sick, more than 95 percent of the world's AIDS patients will die without ever being treated with the antiviral drugs that have made life so much better, and longer, for infected people in the industrialized world.

Although international political pressure has recently caused some pharmaceutical companies to cut the price of anti-HIV drugs in the developing world, most public-health authorities admit that this is "too little, too late." The global AIDS pandemic is not going to slow—much less stop—until we have a safe, effective, affordable vaccine.

Unfortunately, vaccines are not to be found in the storerooms of drug manufacturers. A vaccine is a biological product, not a chemical, and each vaccine must be custom-made to protect against a specific disease. Even though there are many different strategies for designing vaccines, scientists realized early on that protecting healthy people against HIV was going to be very difficult indeed.

When I set out to chronicle the search for an AIDS vaccine in early 1997, I expected to find a classic struggle between scientific ingenuity and an exceptionally wily microbe. But I was in for a surprise. Although the scientific challenges involved in making this particular vaccine are immense, I soon learned that this alone does not account for the absence of a vaccine. Social attitudes toward AIDS, careerism and timidity among bureaucrats, and corporate anxieties about profits and liability have all been roadblocks to vaccine research and development. Far from being a top priority for the scientific and industrial establishment, HIV vaccine research has been a kind of low-prestige backwater that never, until very recently, claimed more than 10 percent of federal spending on AIDS.

Still, hundreds of scientists in dozens of laboratories around the world have worked on vaccines over the past two decades; many more have made scientific discoveries that have advanced the quest, even though they set out to explore seemingly unrelated questions. This account focuses on a subset of scientists, corporate executives, and civilian and military officials whose complex motivations best illustrate the triumphs, and the frustrations, of this long and complicated quest. Some of them are heroes; some are not.

I

THE AGE OF DISCOVERY

April 1984–March 1994

●

I

WHISTLING PAST THE GRAVEYARD

PAUL LUCIW WAS ALONE in his lab at Chiron Corporation in Emeryville, California, on an August evening in 1984. Rush-hour traffic on the nearby Nimitz Freeway had fallen to a dull rumble, the technicians had gone home, and Paul relished the chance to work without interruptions. Then the call came from Kathy Steimer, his closest colleague at the company. "Paul, I've got a problem," she said. "The ultracentrifuge has stopped."

He could picture exactly where she was, all alone in a spooky P3 containment facility—a place where dangerous microbes could be handled in an isolated, specially ventilated room. This lab, a part of the Navy Biosciences Laboratory (NBL), was less than two miles from Chiron. All summer, Paul and Kathy had been loading the huge, heavy ultracentrifuge with samples of virus that doctors had isolated from AIDS patients in San Francisco. Like other teams of scientists in the United States and France, they were racing to unravel the genetic code of the virus and figure out how this tiny killer is organized. Scientists put a premium on this information because it could open the door to diagnostic tests, treatments, or even a vaccine.

When Kathy called, Paul's first thought was that the ultracentrifuge had thumped and bumped itself off balance like an overloaded washing machine, wreaking havoc with its contents while whirling at up to 20,000 revolutions per minute. If this had happened, whoever lifted the lid would find a jumble of metal racks and broken glassware coated with deadly viral goo.

Fortunately, Kathy reassured him, the situation wasn't as serious as that. The ultracentrifuge had simply ground to a halt while she was running a large preparation of virus. What troubled her was the prospect of filing an incident report—required any time something goes awry in a lab—with the central NBL office. Kathy and Paul had been cleared to work in the lab only because a navy researcher, who happened to be an old friend of Chiron's CEO, had lent surplus lab space to the company three months earlier. This made it possible for the fledgling biotech to work on the AIDS virus; at this point, the company hadn't finished building a place where dangerous organisms could be safely handled. As guests of a military facility, working on a virus that terrified most people, the Chiron scientists had kept their heads down.

As soon as Kathy finished talking to Paul, who agreed they had to reveal what microbe was in the broken centrifuge, she called the duty officer for the Biosciences Lab. He immediately notified the commanding officer of the Oakland Naval Depot, where the laboratory was located, to report that there had been an accident with the AIDS virus on the base. The irate commander demanded to see Kathy in his office that very night—not in the morning, but ASAP.

If the base commander was so bent out of shape, what would happen to the viral cultures that she had spent all summer cajoling into lush growth? For all she knew, a hazardous-waste disposal team was already hurtling in her direction, with instructions to confiscate the precious flasks. In a second quick phone consult, Kathy and Paul agreed that it made no sense to wait and see. Within minutes Paul was on his bike, pedaling furiously from Chiron's headquarters in Emeryville, a down-at-the-heels industrial suburb of Oakland, to the navy base. Paul was a short man, only a few inches over five feet tall, but fit in the way of one who shuns cars and walks or bikes wherever he goes.

Once at the Naval Depot, Paul showed his security pass to the armed guards at the gates and pedaled on to the P3 building, a forlorn structure near the base's edge. In the entry chamber, he stripped off his jeans and T-shirt and tossed them into a locker, pulling on a cotton scrub suit, gown, mask, booties, and latex gloves.

As soon as Paul stepped into the ill-lit hallway, lined with derelict freezers and obsolete lab equipment, he began to sweat. His reaction was the same every time he saw the labels on the closed doors of individual labs. The hallway was a rogues' gallery of pestilence: plague, anthrax, slow viruses that eat the brain. God knows what scourges had been handled in this old building and by whom. The only room in use now, however, was the one where he and Kathy had labored fourteen hours a day, six or seven days a week, since May. All that time and they had never seen another person in the corridor.

Kathy had removed the contents of the ultracentrifuge and had lined up the T-150 flasks on the bench. Each contained about one cup of cloudy viral broth, and she was tightening the tops and wrapping them in tape. Working swiftly, the two identically dressed scientists put each flask into a plastic bag, sealed it, then bagged it again. Finally, they loaded the flasks into some of the thick Styrofoam shipping boxes that accumulate in biology labs like coat hangers in a closet. These they sealed with broad strips of plastic shipping tape. The goal was to move the cultures to the small biosafety level-3 room that Chiron had completed only a few weeks earlier. Clearly, they'd have to transport the boxes of virus in Kathy's car, but leaving through the front gate would be too risky: It was now late in the evening, and the guards would surely suspect these civilians of stealing government property. A stealthier departure would be better.

Soon Kathy traded her sterile garb for street clothes, retrieved her car from the nearby lot, and signed out at the guardhouse. A couple of quick turns put her on a service road that hugged the outside of the navy's tall chain-link fence topped with concertina wire. She rolled slowly through the bright pools of the tall security lights, finally dousing the headlights and stopping in a dark patch only twenty yards from the back door of the lab building. She slipped out of the car, taking care not to slam the door.

Paul had been watching, and within seconds he emerged from the lab, looking nervously for the armed sentries who patrolled the base at night. He listened for the crunch of tires but heard only the low whiz of light traffic on the freeway. The air was brackish with the smell of the nearby mudflats of San Francisco Bay. With a box tucked under each arm, he hurried back and forth from the door to the fence until all the shipping containers were out.

Kathy and Paul each took a few steps back from the fence. She was the taller of the two by half a foot, a rangy, flaxen-haired California girl. He was smaller and darker, and his spectacles glinted in the darkness They exchanged furtive whispers and a signal nod before Paul gently lofted the first box, like a square and fragile beach ball, over the fence to Kathy's waiting arms. One by one, she received them. Less than an hour later, all Kathy's precious flasks filled with the AIDS virus were safe on the Chiron campus.

She returned to the Oakland Navy Depot alone to meet with the base commander. He was not a scientist, so Kathy explained calmly and carefully that although a machine had malfunctioned, no deadly organisms had been spilled and nothing had been contaminated. She also explained that she and Paul had been authorized to use the containment facility by the navy scientist in charge of it. The commander did not care what had happened or how it came to be. Only the future interested him. The AIDS virus, he told Kathy, was not the kind of problem he was going to have on his base.

●

In 1981, the same year that doctors in Los Angeles and San Francisco began reporting puzzling and rapidly fatal illnesses among young gay men, the fledgling Chiron Corporation made history by inventing a new kind of vaccine against hepatitis B. Some cases of this viral infection were chronic, untreatable, and ultimately fatal. And like AIDS, it was commonplace among homosexual men and posed a threat to transfusion recipients and health-care workers who handled human blood.

Chiron's founders, William Rutter and Edward Penhoet, were academic biochemists at the University of California campuses in San Francisco and Berkeley, respectively. Both were experts on hepatitis B and other viruses that prey on people. More important, they were charter members of a small club of genetic engineers. They practiced recombinant DNA technology, which basically meant snipping genetic material out of one organism, inserting it into a different organism, and tricking the host into expressing it: churning out the protein specified by the newly transferred DNA. This enabled them to make a large amount of whatever protein they chose, which might hold promise as a preventive vaccine, a treatment, or a laboratory tool.

On Easter Sunday of 1981, Rutter and Penhoet wrote out a wish list of products that their new company might make using recombinant DNA technology. Their goal was not only to solve some real biological mysteries but also to use genetic engineering to improve human health. At the top of their list were vaccines to prevent hepatitis B, herpes, and influenza, as well as tests that could be used to check blood samples for two types of hepatitis—B and the mysterious, newer kind known as "non-A, non-B" (since shown to be several distinct viruses, including hepatitis C).

Rutter's lab at UC–San Francisco had already studied the hepatitis B virus in great detail. At the time Chiron was founded, the East Coast pharmaceutical giant Merck was actively seeking a replacement for its current hepatitis B vaccine, which used a protein derived from the blood of hepatitis B carriers. Making vaccine this way was not only expensive, but the process was also vulnerable to contamination with other blood-borne viruses—including the scary new pathogen responsible for AIDS. Merck wanted a new kind of vaccine that would cost less to make, could be manufactured in a laboratory, and would be free of contamination. This was a tall order, however, and the best ideas for such a product were being nurtured in young biotech companies or in academic labs. Merck invested in several groups racing for the same goal, and one of them was Chiron.

Chiron's main rivals were hotshot researchers at Genentech, the San Francisco Bay Area's preeminent biotechnology company, and a group of Rutter's former collaborators at the University of Washington in Seattle. But it was Chiron's Pablo Valenzuela who got there first. He figured out how to use recombinant DNA technology to make the hepatitis B vaccine of Merck's dreams.

From hepatitis B virus, Valenzuela removed DNA that coded for a protein on the outside of the virus called HBsAg, short for "hepatitis B surface antigen." Then he inserted the DNA into yeast cells, which are cheap and easy to grow, and voilà! The yeast cells cranked out HBsAg that looked like the protein Merck had been laboriously isolating from blood.

This genetically engineered version could be made safely, without any blood or virus involved. By Christmas, tiny Chiron had outdistanced its competitors and licensed this process to Merck. This precedent-setting vaccine, approved for sale by the Food and Drug Administration (FDA) in 1986, does an excellent job of preventing hepatitis B and is used around the world.

●

All vaccines accomplish the same thing: Like a self-defense instructor impersonating a mugger, the vaccine teaches the immune system what to do in an emergency. When a real thug appears, the lesson is recalled and a swift immune response immediately overpowers the attacker. Most traditional vaccines consist of disease-producing organisms that have been altered or killed; the Sabin polio vaccine is made from live attenuated (weakened) virus, for example, whereas the Salk formulation consists of killed organisms. Sometimes nature supplies a vaccine: Credit for eradicating smallpox goes to vaccinia, a pox virus that originally infected cows but in humans evokes a protective immune response to smallpox without causing any harm. Today, recombinant DNA technology offers a wondrous alternative, a wholly new generation of vaccines that are safer and cheaper to make than old-fashioned ones.

The first step toward building a genetically engineered vaccine is to identify an antigen that is always part of the attacking virus. Antigens are simply molecules, usually proteins, that the immune system recognizes as a threat and takes steps to eliminate. Finding the right antigen, as it turns out, can be an enormous challenge.

●

Pablo Valenzuela's hepatitis B vaccine was a cosmic home run for Chiron. Suddenly, anything seemed possible. In order to keep the company's streak going, Bill Rutter and Ed Penhoet drew up lists of scientists they wanted to hire, and most said yes when they were asked. "We were looking for people with a high energy level, dedicated to their work, and who wanted to make a difference," Penhoet recalls. In 1981, the scientists who joined Chiron and other biotech start-ups were turning their backs on stodgy academic tradition and offending many of their mentors.

During the late 1970s, the world of biology was split over the legitimacy of patenting discoveries made in the course of tax-supported research. Old-guard academic scientists saw university-based research as a gentleman's game and looked down their noses at scientists who went into trade by joining a biotechnology company. Today, when professors at elite universities and medical schools race to patent discoveries as soon as they are made, this snobbishness seems as outmoded as the idea that all telephones must have cords. But this attitude was entirely real in 1981. "So we put people on our list that we thought we could actually recruit, and they were all young people," Penhoet recalls.

Virologist Paul Luciw (pronounced "loo-shoo") was thirty-three when he joined Chiron in July 1982. He had just completed postdoctoral training in a UCSF lab whose leaders would win the Nobel Prize seven years later. Rutter, Penhoet, and Valenzuela were a tremendous lure for Paul. Not only were they respected as top-notch scientists, but "they were adventurous, broad in their thinking, yet able to define goals and get things done," he says.

Hiring Paul was a smart move for Chiron because he was an expert on retroviruses—bizarre little organisms that were just beginning to seem relevant to human health. Although doctors weren't worried about retroviruses in the pre-AIDS era, veterinarians were all too familiar with the damage these unusual organisms caused. Feline leukemia virus, known as FeLV, caused many thousands of fatal cancers in domestic cats. There would be a lucrative market for a vaccine against FeLV, and this was Paul's first project at Chiron. He explored two possible approaches at once. One was a classic vaccine strategy, in which protection would come from immunization with a weakened version of FeLV itself. The other, and far more exciting, idea would be to mimic the recombinant hepatitis B vaccine—splicing FeLV genes into yeast cells, so that these cells turn into vaccine factories.

Kathy Steimer had just turned thirty-four when she decided to write to Pablo Valenzuela and ask for a job at Chiron. She and Martin Wilson, a young neuroscience professor she had been dating during the previous year, drafted the letter beside a swimming pool in Davis, California. They had been introduced the previous Christmas by a mutual friend and had since become inseparable. Their lives had begun quite differently, with Kathy growing up as the daughter of a firefighter in Los Angeles, and Martin in a cultured British household where he was immersed in classical music. Both families valued education, however, and each produced a scientist absorbed in the challenges, frustrations, and satisfactions of laboratory research. In addition to falling in love, Kathy and Martin gave each other tremendous professional support. So it was natural for Martin to help her write a job-hunting letter to Chiron.

Like Paul, Kathy was a skilled retrovirologist. Earlier, she had left a biotech company because she was impatient with managerial incompetence, then moved to an immunology postdoc at Stanford, where she grew tired of being patronized by male physicians who were sure they were smarter than any woman with a Ph.D. At this point in her career, Kathy wanted to be respected for who she was and what she knew. During her first biotech job, she'd worked next door to Chiron and had seen Rutter, Penhoet, and Valenzuela in action. Observation told her that they were the kind of people she wanted as colleagues.

The feeling was mutual, and Chiron needed a scientist with exactly Kathy's strengths. An earlier postdoctoral stint at a famous Harvard lab specializing in growth factors—natural substances that signal cells to grow or divide—had made her an artist when it came to growing temperamental cells. At Stanford, which had not been a happy experience on a personal level, Kathy had worked on the cutting edge of immunology. In Chiron's view, she was exquisitely prepared to create new assays for determining how the human immune system responds to experimental vaccines.

Kathy started at Chiron in September 1983. She promptly devised several methods for detecting viruses that proved useful for research purposes, had less success with a crotchety system for automating certain lab tests, and figured out how to synthesize interleukin-2, usually called IL-2, a cell growth factor that was fun to tinker with in the laboratory but didn't appear to have any immediate medical value.

Two months after Kathy started work at Chiron, a thirty-one-year-old molecular biologist named Nancy Haigwood came to the company from another, less-successful biotech in Maryland. At this point there were biotech start-ups on every corner, but in Nancy's mind, Chiron and Genentech were the only two destined for success. A military brat, Nancy grew up on overseas bases where cholera, yellow fever, and the like were commonplace. These early experiences sparked her interest in biology, and in human disease in particular. She joined a biotech company immediately after her postdoc at Johns Hopkins, feeling that the private sector was the place to be if you wanted to develop products that helped people.

On that first job, Nancy met and married a protein chemist who also joined Chiron when she did. Nancy was ambitious, and, in her own words, "I wanted to work in a really high-powered place because I thought it would be fun." She brought important skills to the company. She was expert at site-directed mutagenesis, a technique for introducing deliberate mutations into genes. Another major interest was splicing genes into animal cells, so that they could be turned into protein factories. Although Chiron made its successful hepatitis B vaccine in yeast, some scientists believed that future vaccines should be made in mammalian cells that more closely resemble human cells.

The first generation of molecular biologists thought there was no disease they couldn't conquer, and their dreams were paid for by investors besotted with biotechnology. Dozens of other bright young scientists cast their lot with Chiron in the early 1980s, and they were backed by executives and investors brave enough to risk the time, money, and space needed to tackle major medical puzzles. But it was mainly the brains and determination of Paul, Kathy, and Nancy that enabled the company to create one of the first experimental vaccines for AIDS.

●

The *New York Times* wrote in November 1983 that AIDS cases had been identified in thirty-three countries and on every inhabited continent. By Christmas that year, epidemiologists at UC–San Francisco estimated that one of every three gay men in the city was already infected with the virus that causes AIDS. San Francisco was hit early and hard by the new epidemic, and although cases had been identified among hemophiliacs, transfusion recipients, IV drug users, and a few prostitutes, most people saw it mainly as a gay disease.

AIDS was an ugly way to die. The virus decimated the immune system, leaving the patient vulnerable to opportunistic infections by microbes that aren't normally a problem for healthy people. AIDS patients were disfigured by the purple lesions of Kaposi's sarcoma, wasted by intractable diarrhea, and suffocated by a vicious pneumonia. Microbes swarmed into every orifice; mouths turned mossy with yeast infections and bowels were lacerated by bacteria. Some patients went mad with dementia as malignant lesions swelled in their brains. Doctors prescribed antimicrobial drugs for opportunistic infections, but this was like trying to halt a locomotive with bare hands.

Rutter and Penhoet and their scientists knew about all this. Part of Chiron's business strategy was to maintain close working relationships with UC–San Francisco and UC–Berkeley, where they still had strong ties. The human catastrophe of AIDS was all too evident at UCSF and its crosstown teaching hospital, San Francisco General, which was on the front line of the epidemic. Many of the previously healthy young men who were dying of AIDS were the same people who had earlier been infected with hepatitis B. And this, after all, was the disease that had already made Chiron famous.

Although it would be romantic to think that scientists throw themselves at a new infectious scourge because it vexes their curiosity or stirs pity and terror in their hearts, that isn't how it works. In fact, researchers tackle problems that they believe they are equipped to solve. Rutter and Penhoet figured that they had at least some of the tools needed to study whatever virus might be causing AIDS. At the very least, Chiron might come up with a blood test that could confirm the diagnosis in patients or screen donated blood for signs of virus. The company already had a test for detecting hepatitis B in donor blood, and if it also had a similar one for AIDS, it could package the two and sell the product to blood banks. More important, detailed knowledge of the hepatitis B virus was what enabled Chiron to make the world's first genetically engineered vaccine. If Chiron put its best scientists to work on the AIDS virus, who could say? Back-to-back homers are not unheard of.

●

In 1983, the French researcher Luc Montagnier and Robert Gallo of the National Cancer Institute each reported that he had isolated retroviruses from patients sick with AIDS. Montagnier called his virus LAV, for lymphadenopathy-associated virus. Doctors had noticed that many of their gay male patients suffered lymphadenopathy—chronically swollen lymph nodes—before they developed symptoms of AIDS; Montagnier isolated his virus from some of these patients' lymphoid tissue. Gallo dubbed his virus HTLV-III, because he believed it was the third in a family of what he called "human T-cell leukemia viruses."

Hard on their heels was UCSF virologist Jay Levy, who had also isolated a retrovirus from AIDS patients in San Francisco. He called his ARV, for "AIDS-associated retrovirus." Were these three viruses the same, or were three different viruses on the loose? No one knew. Nor was it clear whether any of them actually caused AIDS, or whether they were among the many pathogens that overwhelmed patients left defenseless by immune-system collapse. These were tough questions that Levy needed collaborators to answer. Not only that, but if the answers were going to make a difference, he needed ties to a company that could convert new findings into clinically useful products. In April 1984, Levy began sending Chiron samples of virus that he had collected from AIDS patients.

●

In addition to the impeccable UCSF pedigrees of Chiron's top guns, this small biotech had three bona fide retrovirologists among its several dozen employees—Dino Dina, head of the vaccine division, Paul Luciw, and Kathy Steimer. Their expertise was crucial because retroviruses are not like other living things, even other viruses.

Most life forms store their genetic code as DNA. When a plant or animal cell divides, this DNA is transcribed into RNA, which in turn tells parts of the cell how to make proteins. These proteins enable living organisms to go about their business. If the human body were a large hotel, proteins would be its bricks and mortar, its plumbing system and telephone wiring, the furnace in the basement, and the stove in the kitchen—even the housekeeping staff that keeps order and hauls out the trash.

The DNA packaged into the nucleus of every cell is the master plan for building and running the hotel. Different types of cells follow different parts of that plan, communicated to them in the form of RNA, and like subcontractors, they follow their specific set of instructions. Some build walls; some install communication systems; others move raw materials from one place to another. Each separate part of these jobs is a protein.

The DNA-makes-RNA-makes-protein pattern also holds true for most viruses. What sets viruses apart from other organisms, however, is that they can't manufacture proteins on their own. So, in order to accomplish this, their DNA must invade another creature's cells and commandeer its subcontractors to churn out more virus. Retroviruses have an even stranger way of perpetuating themselves. Because retroviruses use RNA as their genetic blueprint instead of DNA, they require an extra step not needed by other viruses: A retrovirus uses an enzyme called reverse transcriptase to translate its RNA into DNA. That DNA slips into the genetic code of the infected cell, where it is turned into RNA instructions that direct the cell to make proteins the virus needs to reproduce.

The first hint that retroviruses might be medically important came in the early 1970s, when one of these contrarian viruses was discovered to cause cancer in chickens. Links to leukemia in cats, cows, and other animals soon followed. While it made sense to suspect that retroviruses might also cause cancer in humans, this connection was so difficult to uncover that tired, increasingly cynical researchers called them "human rumor viruses." The jokes were silenced in 1980, when Gallo demonstrated that a retrovirus could cause human T-cell leukemia. Soon afterward, he linked a related virus to hairy cell leukemia. Gallo called these retroviruses HTLV-I and HTLV-II.

Young retrovirologists like Kathy and Paul grew up with these discoveries and couldn't wait to get their hands on the AIDS virus. The leukemias caused by HTLV-I and -II claimed a few hundred lives each year. The human toll of AIDS was already far greater: In 1980 it had been unknown, but by 1984, there were more than 200,000 infections in the United States and more than 1 million worldwide. Fears about personal risk took a backseat to their overwhelming sense that this was the biggest challenge of their careers. The stakes were high for Kathy and Paul, and unlike Gallo and other established scientists, who now spent most of their time at desks, these passionate young researchers were willing to spend long hours at the lab bench.

Which is exactly what Chiron wanted them to do. Bill Rutter, in particular, felt that it was important for Chiron to analyze the virus and generate data that could be patented—paving the way to diagnostic tests and vaccines that Chiron would own. Down the road, when detailed knowledge of the virus had been transformed into marketable products, Rutter wanted his company to be collecting royalties, not paying them to someone else.

Although Chiron had skilled virologists, it didn't have a safe place to work with anything as lethal as the AIDS virus. Fortunately, the company was able to borrow an unused navy P3 lab, which had the isolation barriers and special ventilation needed to contain dangerous pathogens. The Chiron team brought in some new equipment and supplies, turning the old lab into command central for the AIDS project. They set to work on samples of the virus that Jay Levy called ARV, collected from patients in San Francisco and driven across the Bay Bridge in sealed containers.

By May, Kathy and Paul had made an important scientific decision of their own. They decided to study patient samples from a second source, the medical pathology department at the University of California Davis, located ninety minutes away near Sacramento. Although Levy was certain that his virus was indeed the cause of AIDS, Kathy and Paul had been taught to assume nothing. If they studied the virus only in the same group of patients where it had originally been found, they would know only that it occurred in those patients. More patient samples, obtained from an independent source in a different locale, would be essential if they were going to make judgments about the true importance of ARV. The more places it turned up, the more likely it was to be the true cause of the disease.

Paul's most important job was to clone the virus's entire genetic code and to determine the exact sequence of the chemical "letters" that make up the code. Outside of science fiction, most people had never heard of cloning until Dolly the sheep made her debut in 1996. Actually the term has a longer history and broader meaning than the recent interest in copying farm animals. In molecular biology, "clones" are genetically identical copies of a gene, cell, or organism. Cloning a viral genome—meaning its

entire genetic code—involves cutting the genome into pieces and inserting those pieces into a biological system that churns out millions of identical copies. A virus that has been isolated from blood can't be patented;
one that has been cloned and sequenced can be. That's why Paul's work
was so important to Chiron. Kathy's project was also crucial, because her
task was to invent a test that could be used to screen human blood for antibodies to the AIDS virus. The government had already announced that an
antibody test was its top priority for fighting the epidemic, and Chiron
expected this to be its first AIDS-related commercial product.

●

The AIDS virus is the ultimate example of a creature that bites the
hand that feeds it. It penetrates T4 lymphocytes, certain white blood cells
that are essential for a healthy immune system. Once the virus is inside, it
hijacks the T4 cell's machinery to make more of itself. By doing so, the
AIDS virus damages and eventually destroys its host. Sometimes a T4 cell
is killed when millions of virions (baby viruses) explode its membrane
like the skin of an overripe tomato. Other T4 cells expire less dramatically,
when their own metabolic machinery is choked to a halt by wads of viral
genetic material and proteins.

Not only did the AIDS virus's relentless destruction of T4 cells kill
patients, but it was also a major headache for every scientist who tried to
grow it. Whether the setting was Paris, the National Cancer Institute, or
Chiron's improvised lab on the navy base, cultures died as the virus gob-
bled up all the cells in a closed test tube or flask. There was immense pressure to grow great quantities of virus as fast as possible, and the biologists
held their secrets as closely as wine makers.

Unlike the experiments that many people remember doing in high
school or college, where success hinges on little more than the ability to
follow directions, Kathy and Paul had no lab manual to follow. Swaddled
in sterile garb from head to toe, they worked alone in the navy isolation
facility. Paul's cultures were in T-75 flasks, each holding about one-half
cup of material; Kathy worked in T-150 flasks twice that size.

They moved slowly, carefully, like dancers, not wanting to break or spill
anything or even to breathe the air that was released when they pulled the

stopper out of a flask. "Kathy and I trusted each other," Paul would later say. "If there had been more people in the lab, there would have been the element of mistrust, of wondering whether others were being as careful as you are. That adds a lot of tension." Neither Kathy nor Paul was willing to expose Chiron lab technicians to such a dangerous microbe. In 1984, it was clear that the AIDS virus could be transmitted by blood, but virologists didn't know whether it might also be spread by aerosols—tiny infectious particles that could be breathed into the lungs. Not only that, but how could the scientists tell technicians what to do when they were improvising every move?

Kathy and Paul fed the cultures with biologic broths that they hoped would nourish the T cells and keep the virus growing. They added dribs and drabs of this and that: chemicals called growth factors, which stimulate cells, and chemicals called cytokines, which cells use to communicate among themselves. They used different T cell lines—some they'd purchased from a biological supply company, some they'd gotten from Jay Levy. For more than a month, they couldn't get a culture established no matter what they did. When they talked, it was about what to try next. Finally, in early June, all their conscientious tinkering paid off: The virus grew happily in a T cell line that had come from Levy.

Now Kathy and Paul were excited and spent more time in the lab than ever. Martin Wilson, who later became Kathy's husband, remembers that a typical Saturday night date during this period involved going with Kathy to the eerily deserted navy containment facility, suiting up in scrubs, and watching Kathy pour supernatant, the liquid from the flasks, into containers that she spun in the centrifuge. "It scared the shit out of me. I always thought, give me one little bit of aerosol here, and who knows what can happen?" Martin said.

On the small television in the corner of the navy lab, the games of the Twenty-third Olympiad played out as Kathy and Paul cultivated increasing quantities of the AIDS virus and began experimenting with it. Most of the time they were intensely busy. But sometimes they were forced to wait while the centrifuge spun or the electrophoresis gels worked their magic. In these small boxes of translucent gelatin, droplets of liquid were lined up like sprinters in the starting blocks. Drawn from one end of the box to the other by the invisible pull of a tiny electrical current, the distance traveled by each sample told the researchers exactly what it was. These little races were slow and painstaking and had to be run again and again to make sure the results were right. Each time they looked up to see Carl Lewis winning yet another gold medal, it was a reminder that sports was gloriously simple compared to science. Or at least faster.

●

The pressure to make progress against AIDS was intense in 1984. Rutter and Penhoet could stand in their offices on the third floor of 4560 Horton Street in Emeryville and see San Francisco's skyline across the Bay. The disease was rampaging through the city's gay community, and there was a huge brouhaha about shutting down the bathhouses where men went for anonymous sex. In Atlanta, the U.S Centers for Disease Control (CDC) announced that most of the nation's hemophiliacs were already infected with the virus and that the number of cases related to blood transfusions had quadrupled in four months. There was widespread panic about AIDS in donated blood, and the National Institutes of Health (NIH) was ready to pump money into tests that blood banks could use to protect the "general population"—an unsubtle way of saying heterosexuals who didn't inject drugs.

Although Kathy and Paul had worked incredibly hard to grow the virus, when they returned to Chiron headquarters the pace was so intense that their time at the navy P3 facility seemed tranquil by comparison. The ultracentrifuge accident ended their stay in the deserted Naval Biosciences Laboratory, and now they were buffeted by noise and distractions on all sides. Chiron was housed in an old research building that had been used by Shell Oil, then abandoned in Emeryville's industrial flatlands until Chiron had dusted it off and reopened it in 1982. On one side of the long third-floor corridor were Chiron's executive and administrative offices; on the other side was a row of large open laboratories, facing not the Bay but the Berkeley Hills.

There was no air conditioning or heating in the labs, and on hot days, when the tall windows were open to catch a breeze, the air was heavy with the stench of a nearby plant where cattle were rendered into hides, fertilizer, and the like. Grit and pollution from the busy freeway feeding the

Bay Bridge settled on the lab benches and had to be constantly wiped away. The Ph.D.-level scientists and their lab technicians, many of whom were fresh out of college, wore jeans and listened to the radio while they worked. What set the techs apart was that they worked only eight hours a day.

Paul lived in a large condominium complex on the edge of San Francisco Bay, a short walk or bike ride from Chiron. He didn't have a phone in his condo because he was rarely there. Paul usually started work around 10:00 or 11:00 A.M. and left around 2:00 the following morning. Kathy and Paul shared a small office next to the lab, and sometimes she would come in at her usual starting time, around 9:00 A.M., and find him asleep on the office floor.

Nancy Haigwood's lab was just down the hall, and although she wasn't working on the AIDS project yet, like all Chiron scientists she was constantly in overdrive. "We worked all the time. It was rare to take a whole weekend off. We worked really hard because the company's survival depended on us and we were really into what we were doing." Most of the scientists were young and few had children, so there was nothing to stop them from working a full day, taking a break for dinner at one of the neighborhood dives, then going back to the lab until 10:00 P.M. The influx of biotech companies had not yet changed this run-down industrial area, and during Chiron's early years, it wasn't unusual to see empty wine bottles or used syringes in the gutters.

●

In September 1984, Pablo Valenzuela promoted Kathy from staff to senior scientist. One of her great strengths was her excellent grasp of immunology, a discipline essential for development of a vaccine to defend against AIDS. Stripped down to its basics, immunology is the study of how the body determines whether something is "self," and therefore harmless, or "non-self" and potentially dangerous. The basic ability to identify something as foreign is the first step toward a protective response against threats as minor as a splinter or as potentially lethal as the AIDS virus.

Paul cloned Levy's virus and determined its full sequence in September. This was a landmark accomplishment, and Chiron filed for a patent on the genetic sequence of the virus and the general arrangement of its genes. Having staked this claim, Chiron wanted to move fast on products. Kathy was whipsawed from one task to the next, trying to do everything at once, sometimes collaborating with Paul and sometimes working only with her five technicians. Chiron identified two genes that coded for parts of the envelope glycoprotein—a protrusion on the surface of the AIDS virus and on infected cells. Glycoproteins were important antigens in experimental vaccines against feline leukemia virus, influenza in mice, and of course the successful hepatitis B vaccine being used in humans.

Confronted with the AIDS virus, the body's first response would probably be to make antibodies against this knobby glycoprotein. If blood-bank technicians could detect these antibodies in donated blood, they would know which units to throw out. Certain parts of the envelope protein elicited stronger immune responses than others, and Kathy performed a series of experiments to pinpoint the most reactive parts. She picked away at genetic sequences to figure out which peptides, or small proteins, kicked antibody production into high gear.

As important as this work was to the company's future, there were other demands on Kathy's time as well. She was working with Paul, Jay Levy, and Dino Dina on the journal article reporting the cloning of the virus. There was a mad dash to get it into print before their competitors did, and on September 22, 1984, they finally shipped it off to *Nature*, a famous scientific journal edited in London. But there was no time to relax. The Chiron team worked on inserting the glycoprotein genes into yeast, so that the yeast would make viral proteins when it reproduced.

Protein production is difficult to measure in cultures of yeast cells, and Kathy's group worked nonstop to accomplish this. During this intensely demanding period, Martin Wilson saw a side of Kathy Steimer that she kept well hidden at work. By that time they were renting a house together in Benicia, a bucolic waterfront village on the Carquinez Strait, which joins the Sacramento River and San Francisco Bay. Benicia was a geographic compromise for this two-career couple, located halfway between Chiron's Emeryville headquarters and the campus of UC–Davis, where Martin worked.

Kathy struggled with long bouts of depression, during which getting herself off to work was a major exercise in emotional weight lifting. And the longer her workdays, the more sleep-deprived she became, and the less able to sleep. And when this happened she drove herself onward with an unnatural, manic energy until finally Martin would force her to go away with him for a few days, usually to a favorite spot in Baja California. Photographs from these trips show a handsome couple, his short hair spiky with seawater and hers wild and blond, tanned arms hugging each other against backdrops obliterated by sun. In Baja, Kathy stepped off the treadmill.

●

In April 1984, Secretary of the U.S. Department of Health and Human Services Margaret Heckler told a Washington press conference that a vaccine against AIDS would be ready for testing in two years. A former Republican congresswoman from Massachusetts, Heckler had no science expertise and on this occasion was suffering with a rotten cold. Minutes before stepping on stage, Heckler asked Bob Gallo, whom she was just about to hail as the discoverer of the virus that causes AIDS, what to say if anyone asked about a preventive vaccine. Gallo pulled a number out of the air. Although this sadly wrong prediction has been attributed both to Heckler's ignorance and Gallo's legendary arrogance, it may simply have reflected the optimism that ruled early in the biotech era.

Researchers in government laboratories, biotech companies, and universities were bursting with ideas about how to make an AIDS vaccine. Jonas Salk was convinced that it would be possible to protect against AIDS with an inactivated version of the virus—an updated version of the paradigm for his successful polio vaccine. Largely on the strength of his name, Salk quickly raised $20 million to start a biotech company—a move that many investors would later come to regret as stock prices fluctuated wildly. A Harvard primate researcher and a Cambridge biotech company jumped on the live-attenuated bandwagon early, even though most experts believed that a live vaccine for AIDS would be too risky. Other start-ups set out to create AIDS vaccines from synthetic versions of antigenic peptides, short chains of amino acids that some predicted would safely elicit powerful immune responses. Everybody had an idea.

Chiron's big score had been the hepatitis B vaccine—a protein subunit expressed in yeast. "Clearly the potential for using this technology to make [an HIV] vaccine seemed relatively straightforward," Ed Penhoet said years later, shortly after he left Chiron to become a university dean. "This is one of those cases where ignorance was bliss."

Kathy's mission was to find out everything she could about gp120, the envelope glycoprotein that would be—in one form or another—the antigen for Chiron's new vaccine. Early on, Kathy agonized that she would never figure out exactly what this antigen should look like. For months she worried that some other scientist, in some other lab, had a surefire way of making a vaccine against AIDS. Gradually, Martin recalls, she came to see that none of the other aspiring vaccine designers and entrepreneurs knew any more than she did. "Nobody knows how to make AIDS vaccines," Kathy told Martin. "We really don't understand the basic immunology that goes with this."

In her lab, Kathy studied the blood of AIDS patients in minute detail. By carefully analyzing their antibodies against HIV—as the AIDS virus was officially named in 1986—Kathy hoped to determine exactly which parts of the virus elicited the strongest immune response. If a vaccine was based on the most powerfully antigenic bits, perhaps it could stimulate a response strong enough to protect people who later encountered HIV in the wild.

Kathy missed being able to talk with Paul, whom she greatly respected as a scientist, as she tried to pick the right antigen. But Paul was gone. In mid-1986, when Chiron was becoming less like an academic lab and more like a business, he had left the company for a faculty position at UC–Davis. Paul wasn't really a corporate type of guy, and he had become less interested in making products and more inclined toward laboratory research on HIV and similar primate viruses. His main focus was using animal models to test HIV vaccines, and over the years, he's built a distinguished career and mentored dozens of young researchers.

Back at Chiron, Kathy and Nancy Haigwood worked together to refine gp120. In the lab they chiseled off epitopes (tiny parts of the antigen) that they thought might interfere with the powerful immune response they were seeking. Because Nancy's special expertise was in expression systems, which harness ordinary cells to make foreign proteins, her role was to make larger quantities of the gp120 pieces Kathy judged most promising.

Just how gp120 should be made was a hotly debated issue at Chiron and elsewhere. The question was whether yeast or animal cells should be used to manufacture gp120, and a growing number of scientists were coming to believe that gp120 grown in cells from mammals would more closely resemble the knobby protrusion on HIV. But Chiron's forte was making proteins in yeast cells, so they stuck with that system.

●

Once a week, Kathy and Nancy scheduled a working lunch. On pleasant days they would leave Chiron and walk to one of the new cafés that were cropping up now that scruffy Emeryville was beginning to gentrify. Both were blonde and blue-eyed; Nancy was three years younger, a tad shorter, and prettier in a more conventional way. Both were being promoted up the corporate ladder in the late 1980s and had traded jeans for a softer, more corporate look. Nancy was ambitious and self-assured, and for the most part she shrugged off adversity or criticism.

Although she tried to hide it at work, Kathy was by far the more sensitive of the two. When Kathy traveled to conferences at Cold Spring Harbor Laboratory in Long Island and other temples of the East Coast scientific establishment, she was surrounded by men who never lost sleep wondering whether they were wrong about anything. When she rose to question an experimental procedure, she was often dismissed and sometimes even attacked. Kathy told her close friend Kathryn Radke, also a retrovirologist who knew the major players, that she didn't know whether she could ever go to another AIDS conference "where all the big egos and high rollers were jockeying with each other for glory." This may have been after the meeting where a famous Duke University researcher loudly propositioned Kathy while his inebriated dinner companions egged him on.

As upsetting as these East Coast meetings were to Kathy, life was good in California. At Chiron, Kathy was beginning to bring in outside funding for AIDS vaccine research. She started small, in 1987, with a $500,000 National Institutes of Health grant to work on genetically engineered vaccines. In 1988, Kathy and Nancy were co-principal investigators on a $3.1 million AIDS vaccine grant from the state of California; Kathy soon got an additional $1.3 million from the NIH on her own. Chiron had also begun manufacturing gp120 in mammal cells instead of yeast.

Lunching in the California sunshine, talking about the temporary setbacks and ego battles that are inevitable in any kind of work, Nancy and Kathy never doubted that genetic engineering would enable science to win the war against AIDS. With the recombinant hepatitis B vaccine as a precedent, how could they fail? "There were so many ways that we could make this vaccine, it was just a matter of who was going to get there first," Nancy recalled a decade later. Sure, there were difficulties along the way, but they were going to prove that they could beat the virus.

Kathy's personal life was also on the upswing. She and Martin had been together since 1982, and in 1987, they moved from their rental house in Benicia to a quirky, dramatic home designed just for them. On the outside it looked like a modest frame house onto which a boxy, two-story concrete addition had been grafted; inside, the space was airy and coherent. The site commanded a spectacular view across the Carquinez Strait to the hills of Port Costa, a small town on the opposite shore.

Kathy and Martin gardened with a passion, planting great rosemary hedges and fruit trees with a special fenced enclosure for Leroy, their black standard poodle pup. Photos from that time show the two of them with a dog as dark as an inkblot squeezed in the middle. With the house and dog in place, the absence of the child they had been trying to conceive for years became acute. Finally, they began to investigate adoption, only to discover that agencies favored couples who were married—which they weren't. They simply hadn't felt the need to make it official. Each had been married before, in Kathy's case a graduate-school misjudgment that had lasted less than one year. Martin's first marriage had lasted longer and had a more amiable parting, but with Kathy he had not felt that a wedding was needed to cement their bond.

Now it appeared that if Kathy and Martin wanted a child, which they did, they would have to tie the knot. So in December 1989, they went to Tijuana with Kathy's father, Harry Steimer, and his lady friend, Sandy Davis. "We paid a guy $5 to make sure that the hubcaps didn't get stolen off the car, while we went into one of those places with a big sign out front saying 'Marriages and Divorces.' It seemed like it would be much more fun than to have a big production," Martin recalled. Afterward, the four-some went out for margaritas. Harry and Sandy took the Tijuana Trolley back to San Diego, while Kathy and Martin took a road trip through Baja.

They returned from their honeymoon to find an answering machine message from a young woman who thought they sounded like good adoptive parents for the baby she was carrying. Kathy's date book for early 1990 was crammed with appointments with lawyers, doctors, social workers—all the people who become involved when an adoption is being arranged. On March 25, Kathy and Martin were at the hospital when the baby they named Acacia Lynn was born. She went home with them to Benicia the following day.

Kathy took a month off from Chiron, although now and then she went to Emeryville for a day jammed with meetings. Both she and Martin worked part-time for six months, and Casey—as the baby soon came to be called—was the center of their lives. For the first time, Kathy stayed up late with an infant instead of an experiment. Except for the addition of the baby, their overall domestic arrangements were the same as ever; Kathy handled all the financial accounts and Martin—an expert and talented chef—did all the shopping and cooking.

Meanwhile, Nancy, who had been made co-leader of the HIV vaccine project and associate director for virology in early 1990, ran the show while Kathy was on leave. By this point she was using mammalian cells to make GMP lots—large batches of vaccine that meet federal standards for Good Manufacturing Practices. Before the U.S. Food and Drug Administration will agree to let a vaccine be tested in humans, it demands that the safety of the product has been demonstrated in animals, that the identity and purity of the product can be assured, and that the product will be stable during the course of a clinical trial.

During the summer of 1990, Nancy and other Chiron representatives met with NIH officials in Bethesda to talk about a government-supported trial for gp120. The prospects looked good, and Chiron submitted an Investigational New Drug (IND) application for its recombinant gp120 vaccine to the Food and Drug Administration. The IND described in

great detail all the cutting-edge molecular biology, all the novel manufacturing techniques, that had gone into the making of this new vaccine. As
dazzling as all this high-tech wizardry was, there was still only one way to
prove whether it would actually protect people against AIDS: immunize
volunteers and see what happened.

2

ARE WE NOT MEN?

WE ARE GENENTECH

I N THE SPRING OF 1980, Jack Obijeski was headed for Cold Spring
Harbor until Denny Kleid talked him out of it. A ten-year veteran of
the Centers for Disease Control in Atlanta, Obijeski was a self-
described "gumshoe virologist" who had become fascinated with using
the new tools of molecular biology to track the spread of poliovirus and
other organisms. He was especially interested in rabies, and in the possibility of making a vaccine that might protect people against it. For
starters, he was slowly sifting through the genetic material crammed into
the nucleus of the rabies virus, hoping to identify individual genes that
could be cloned and used in a vaccine.

Obijeski needed technical help, however, and for this he was planning
to rely on experts at the Cold Spring Harbor Laboratory, an elite, 100-
year-old institution on the North Shore of New York's Long Island. It had
become quite famous for genetic research under the leadership of James
Watson, who shared a Nobel Prize with Francis Crick for discovering the
double helix structure of DNA.

When Obijeski mentioned his travel plans to Dennis Kleid, a top scientist at Genentech, the response was swift and dismissive. "Denny said,
'Lookit, you don't want to go to Cold Spring Harbor. They don't know
what the hell they're doing. You've got to come to the West Coast to do

really good recombinant DNA technology.'" Although this sounded like braggadocio, Kleid had earned the right to swagger: only fifteen months earlier, he and his younger colleague, Dave Goeddel, had triumphed in a fierce, dog-eat-dog race to clone the gene for human insulin. Their upset victory over more famous competitors from Harvard and UC–San Francisco had catapulted Genentech to the front ranks of biotechnology.

So instead of heading north from Atlanta, Obijeski went west. As a guest investigator hosted by Kleid, he would spend three months learning to clone rabies genes at the rapidly expanding laboratories of Genentech, located in industrial South San Francisco. Undoubtedly, Obijeski made the right choice; besides having the scientific expertise he needed, Genentech offered an atmosphere more congenial than Cold Spring Harbor to a fellow with Obijeski's unpretentious and outgoing personality. The Long Island institution has been heavily influenced by Watson's reverence for all things British, and its genteel campus is perfumed with a blend of old money and abundant apple blossoms. Genentech was more like the locker room of a pro sports team, ringing with loud male voices and redolent of competitiveness, testosterone, and the certainty of glory. At thirty-nine, Obijeski was a big, optimistic guy built like an inverted wedge—with broad shoulders and slim hips that had to have served him well when he played football at the University of Connecticut, twenty years earlier. Once Obijeski got to Genentech, it was a hard party to leave.

●

Biotechnology. Genetic engineering. Recombinant DNA. Gene splicing. DNA recombination. These are among the many terms for the revolutionary technology birthed by Herbert Boyer, Genentech's cofounder. In 1972, when he was a young assistant professor at UC–San Francisco, Boyer worked on restriction enzymes, a group of chemicals that bacteria use to fend off attacking creatures by chopping up their genetic material. Boyer and his colleagues had made two fascinating discoveries about these enzymes: First, they cut strands of DNA only where they encounter a specific genetic sequence; second, the snipped strands have "sticky ends" that will lock onto a complementary sequence. These findings suggested that DNA from two wildly different organisms—such as a deadly virus and a harmless yeast—could be joined together if they had earlier been snipped with the same restriction enzyme. A virus and a yeast were never intended to adhere to each other, but they will—just as a Velcro watchband will stick to a Velcro shoe closure if complementary sides come into contact.

Boyer's work caught the attention of Stanley Cohen, a Stanford University scientist who studied bacterial plasmids—minuscule rings of DNA drifting around outside the nucleus that contains the creature's essential genetic code. Cohen had figured out how to remove these tiny DNA donuts from bacteria and then stick them back in. Once he and Boyer began to talk, they quickly guessed that if the same restriction enzyme was used to snip the plasmid circle and to excise a useful gene from a different organism, the two would have complementary sticky ends that could be used to glue the gene into the loop—sort of like attaching a sports watch to a running shoe.

Using the altered plasmid as a molecular handle, Boyer and Cohen expected that they would be able to put the gene into bacteria, yeast, or other rapidly growing cells, much as a hobbyist might insinuate a miniature ship into a bottle. As these cells divided, they would make clones, or identical replicas, of the original material spliced into the plasmid. If this worked, scientists would be able to produce large quantities of proteins at will, instead of painstakingly purifying minute amounts from crushed cells or tissue.

And work it did, as Cohen and Boyer proved in an experiment published in *Proceedings of the National Academy of Sciences* in November 1973. They inserted a bit of genetic material from a toad into *E. coli*, the ubiquitous intestinal bacterium, which obligingly copied the toad gene sequence. It is no exaggeration to call this one of the most influential experiments of all time. In addition to allowing scientists to do more and better laboratory experiments, this discovery changed the lives of children and adults worldwide. Today, hundreds of thousands of people with heart disease, cystic fibrosis, diabetes, hemophilia, and other diseases owe their lives to genetically engineered drugs made possible by Cohen and Boyer's invention.

Although Cohen was content to remain in academia after this triumph, Boyer was restless. As a scholar-athlete in high school, back in the small Pennsylvania town where he was a football star and class president in the early 1950s, Boyer aspired to be a successful businessman. He got the chance in 1976, when he was approached by Robert Swanson, an ambitious twenty-eight-year-old who worked for a venture capital firm in San Francisco but was itching to strike out on his own and start a company. Boyer was a scientist who wanted to be in business, and Swanson was an MBA who wanted to be in science. It was an improbable yet perfect match between a guy who rarely wore anything but blue jeans and one who lived in a suit and tie.

One year after the company was formed, a Genentech team astonished the scientific world by cloning and expressing somatostatin, otherwise known as human growth hormone, or hGH, in *E. coli*. This meant they had stuck a human gene into a simple bacterium and induced that bacterium to copy itself, over and over, each time making more hGH. Although this exact method would not be practical for making large quantities of this hormone, it was a coup that enabled Swanson to raise venture capital for the fledgling company's next project.

He and Boyer had decided to bet everything on the cloning and expression of human insulin, which, if it worked, would yield a product with enormous profit potential. The U.S. market consisted of 1.5 million diabetics who were relying on insulin derived from beef and pig pancreases, raw materials that would eventually fall short of future demand. The worldwide potential for this drug would be huge.

For the insulin project, Swanson rented lab space in an old warehouse in South San Francisco and hired Dennis Kleid and Dave Goeddel, brilliant "clone heads" from the Stanford Research Institute in Palo Alto. In a go-for-broke effort that pulled in scientists from Boyer's UC–San Francisco lab and researchers from the City of Hope Medical Center in Duarte, California, Kleid and Goeddel accomplished the task in an astonishingly short nine months. In September 1978, Genentech held a press conference to announce that it had successfully produced human insulin in *E. coli,* now recognized as the bacterial workhorse of DNA science. The technology for making recombinant human insulin was soon licensed to the giant drugmaker Eli Lilly & Co.

On October 14, 1980, Genentech stock was first offered to the public at $35 per share. Before the end of the day, the price had soared to $89, an unprecedented high in that innocent, pre-Internet era. Although the company did not yet have a single product on the market for human use, it was gaining a reputation as "the Tiffany of the biotechs."

●

When Jack Obijeski came to Genentech in the spring of 1980, he entered a world that was a lot more like a rathskeller than a luxury jewelry emporium. Tall, rangy Dave Goeddel sported a T-shirt emblazoned with the words "Clone or Die." The place was dominated by jocks with brains, guys who shot hoops and spiked volleyballs while they were waiting for their experiments to run. During the mad dash to clone the insulin gene, Kleid and Goeddel spent their downtime in personal angling derbies, competing to see who could catch the biggest striped bass off Point San Bruno, a short hike from their lab. In whatever spare time he had left, Goeddel climbed mountains for fun.

Not only was Swanson serious about creating products that would boost Genentech into the big leagues of the drug business, but he also seemed determined that his company not be snickered at as a bunch of eggheads. In the early days, Swanson began staging Friday afternoon beer bashes, events he called, with a kind of forced cheeriness, "Ho-Ho's." Sometimes he put on a ridiculous rented costume—a giant bumblebee outfit made an indelible impression—over his business suit.

In a 1979 talk that he gave to a group of business analysts, Swanson said, "We should all have people working for us who work like microorganisms. They divide every twenty to thirty minutes and work twenty-four hours a day—just for room and board. What's more, they make the ultimate sacrifice—they die making the product for you." He was joking, of course, but nevertheless, many of the young scientists would down a couple of beers on Friday, scarf down some pizza, and go back to the lab.

Jack Obijeski fit right in at Genentech, and in 1982, he officially resigned from CDC and cast his lot with the company. He was hired by Goeddel, now thirty-one years old and the company's director of research, to head its nascent vaccine program. "I still loved CDC," Obijeski recalls, "but this is where the action was in biotechnology. This is the hotbed of stuff. Every week was something new happening." Meanwhile, back at CDC in Atlanta, his old colleagues were absorbed in tracking a new disease that had begun killing gay men in big cities.

This was an exhilarating time to be part of Genentech. "We hired the best and the brightest. At first there was this reluctance, you know, you don't want to work in industry. But then academics found out that every time they wanted to get their hands on some material like interferon, or hepatitis B surface antigen, or tissue plasminogen activator, or human growth hormone, we had it," Obijeski says.

Although Chiron had beat Genentech in the race to win U.S. Food and Drug Administration approval for a hepatitis B subunit vaccine, Genentech's version had been licensed for sale in other parts of the world. Now Obijeski's group turned to other projects. Among them were vaccines for rabies, his original interest, and herpes—a high-profile, sexually transmitted viral disease that was striking people who would be willing to use a vaccine if one were available and who would be able to pay for it.

•

Phil Berman grew up in Los Angeles and played defense for his high-school football team. But it was the mid-1960s; the Beach Boys ruled in Southern California, and when Phil got fed up with being bruised and sore, he swapped his shoulder pads for a surfboard and took to the beach. He went to college at UC-Berkeley, where antiwar activists took precedence over surfers, then decamped for Dartmouth Medical School in New Hampshire. At the most macho of the Ivies, Phil earned a Ph.D. in protein chemistry and immunology.

In 1982, Phil Berman was thirty-four years old and wrapping up a postdoctoral fellowship in Herb Boyer's laboratory at UC-San Francisco. Boyer's fascination with business had proved short-lived, and he had returned to academia after Genentech went public and money was no longer an issue. Phil was at UCSF because he'd had an epiphany just as he was finishing a postdoc in immunology and neurology at the Salk Institute for Biological Studies in San Diego. Phil abruptly changed course after a lecture by a Genentech scientist who explained how manipulating DNA enabled the company to synthesize human growth hormone. "I realized that the world would never be the same, and so I went to Herb

Boyer's lab to do a second postdoc," he remembers. At UCSF, he worked to clone herpes genes and to express them in *E. coli*, an undertaking that was clearly relevant to Obijeski's vaccine project.

The early 1980s were a buyer's market in the life sciences, and Genentech's fledgling personnel department was overwhelmed by hundreds of applications that poured into the red-hot company every week. Phil sent his curriculum vitae several times, only to have it lost in the shuffle. Boyer buttonholed Obijeski on one of his consulting visits to South San Francisco. "Hey Jack—God, this guy Berman is great. Are you gonna hire him?" Obijeski had to admit that he'd never even seen Phil's CV. On a later visit, Boyer hand-carried a copy to Obijeski and told him, "Don't lose this." Obijeski hired Phil right away.

The vaccine team worked mainly on herpes for the next couple of years. At one point, Obijeski says that Phil and another young molecular biologist, Larry Lasky, got tremendously excited about using a portion of a herpes surface glycoprotein, known as glycoprotein D, or gD for short, as an antigen in a vaccine. Recalling what he had learned during his CDC years, Obijeski told them that earlier efforts to incorporate pieces of surface proteins into other viral vaccines had failed. When scientists shortened a protein to separate it from the rest of an influenza virus, for example, they watched it "unwind like a clock spring." Once this protein had changed shape, the immune system made antibodies against it that were powerless against the tightly coiled protein found on the virus itself.

"So I told them that it might not work," Obijeski says. "But Phil and Larry didn't know any better, so they just did it!" His voice rises and his eyes widen as though he is describing a sixty-yard field goal or an astonishing hole-in-one. "So they truncated the protein and it worked! I would never have predicted it. I would have been petrified by my previous thoughts of being a virologist, where they had no ax to grind. They just didn't care. They just did it." As exciting as the making of this protein was, it would not get far on the long road toward testing as a vaccine.

●

In September 1984, a Genentech scientist named Dan Capon sequenced the genome of a different AIDS virus than the one studied at

Chiron. This particular AIDS virus, known as HIV_{LAI}, had been cultured by government scientists at the National Institutes of Health, where its nucleic acids, which encode its genes, had been extracted and shipped to South San Francisco. In this form, Genentech scientists felt they could handle it without the special precautions that Paul Luciw and Kathy Steimer had used when they cultured virus samples from HIV-infected patients. Because those patients lived in San Francisco, the virus sequenced at Chiron was dubbed HIV_{SF2}.

In contrast to the hands-on approach that prevailed at Chiron, Genentech had never allowed live, disease-causing microbes on its premises. When the Boyer-Cohen experiment with the toad genes and *E. coli* was first announced in 1973, there was a tremendous public uproar over the possibility that DNA recombination would spawn frightening and uncontrollable new life forms. This controversy had settled down by the early 1980s, but Genentech was still leery about linking genetic engineering with scary pathogens. It would be bad PR, and that would be bad for business.

Human growth hormone, or hGH, was a central concern. The corporation's lawyers didn't want pathogens anywhere near the place where hGH was manufactured. Because its target users would be children who were healthy except that their pituitary glands couldn't generate sufficient hGH, this costly, growth-promoting chemical needed to appear as safe as milk. The lawyers shriveled at the thought of being sued by parents claiming that hGH shots had infected their child with herpes, rabies, or—even worse—with AIDS. Never mind that by 1984 Genentech's research and manufacturing operations were under separate roofs, and that its 1,000 employees worked in eight different buildings.

"There was never any virus here, it was always the [harmless] nucleic acid," Obijeski recalls about Genentech in the 1980s. "It was like we were fighting the battle against HIV with one hand tied behind our back." This situation was frustrating to someone who had been at the CDC, where part of an epidemiologist's job was bagging samples of potentially lethal organisms and bringing them back for analysis. But it was probably fine with young molecular biologists who had not grown up amid dangerous pathogens and who might prefer to deal with bits and pieces of virus, instead of organisms that are intact, infectious, and hungry for a host.

Dan Capon cloned the AIDS virus at a time when Genentech's herpes vaccine effort was limping along, due to a lukewarm response in the executive suite. Unlike Chiron's founders, who made vaccine development a top priority from the start, Swanson and Boyer had always emphasized therapeutic drugs over vaccines. If company scientists already had some expertise on a pathogen, such as rabies or herpes, the company would support vaccine research up to a point. Because a pill that is taken daily will always earn more than a vaccine that is administered every few years, however, the top executives were not scanning the horizon for new diseases to prevent.

As head of molecular biology research, Dave Goeddel had to decide what to do with the sequence of the not-yet-named AIDS virus once it was in hand. Having won the race for human insulin, he was now in the starter's box. His top priority was to find a treatment based on the new genetic information, and a high-powered research group immediately went to work on this. But Goeddel also set up a "clone or die" contest that pitted teams of scientists against one another in the quest for a possible AIDS vaccine. Phil Berman and Larry Lasky joined forces to try to make a recombinant surface protein like the one they'd created for herpes. Dan Capon and Tim Gregory, whose usual line of work was process development, set out to make inactive virus particles that might be used for immunization. Other teams chased other ideas. Years later, one of the combatants summed up the experience: "It was a typical Dave Goeddel competition. It was okay, whoever gets the vaccine first gets promoted and the others are shit. That's it. The winner takes all."

When the dust settled, Berman and Lasky had come out on top. They had two possible vaccine candidates—a recombinant gp120 protein, similar to the one that Chiron was pursuing but derived from HIV_{LAI} instead of HIV_{SF2}—and a larger surface protein called gp160. Before these ideas could go much further, larger quantities would be needed for experiments with animals and, in the more distant future, with people. Tim Gregory's job in process development was figuring out "how to actually *make* what comes out of research," which made him a natural to join the AIDS vaccine team.

Like Berman, Tim had come to Genentech in 1982. He was thirty-one at the time, and instead of stretching out his years in academia, as Phil had done, Tim went straight from his Ph.D. program at UC-San Diego to Syntex, a pharmaceutical company in Palo Alto that did pioneering work in hormonal contraception. There he studied neuropeptides, tiny molecules that brain cells use to communicate among themselves. Tim didn't feel that this research was leading anywhere he particularly wanted to go, so when he heard about an opportunity in Genentech's process development operation, he jumped at it.

●

Drag queens trailing feather boas, sex education posters showing hunky guys in leather, and a roaming character dressed as a life-sized "Mr. Friendly Condom." The medical conventions that usually populated the cavernous, frigidly cooled Georgia World Congress Center in Atlanta had none of the flamboyant touches that made the world's first international scientific meeting on AIDS an unprecedented event. Of the 2,000 people who poured into the hall April 15–17, 1985, many were wearing the contemporary uniform of the physician—a sports coat and Hush Puppy lace-up shoes. But hundreds were not, as young and overtly gay men (and a smattering of lesbians and fag hags) attended their first scientific conference, upping the anxiety level for doctors and scientists accustomed to discussing diseases out of patient earshot. This marked the first time, although certainly not the last, that large numbers of patients and advocates sat in on a scientific conference.

At the World Congress Center, the face of AIDS was gay and most likely white, despite mounting reports that the virus was spread by heterosexual contact, that it was more widespread in Africa than in the United States, and that it was also being transmitted by IV drug use, blood products, and by birth itself. The powerful association between AIDS and male homosexuality gave many Reagan administration officials and others all the excuse they needed to move slowly against the unfolding public-health emergency. In a 1985 cartoon, Jules Feiffer lampooned one rationale for inaction: "Lung cancer is God's punishment on smokers," one character says to the other, only to be met with an astonished "What?!" The exchange continues: "And heart disease is God's punishment on joggers." "Are you kidding?" "And diabetes is God's punishment on sweets eaters." "Are you crazy?" "And hunger is God's punishment on Ethiopians." "You are sick!" "And AIDS is God's punishment on homosexuals." "You said it! You better believe it! Serves 'em right."

In her keynote address to the conference, Secretary of the U.S. Department of Health and Human Services Margaret Heckler repeatedly insisted that "AIDS is our number-one health priority." Reporters who had been handed the text in the press room were stunned when Heckler, who had been sticking closely to her script, inserted an ad-lib in the penultimate paragraph. "For individuals in every country who fall within the risk categories, AIDS is an enormously serious disease. We must conquer it for their sakes. We must conquer it, as well, before it affects the heterosexual population and threatens the health of our general population." In a flash, the head of the nation's vast health establishment made it clear whose well-being *really* mattered.

The message was not lost on the activists who heard Heckler's words, and the next day they passed out a reply in the corridors. "We point out that gay men, hemophiliacs, intravenous drug users, Haitians and people with AIDS are also among the general public, and failure to acknowledge this is a denial of our basic humanity." Right from the start, it was clear that AIDS would never be just another infectious disease and that it was not going to be treated like one by the nation's public-health establishment.

One of the most controversial figures at this landmark AIDS conference was Don Francis, a virologist at the Centers for Disease Control who had been raising a ruckus with outspoken pronouncements about what gay men—and the CDC—should do in the face of the growing epidemic. At forty-three, he was a handsome, tawny-haired California native who didn't seem to care whom he offended. Gay leaders were mad at him for urging homosexual men to seek out the newly available antibody test and to have sex only with people whose status matched their own. His CDC bosses were nettled by Don's willingness to recommend such a specific, aggressive measure for slowing the spread of AIDS. The agency itself had not generated any explicit recommendations about how individuals might protect themselves, reportedly because the Reagan administration believed that educating people about risky behaviors would encourage them to take more risks. A real sore point with Don and others was CDC's foot-dragging over publication of a report indicating that a common spermicidal jelly—available in drugstores everywhere—could kill the AIDS virus.

Clearly, Don was out of step with the CDC leadership, which was wary of doing anything that might offend the White House. By the time the international conference took place, Don had asked for a transfer from CDC's Atlanta headquarters to San Francisco. Some of his colleagues said this was the CDC equivalent of exile in Siberia, but Don genuinely believed that he could have more impact on the epidemic as a special adviser to the State of California than he could from his post in Georgia. The transfer was approved, and in July 1985, Don and his family moved from Atlanta to the San Francisco Bay Area. Don, the son of two physicians, had grown up in Marin County, at the northern end of the Golden Gate Bridge. He had crossed the Bay to spend his undergraduate years at UC-Berkeley, before going to Chicago for medical school and then chasing infectious diseases around the world. He was coming home, and home was a mess.

●

Jack Obijeski and Don Francis knew each other from CDC, where both had worked on the eradication of smallpox in the 1970s, so it was natural for them to renew their friendship after Don came back to San Francisco. Scientists often gave guest lectures at biotech companies, just as they did in university departments, and Obijeski added Don to Genentech's schedule. At the time, Don was obsessed with San Francisco's popular gay bathhouses, which he saw not as symbols of post-Stonewall gay liberation but as lurid, highly commercial "amplification systems" for the AIDS virus. Don had studied animal retroviruses at Harvard, and he knew that, given the chance, they race from host to host as fast as summer lightning.

"He'd come and give seminars about the bathhouses, and people would be sitting in their chairs and going, 'Ewww,'" Obijeski recalls. He mimes men squirming nervously in their seats, as if they expected a big guy in leather to sneak up from behind and do something unspeakable to them. The majority of the listeners were straight men, because Genentech had few female molecular biologists, and if there were any gay men present, they kept it to themselves. Although frank talk about homosexuality made individual scientists fidget, they nevertheless understood that the AIDS epidemic was a genuine public-health emergency. "We'd come out of the session and say, 'Hey, this is an important problem. We need to be working on important medical problems and seeing if our technology can help.'"

Obijeski wanted Genentech to hire Don for its AIDS projects, which included efforts to discover both therapeutic drugs and vaccines. The company had just recruited pediatrician Art Ammann, a pioneering researcher on infants and children with AIDS, from UC-San Francisco. But Don wasn't ready to leave CDC until he'd passed the twenty-year mark and qualified for his pension, Obijeski recalls, so he kept plugging away in public health.

●

"Lookit, when you think about recombinant vaccines, what you think about are envelope proteins, because those are the ones that come in contact with the immune system." That's what Jack Obijeski believed, and many other scientists agreed. By this point, at least a half dozen other biotech companies were working on vaccines that mimicked some part of HIV's outer shell.

Obijeski was the main cheerleader for the gp120 project at Genentech. In the lab, Phil had struggled to make a protein that was shaped like the natural protrusion on the virus's surface. Once he and Tim Gregory had made what looked like the right protein, the next step was to inject it into mice. After a series of inoculations, blood drawn from the mice would be mixed with a sample of a laboratory-grown AIDS virus. If the blood contained enough of the right antibodies, the virus would be neutralized— which is lab-speak for "killed"—and the experiment would be a success. In late 1985, they felt very successful indeed.

"That was our first big experiment, showing that you could make antibodies that neutralized virus by immunizing animals with gp120. No one had ever done that before," Phil says, remembering the excitement that he and Tim had felt. "It worked great in small animals and in test-tube experiments, and then we rushed to test it in chimpanzees." Phil had good reasons for wanting to test his new product in chimps. In 1984, Bob Gallo and his colleagues had deliberately infected several chimps with HTLV-III, the AIDS virus identified in his lab at the National Cancer Institute. The animals mounted an immune response and some developed swollen lymph nodes, a condition often seen in patients who later develop AIDS. A good animal model requires that the human pathogen cause signs and symptoms that mirror human disease, and in 1985, chimps seemed to meet these criteria. Beyond that, Phil also knew that encouraging results in chimps had kept development of recombinant hepatitis B vaccines alive in several companies that might otherwise have dropped them.

Before Phil and Tim could test gp120 in large animals, they had to have more of it. Genentech needed recombinant gp120 not only as a possible vaccine but also because it was an essential reagent, or test material, in experiments with soluble CD4, a radical new drug that might be able to treat AIDS. A key element in making gp120 turned out to be a plasmid called "Big Dude," named after—what else?—a hulking Genentech employee who had once played center on a football team.

Phil and Tim used Big Dude to shuttle the gp120 gene into immortalized Chinese hamster ovary cells, referred to in the lab as CHO cells. Because they don't wear out and die when normal cells would, the immortalized CHO cells tirelessly churned out gp120. This was the same type of cell that Nancy Haigwood, on the other side of the Bay, wanted to use for Chiron's version of a gp120 vaccine.

Tim's next challenge was purifying the gp120 protein so that the vaccine would be as clean as possible. This meant popping the CHO cells open, then sifting through the debris to separate the gp120. Tim knew his production process wasn't perfect and that the gp120 he was making in the lab wasn't as consistent or as pure as he would have liked. But he and Phil never forgot for a moment that they were in a head-to-head competition with major pharmaceutical companies and hungry young biotechs staffed by competitors who were very smart and very aggressive. It felt like fourth down and four, with only seconds to go. As soon as they could scrape together enough gp120, Phil and Tim lunged for the goal.

●

The Southwest Foundation for Biomedical Research is one of several private facilities in the United States where pharmaceutical researchers can exchange large sums of money for the opportunity to experiment on chimpanzees and other nonhuman primates. The practice of testing drugs and vaccines on apes and monkeys has long been the center of an ethical maelstrom, and in 1986, the battle was especially intense. That year, animal rights activists breached a government research facility in Rockville, Maryland, and circulated highly inflammatory pictures of some of the 500 primates caged there.

As soon as Phil had a sufficient quantity of the gp120 vaccine, he personally traveled with it to San Antonio. Located on Military Drive, not far from San Antonio's version of the beltway, the entrance to the Southwest Foundation is marked only by a low-profile sign. A nondescript road leads to a guardhouse, and the sprawling facility is a mix of large outdoor cages, where troops of macaques live and breed, and buildings of various sizes. Although chimpanzees that aren't actively being studied also live in groups, research animals are housed individually like dogs in a boarding kennel—each cage has an indoor room and an outdoor run.

Once Phil dropped off the vaccine, Southwest staff immunized four chimps on a rapid-fire schedule, three quick doses of gp120 over a few weeks followed by a large "challenge" dose of AIDS virus. The vaccine's effects were measured not by looking for symptoms of AIDS, which chimps didn't appear to develop, but by drawing blood and checking it for immune activity and the presence of virus. These tests revealed that all the animals were infected. The chimps immunized with gp120 might as well have been injected with tap water.

When news of these disappointing results reached South San Francisco, Genentech's top brass responded by dismantling Phil's lab and reassigning him to work on anti-inflammatory drugs. The vaccine was clearly a loser, and they weren't going to throw good money after bad. Tim continued making gp120, but only because it was needed for experiments with soluble CD4, a novel AIDS treatment that was the company's best hope as an entry into the AIDS sweepstakes. Gossip about the infected chimps spread swiftly from Genentech to scientists working on possible AIDS vaccines at other companies and in universities. "A huge wave of darkness rolled over the whole field," Phil recalled. "There was all sorts of unwarranted pessimism."

When Tim thinks back on the disastrous chimp experiment and its fallout, he blames that calamity on his generation's ignorance about vaccinology. After polio was defeated in the United States by two highly effective vaccines, the focus of biomedical research swung away from infectious illnesses and toward heart disease and cancer, the two leading killers of adults. As a result, vaccine research fell off the scientific agenda during the 1960s and 1970s. When hepatitis and AIDS came along, "there were not more than a handful of people around who really had serious vaccine experience, and none of the vaccinologists were in the biotech area," Tim said years later. "We were just young and foolish and in a competition, rushing blindly ahead. That was the whole spirit of the early days of biotechnology. Damn the controls, full speed ahead."

•

Phil and Tim's failure to protect chimps against HIV infection came at a time when pharmaceutical companies regarded preventive vaccines as categorically less attractive than drugs aimed at treatment. One concern was that vaccines always come bundled with more liability than treatments. People who have been ill are probably not going to sue over minor side effects if a drug has relieved or cured their original complaint. Healthy people, on the other hand, have been known to blame vaccines for all sorts of problems that crop up long after they've gotten a shot, whether or not there is any plausible connection between the illness and the vaccine. As far as these folks are concerned, they took the vaccine in order to stay healthy—so if they don't feel well, the vaccine maker is at fault. Executives could develop palpitations just thinking about the hot-button issues tied to a vaccine for AIDS, a highly stigmatized ailment that killed everyone it touched. Any company that made a seemingly unsafe AIDS vaccine would not have to ask for whom the bell tolled.

Another disincentive is that vaccines cost more to bring to market than drugs. Initial discovery and preclinical development costs are generally higher for vaccines, and clinical trials are always more expensive. Although the efficacy of a treatment is often obvious after a few weeks or months of testing in fewer than 2,000 patients, many vaccine efficacy trials require tens of thousands of people and last for several years. Genentech couldn't afford this sort of undertaking and couldn't count on the federal government to pay for huge, expensive studies. And what is the reward if an AIDS vaccine finally proves effective at the conclusion of a large and lengthy Phase III study that determines efficacy? A product that is injected once in a great while will never be as lucrative as a treatment, which, in most cases, must be used every day. There was also an increasing likelihood, based on horror stories that were already emerging from Africa in 1986, that the people most in need of an AIDS vaccine would not be able to pay for it.

Genentech's own experience in the late 1980s showed that drugs were a better bet. In 1985, the FDA approved the company's recombinant human growth hormone as a treatment for children with pituitary dwarfism, which is caused by the inability to generate sufficient hGH. Although there were only about 7,000 of these children in the United States, physicians were free to prescribe hGH for other short children. Within a few years, at least 20,000 kids were being given hGH treatments that cost $20,000–30,000 per year. On top of that, Genentech's clot-dissolving recombinant tPA made a spectacular debut in November 1987. When the drug was given promptly to people having a heart attack, it reduced by half the risk of dying during the next few days. In addition to sparing thousands of lives, in many cases tPA saved the heart muscle from permanent damage—enabling people to recover fully from heart attacks that might otherwise disable them for life. Physicians embraced tPA, even though a single dose cost $2,200. Of this amount, industry analysts estimated that $1,800 was pure profit for Genentech.

Genentech had sound business reasons for making AIDS treatments a higher priority than vaccines that might prevent it. And the gee-whiz nature of Genentech's entry into the therapy sweepstakes made a tremendous media splash in August 1988. In the *New York Times,* Nobel laureate David Baltimore sang the praises of "rational drug development," which Genentech's soluble CD4 exemplified. Using the gp120 made by Tim Gregory as a key, researchers created a lab-made molecule that mimicked the CD4 receptor on the surface of human T cells. In essence, the researchers synthesized a lock that fit Tim's key. And this lock is the primary portal that HIV uses to enter these cells, where the virus replicates before popping open the cell and sending virions forth to hijack and kill more T cells. If the patient's system was flooded with fake CD4 receptors, the theory went, then the virus would cleave to them instead of the real thing.

Baltimore and others, including some of the top administrators at the National Institutes of Health, were bedazzled by this approach to drug design. Traditional drug development was messy and serendipitous, and it meant rummaging in chemical storage closets or pawing through dirt and fungus samples, in the hope of stumbling across something that would kill a dangerous organism. The concept of rational design, of figuring out what's needed and building a molecule to fit that function, was hugely appealing. People could save the world without stepping outside a clean, well-lighted lab.

If only life were that simple. In AIDS patients, it turned out that virus and cell reached for each other with the sad and practiced precision of expert tango dancers. Apparently, it was hubris to think that the virus would embrace a stranger substituted for its familiar partner. This virus was not easily fooled, and soluble CD4 failed utterly in its first clinical trial.

●

So long as CD4 was riding high, Tim was authorized to keep making gp120. Phil, on the other hand, had been told to lay off HIV vaccines. Tim remembers, "I kept plugging along because I was up to here in HIV stuff anyway, and the technology was important. Phil was much more dedicated to the success of the vaccine per se." Like all Genentech scientists, Phil had been encouraged to spend a small percentage of his time on discretionary research. For the next year or so, Phil used his spare time to make different versions of HIV surface proteins and to figure out how CHO cells could be induced to churn them out more efficiently. He was certain that if he just kept at it, he could make a protein subunit vaccine that would work. Once Phil was satisfied that he had made progress, he and Tim came up with better ways to purify the protein.

While they refined their processes for making antigens, Phil and Tim also tried to step back and take a broader look at what had gone wrong in the chimp experiment. On their own, they realized that they had injected gp120 that was only about 50 percent pure. When they sought advice from the vaccinologists of the previous generation, Phil and Tim saw that their immunization schedule was all wrong. "Jonas Salk told us later that it was stupid," Tim recalls. They weren't waiting long enough between injections, nor had they let enough time pass before challenging the animals with virus. No wonder the HIV, which was notoriously quick on its feet, waltzed right into the cells of the poorly protected chimps. Now Phil and Tim saw the error of their ways, and they wanted to try again.

In many pharmaceutical companies, the word of a corporate vice president is law: Young scientists told to abandon a project would stop immediately. But this was not the Genentech way. "From the early days, whether it was three people, thirty, or 3,000, there was never a concept of the boss," according to Jack Obijeski, who initially hired Phil. At Genentech, scientists barely bothered to hide their contempt for what they called "approvatrons" in the executive suite. When top executives lost interest not only in HIV but in all vaccines, gutting Obijeski's department, he thought they were dead wrong. And he still thinks so. "Don't assume that the business people and the lawyers that you hire at a company are as smart and creative as the scientists. They clearly were not. All they had were the pretty faces and the straight teeth and Brioni suits."

Before business writers were mesmerized by Silicon Valley, they ate this stuff up. They went gaga over Genentech's beer busts and its freewheeling corporate style, which was dignified by the label "postindustrial management." At their most defiant, Genentech researchers resembled a cadre of feral postdocs, willing to practice guerrilla science rather than kowtow to authority figures—especially pretty boys in suits. Scientists who didn't fit this macho mold, some because they were women and some who just weren't jock enough, quickly moved on to other companies. One disaffected former employee says of his Genentech experience, "It is like having your car break down in Appalachia, where everyone is named Jones, looks the same, and has some problems as a result of incestuous breeding."

●

By late 1988, working below the radar of their nominal bosses, Phil and Tim had generated a recombinant gp120 that was 95-percent pure, a great improvement over the messy, rough draft of a vaccine that had been shot into the chimps in 1986. They were even more excited about a new gp160, a full-length version of HIV's surface protein that they hoped would stimulate a more powerful immune response than the smaller gp120. In order to find out whether they were any closer to having a vaccine, the two researchers needed chimps.

In late 1988, the rumor was that another research group at Genentech had reserved five chimpanzees at the Southwest Foundation in San Antonio, but wasn't ready to use them. "It cost about $300,000 to reserve these chimps, and if they weren't used in an experiment by December 31, the company would lose them. We heard about this between Christmas and New Year's, so we approached some VPs and said that the company already paid for these, why not let us use them," Phil says. The huge down payment covered the care of the chimps for the coming year, and two sympathetic vice presidents finally agreed to sign the paperwork that gave Phil and Tim another chance to try for an AIDS vaccine.

Now they had to get going before the December 31 deadline. Immediately, they asked the Southwest Foundation to draw blood from the chimps for pretest studies of health and immune function. Because Phil couldn't travel to San Antonio for a clandestine experiment, he shipped the vaccines. On January 3, 1989, technicians at the Southwest Foundation injected two chimps with gp160, two with gp120, and one with an inactive placebo. Unlike monkeys, which must be sedated before they can be injected or have blood drawn, chimps are taught to hold out their arms. The animals were immunized again in early February and for the third time in early August, eight months after the first shot. Three weeks later, on September 6, they were injected with a large dose of HIV_{LAI}, the same strain that Phil had used to make the vaccine. Soon the results began rolling in: "The controls became infected, the gp160-immunized animals became infected right away, but the gp120 animals didn't show any signs of infection. We waited for month after month, and thought, holy shit, we might have protected the animals," Phil says.

Phil and Tim went about their daily business at Genentech, their secret swelling inside them with each passing week. More blood samples were taken from the chimps, and again and again the animals tested negative. The AIDS virus could not be found in their blood. Phil became increasingly certain that the new gp120 vaccine had protected the chimps, but he was afraid that he would be fired on the spot if he told anyone. And he had good reason to be worried. "The head of the company, people very high up in the company, thought that they had killed this project a long time ago," Phil said.

Phil and Tim became increasingly elated about positive results, and in March 1990, they couldn't keep the secret any longer. But neither were they ready to march into the executive suite. Phil telephoned Jack Obijeski at his vacation home on the coast of Washington, where Obijeski hung out when he wasn't working at Genentech as a part-time consultant. Obijeski had the ear of top executives, and Phil asked him to hint that good news about a vaccine might be on the way. Obijeski was as excited about the chimp results as the two researchers, and he "raised the flag a little bit." Once the top brass had been softened up, Phil and Tim told them what had happened in the chimp experiment. The result was that chutzpah paid off: Vaccine development was once again on the corporate agenda, and Phil became known as a guy who did it his way. At a different company, with a different ethos, he probably would have been canned.

●

In Phil's view, "the successful chimp results lifted the cloud and brought in an era of unbelievable optimism." That was certainly true at Genentech and at other biotech companies, where vaccine researchers were predisposed to take the chimp results seriously. When experimental hepatitis B vaccines had been tested in these great apes in the early 1980s, vaccines that elicited antibodies in chimps later protected people in clinical trials. Chimps and humans have nearly identical immune systems, and both can be infected with hepatitis B or HIV. Unlike people, however, chimps don't get sick when they're infected with either of these viruses. This is a difference that corporate researchers were willing to overlook, because they had laboratory tests that could detect infection in animals with no symptoms.

Elsewhere in the scientific world, Genentech's successful experiment made barely a ripple. Although Bob Gallo and other leading basic researchers had initially viewed chimps as the best model for studying AIDS, by 1990 many had abandoned chimps and had transferred their allegiance to macaques and other smaller primates. Five years of experience showed that chimps, in addition to being scarce and expensive, were much better than humans at fighting off HIV infection. After infection, the virus doesn't grow well in chimp cells, the animals don't get sick, and the virus often disappears from their bodies if you wait long enough.

Basic scientists were also skeptical about the chimp protection study because many strains of HIV had been identified, and these could be as different as poodles and pit bulls. Phil had immunized the chimps with gp120 modeled on the surface protein of HIV_{LAI}, one of the earliest strains that thrived in laboratories, and had challenged them with a walloping dose of the same strain. Elsewhere, researchers had discovered that HIV_{LAI} wasn't as virulent as other HIVs, meaning that it had a harder time penetrating host cells. Other experiments showed that chimps infected with HIV_{LAI} cleared it from their systems—without any immunization or treatment at all—in about one year.

Regardless of where they stood on the chimp question, Phil and everyone else in the field took notice of an article that appeared in *Science* in 1990. The lead author was John LaRosa, a scientist at a Massachusetts biotech company also working on genetically engineered AIDS vaccines. LaRosa showed that antigens from HIV_{LAI} stimulated antibodies against only a small percentage of viral strains found in AIDS patients, whereas those from another virus, known as HIV_{MN}, reacted with a majority of patient samples. Phil immediately got a sample of MN from the National Institutes of Health and made a new version of gp120.

This time he didn't have to sneak around to test it in chimps, and again the immunized animals were protected. Because the NIH hadn't been able to generate MN in a form that could be used to challenge chimps, the animals were instead exposed to HIV_{SF2}, the strain originally sequenced at Chiron. Protection against a strain other than the one used to make the vaccine was considered a very promising result indeed, at least in the world of corporate science. Clinical researchers had isolated many different HIV strains from patients in San Francisco and other hard-hit cities, and clearly HIV was a Mafia family rather than a lone serial killer. An effective vaccine would have to protect against as many strains as possible if the epidemic were to be slowed or stopped.

●

Although Genentech resuscitated its HIV vaccine effort after the successful chimp experiment in 1989 and pumped in more money during 1990, this did not mean the sky was the limit. The company still had sound economic reasons for favoring therapeutic drugs over preventive vaccines, and the challenge for the in-house vaccine loyalists was to get around this attitude. Obijeski, who had originally come to Genentech to work on vaccines, decided to pitch gp120 as a treatment for AIDS. Early in his scientific career, Obijeski had worked at an army research facility in Maryland, and he was still well-connected to military researchers. He knew that army scientists, back on the East Coast at Walter Reed Hospital, had taken a radical step by using vaccines not to prevent illness— which was their time-honored role—but to treat people who were already sick. The idea of a therapeutic vaccine was completely new, and the first experiments used a gp160 vaccine that army researchers hoped would boost the flagging immune systems of AIDS patients. Preliminary results weren't encouraging, the manufacturer was a pain to work with, and the army was reportedly looking for additional products to test.

Obijeski saw no reason why Phil's gp120 shouldn't be the next candidate, and if the army took it on, it would pay for clinical testing. "We're into therapy. Look at all the money we can make," Obijeski told Genentech's corporate leadership. "[Army researcher] Bob Redfield thinks that because there's a long, protracted disease process you can use a therapeutic vaccine." The executives liked this idea. Phil himself wasn't really interested in treating patients; he wanted to make a vaccine that would protect healthy people. But he could not afford to turn his back on free clinical testing.

The main sticking point for corporate vaccine developers is the cost of proving that their product is efficacious—that it keeps people healthy. Like drugs, vaccines start out in small Phase I trials. Here the measure of success is that the vaccine doesn't hurt anyone and elicits an immune response that seems desirable. Next comes a Phase II clinical trial, which typically enrolls hundreds of patients (for a drug) or healthy volunteers (for a vaccine). If an experimental drug treatment looks good at this stage, "then you're about 90-percent sure that the stuff is going to work and it's worth putting out the big money to do a Phase III trial," says Tim Gregory, who supervised production of dozens of drugs and vaccines at Genentech. Vaccines are a different matter, however, because protection is never clear until the product has been tested in a Phase III study that involves not 1,000 or 2,000 volunteers, but tens of thousands.

"People throw around the idea that an HIV vaccine would be worth a billion dollars," Tim said. "But first you've got to invest several hundred million dollars in a lottery ticket versus putting $100 million into a Fidelity Magellan Fund." For companies with both treatments and vaccines in the hopper, the choice isn't difficult when their own money is being put at risk. What drove Genentech to pursue an HIV vaccine, back in 1990, was the expectation that the army and the National Institutes of Health—not the company itself—would pay for clinical trials when the time came. They were banking on it.

3

NAKED CAME THE DNA

J UST FOR A LARK, a group of journalists once decided to write a
trashy, sex-laced novel, with each person contributing a chapter. The
writers revised one another's work just enough to provide a mod-
icum of continuity, chose a silly, provocative title and a nom de plume,
and submitted the manuscript to a publisher. The result far exceeded the
journalists' expectations: When *Naked Came the Stranger* appeared in
1969, it was one of the year's ten best-selling works of fiction. And the
nonexistent Penelope Ashe, the purported author, was in huge demand
with talk-show hosts across the country.

Although many in publishing industry cried foul, the authors were
unrepentant. They had pulled off a wicked practical joke, in the process
demonstrating that collaboration and revision can yield startling results.

Collaboration and revision are what writers—and scientists—do.
Sometimes the result is a naked stranger. Sometimes it's naked DNA.

•

In August 1989, Chiron was using yeast cells to generate the gp120 protein that it was developing as an AIDS vaccine. As a pet project of their

own, Chiron biologist Nancy Haigwood and a colleague had created a plasmid that could galvanize hamster cells, called CHO cells in the lab, into generating larger quantities of gp120 than anyone would have thought possible. A plasmid, also referred to as a vector, is a biological handle that lets a scientist pick up a piece of DNA material and move it into a target cell. Nancy's invention was the hottest vector that the young field of genetic engineering had seen so far, and other scientists were excited about the high levels of protein it could induce mammalian cells to express. There was less excitement about it at Chiron, where the primary focus was on making vaccines in yeast cells.

Nancy was surprised when she received a phone call from Philip Felgner, a biochemist at Vical, a biotech start-up in San Diego. Although the two had never met, Felgner had heard rumors at a recent scientific conference about Nancy's remarkable high-expression vector. His company had been eagerly seeking just such a plasmid, he said. If Vical had a vector as jazzy as Nancy's, they could move forward with what Phil promised would be an entirely new concept in immunization.

"You'd better make an appointment to come up here," Nancy told him.

When the day arrived, Nancy and her colleagues and bosses gathered in a Chiron conference room. Before them stood thirty-nine-year-old Phil Felgner, a Ph.D. in biochemistry who had pioneered the idea of gene therapy at Vical. Phil came from a small German town in Michigan and had spent a decade at Michigan State as an undergrad and graduate student. He was a good-looking man of medium build, with wavy hair and eyes that crinkled when he smiled, and he spoke with the flat accent of the upper Midwest. With him was Gary Rhodes, at forty-six a burly, gray-bearded bear of a fellow who looked like central casting's idea of a classic mountain man. The two were a study in contrasts, with Phil as the smooth, articulate front man and Gary as the guy who would do the heavy lifting if the companies agreed to collaborate. One thing was certain: If they struck a deal, Nancy's plasmid was going on an adventure that she had never imagined when she made it. In Phil's hands, it would dramatize the power of DNA vaccines.

The story that Phil unfolded on that ordinary August day was spiced with serendipity and high hopes, and the Chiron scientists and executives listened attentively.

●

Vical was one of hundreds of biotech companies that academic scientists scrambled to form once they decided that business was not a dirty word. A group of AIDS researchers at UC-San Diego founded Vical in 1988, one year after the antiviral drug AZT was approved as a treatment for AIDS. Already doctors were reporting that AZT, which was given in pill form, had serious side effects and didn't work for everyone. AIDS cases in the United States had soared from nearly 50,000 in 1987 to more than 80,000 by the end of 1988, and the demand for new treatments was intense.

AZT works by inhibiting reverse transcriptase, the enzyme that HIV uses to translate its RNA genetic code into DNA, the programming language that human cells understand. Vical's founders knew of similar compounds, which they thought would be more clinically effective packaged in man-made beads of fatty acids, called liposomes, and given to patients as injections. They based this reasoning on earlier experiments showing that liposomes seemed to be easily taken up by certain types of cells.

Phil Felgner and his wife, Jiin, a pharmaceutical chemist, were among Vical's earliest hires, even though neither had any experience with AIDS research. Phil had been interested in cell membranes since he was a postdoc and for the past six years had been packaging DNA in a special kind of liposome he invented while working for a larger company. These fatty packets were made of fats with a positive electrical charge, called cationic lipids. They had two advantages over garden-variety, negatively charged fats. First, he found that if cationic lipids were tossed in a test tube with DNA, they wrapped the DNA into neat little packages without further human intervention. So the labor costs would be low. Second, he hoped that cells—whose negatively charged membranes ordinarily repel negatively charged DNA—would draw positively charged liposomes right in.

When Phil arrived at Vical, he spent part of his time packaging possible AIDS drugs in liposomes. But he was more interested in exploring how these DNA-lipid complexes could be used for gene therapy, especially against cancer. If liposomes could ferry carefully chosen DNA into tumors, the cancer cells should manufacture the protein encoded by the

DNA. Then, if everything went well, the patient's immune system would recognize the protein as an intruder and attack it, thus destroying the tumor cells. Although Vical's founders were still mainly interested in new ways of delivering AIDS drugs, they encouraged Phil to pursue gene therapy for cancer.

Encouragement is one thing, Phil soon discovered, and material help is quite another. Vical was a tiny company that spent its first nine months at General Atomic, a defunct nuclear research facility that became a famous biotech incubator by renting lab space to start-ups. Like starstruck kids, Phil and his coworkers watched the legendary Jonas Salk come and go from his infant AIDS vaccine company, Immune Response Corporation, which was right next door. They marveled that Salk had raised $100 million in his company's initial public offering (IPO), an amount they could barely dream about. At the time, Vical didn't have anything to do with AIDS vaccines. If they'd had a crystal ball, Phil and his coworkers would have been surprised to find that a vaccine they pioneered would have more staying power, and become more scientifically respectable, than Salk's.

When Phil gave his presentation at Chiron in August 1989, he described making a new generation of lipids that zipped genes into cells more efficiently than his earlier creations. Inside these liposomes he inserted one of several gene "markers." Researchers love gene markers because they light up when exposed to radiation. And when researchers see this glow, which constitutes a "positive result," they know that the gene got into the cell and made its product.

Phil could see the glow of radiation in vitro, meaning in test tubes, but this was only the first step. What he needed was to demonstrate this same effect in living tissues, that is, in vivo. But at the time, he couldn't take this next step because Vical wasn't equipped to do animal experiments.

Just before Christmas in 1988, Phil went to visit a UC-San Diego professor who worked on gene therapy. The professor was away, and Phil instead struck up a conversation with a young postdoc named Jon Wolff, who was leaving in a few weeks for the University of Wisconsin. Wolff had been packaging marker genes in his lab chief's retroviral vectors, injecting them into mice, and looking for proteins coded by the marker genes. If he saw the proteins, he would know that the genes had been expressed in the cells. Now he was going to have his own lab at Wisconsin, complete with animal facilities. What Wolff did not have was a project, and here stood Phil, an interesting guy with a provocative idea but no way of doing immunology experiments in mice. Clearly, it was a match.

"We decided that we would make all the formulations at Vical, and then ship them to Jon and he would inject them the next day and analyze the tissue," Phil recalls. They agreed to use a marker gene known as CAT, whose protein product glows brightly on radioactive plates. As soon as Wolff had photographs of the images in hand he would fax them out to Vical.

Wolff injected the first batch of mice right after New Year's Day 1989. Because he didn't know which tissues might be most receptive to the CAT-carrying liposomes, he injected into legs, tails, ears—pretty much anywhere he could insert a needle. A few days later he sent the results to Phil, who was hovering over his fax machine in San Diego. "The very first week, the very first experiment, all these tissues were showing *spots*," Phil says, his voice rising excitedly even ten years after the fact. "We were able to observe expression in vivo and we were thrilled." If the liposomes and their DNA cargo had not gotten into the cells, and if the marker gene hadn't been able to make its protein, the sheets in Phil's hand would have been a flat, uniform black.

But the following week, things got screwy. Again Phil sent Wolff vials of liposomes loaded with the CAT gene, but this time he also sent others containing nothing but the plasmid that had been used to insert CAT into the liposomes. These plasmids, which Phil and his colleagues thought of as "naked" DNA, were included as a negative control, a supposedly inert material that should not light up on the assay. Their only purpose was to make the ever-so-promising liposomes look good. The naked DNA sheets should be basic black and the liposomes should show up as white polka dots.

When the second week's results emerged from Vical's fax machine, Phil and his colleagues were flummoxed. Every page showed bright spots against a dark background, sure signs that the CAT gene was being expressed no matter which vial of material had been injected. They called Wolff immediately. "This can't be right," Phil told him. The collaborators agreed that there was some mistake: The samples had gotten muddled, there were liposomes in all the vials, or somehow lipids from Vical's lab had contaminated the samples of naked DNA. So Phil's lab prepared another set of vials and sent them to Wisconsin. But the results were the same.

By the third week of January, Phil recalls, "we started doing experiments without any lipid involved. And then we got convinced that this was actually a naked DNA effect." Although biologic principles dictated that the negatively charged membrane of mouse cells should repel negatively charged DNA, obviously some cells not only invited the DNA inside but also made whatever protein it encoded. This was a mind-blowing result.

Phil saw the business implications immediately: If Vical hitched its star to liposomes, it would be forced to compete with larger, richer companies that were also seeking patents on liposome technology. "But as soon as we got the naked DNA results, we knew that this was quite different from a business and from a patent perspective. Nobody was doing anything with naked DNA, so we had a blocking position that was very broad. And when you start a biotechnology company, that's what you're looking for," Phil said.

If they did nail down a broad patent on naked DNA, what would it be good for? The mouse cells were making some proteins, but not in quantities large enough to treat a disease like diabetes or cystic fibrosis, in which the absence of a crucial protein causes chronic illness. Treating such a condition would require proteins by the teaspoon, not by the drop. Small doses of protein might be useful as a vaccine, Phil thought, and this was worth pursuing.

Gary Rhodes, who had been doing immunology research at nearby Scripps Clinic in San Diego, was swiftly brought in to explore whether naked DNA had a future as a vaccine. His task was to determine, as fast as he could, whether protein levels would be high enough to elicit immune responses that might protect against an infectious pathogen. Gary's early results suggested that this might work, and from practically his first day on the job, he was funneling his data to Vical's lawyers.

"They spent more money on patent attorneys than on scientific research when I was there," Gary later said, with more than a touch of acid, "and they got what they paid for." On March 23, 1989, Vical applied for two extremely broad patents. One covered direct administration of naked DNA for protein expression in mammalian cells, and the other claimed direct administration of naked DNA for immunization. Both drew this new technology with a paint roller, filling in no details about the plasmids they were using or how they were being administered. Like a yard dog that wants to scare off rivals, they were trying to mark every tree. How well they succeeded would not be known for many years.

●

When Vical and Chiron representatives met for the first time, about five months after Vical applied for its key patents, Phil gave a glowing account of his group's remarkable discovery. Although he presented experimental data suggesting that naked DNA held promise as a vaccine because it could stimulate immune responses, he could sniff skepticism in the air at Chiron. But Phil and Gary did not slink out of the room. They insisted that Nancy's plasmid, known to express tremendous levels of HIV gp120 protein in hamster cells, would be the most efficient and dramatic way to discover what naked DNA could accomplish in animals. And if the gamble paid off and Chiron's plasmid elicited a strong immune response, then Chiron's leadership in AIDS vaccines would be solidified and Vical would become a player.

Nancy was willing to allow Vical to use the plasmid, known around the lab as 6a, for six months. Vical was authorized to use 6a only to try to demonstrate the principle of naked DNA immunization and in return agreed to send blood samples from the animals to Nancy's lab for independent testing. The agreement was signed on October 11, 1989.

It was a win-win situation. Chiron was riding high and growing fast in late 1989: Although it had yet to earn a profit, the Food and Drug Administration had just approved its blood-screening test for hepatitis C, and stock analysts were impressed by its joint ventures with international heavy hitters like Ciba-Geigy and Merck. Phil was confident that DNA vaccines would put Vical on the map and that Nancy's expression vector would make this happen.

By now Vical had set up its own animal facility, and Gary immediately began immunizing mice with the Chiron plasmid. It didn't take long for him to detect antibodies to the HIV gp120 in blood samples. Next, Gary looked for a cellular immune response, a task that required more elaborate lab assays, and found signs of killer T cell activity against HIV. But that was as far as he could get in this animal model, because nature has made mice safe from AIDS. Just as plants require certain conditions to thrive, viral infections can only be sustained by certain types of cells. And mouse cells won't support HIV infection long enough for AIDS to develop. Gary wanted to work with chimps or better yet with monkeys, which can develop AIDS-like disease, immunize them, and see how well they were protected when exposed to virus.

Gary and his colleagues wrote up their mouse results and submitted the article to a series of scientific journals, only to be rejected time and time again. "We got the usual runaround: this can't be true, and even if it was true you people couldn't do it." Some of the article's peer reviewers, outside scientists who advise editors about what they should print, grudgingly admitted that the mice did seem to mount an immune response. But this meant nothing unless protection could be shown in a challenge experiment.

Chiron did not have the enthusiastic response to Gary's experiments that he and Phil had hoped for. In early 1990, when the six-month agreement between Chiron and Vical expired, it was not renewed. Vical would have to look elsewhere for money and support.

●

Phil Felgner was wrong in assuming that he was the only one vaccinating mice with naked DNA. In fact, just as Jon Wolff's riveting results were emerging from Phil's fax machine in San Diego, a nervous young immunology researcher on the East Coast was telling a renowned scientist about this very same idea. It was early 1989, and on short notice, thirty-four-year-old David Weiner found himself in an elegantly appointed private dining room at Philadelphia's famous Wistar Institute, describing DNA vaccines to Hilary Koprowski, one of the grand old men of virology.

Less than an hour earlier, Dave had been across the street in his laboratory at the University of Pennsylvania's medical complex, where he was a lowly research assistant professor of medicine. He was working under a flow hood, which looks like a fancy kitchen exhaust hood. Clad in a protective gown, mask, and gloves, Dave was mixing blood from immunized mice with samples of HIV-infected human blood, hoping that the mouse blood would kill the virus in a test tube.

This was not the best time for Dave to stop what he was doing and take a phone call, but when he was told that Koprowski was on the line, he shed his gear immediately. Koprowski was a member of the prestigious National Academy of Sciences, a legendary vaccine developer at Lederle Laboratories and elsewhere, and for more than three decades director of the Wistar Institute, which had grown and thrived during his regime. Dave knew him only as a larger-than-life figure who showed up at meetings, someone who should always be greeted politely. They had never exchanged more than a few pleasantries.

"How are you? Why aren't we getting together more often?" Koprowski spoke to Dave as though they were old friends.

"I'd love to get together more often," Dave said, somewhat puzzled.

"Good. I'll see you in fifteen minutes for lunch." Click.

Fifteen minutes later, Dave was seated in Koprowski's executive dining room, eating a lovely meal prepared by the great man's chef and explaining how he got involved in DNA vaccines, a concept that was unknown to most scientists and not taken seriously by the rest. Even at Penn, nobody paid much attention to this idea except the people who worked in his lab. Dave's DNA brainstorm had come during a cancer seminar, where researchers described how they put genes associated with cancer, called oncogenes, into plasmids that could sometimes penetrate animal cells and turn them malignant. In these experiments, one way to tell whether an oncogene had reached its target was to look for antibodies to it in the animal's bloodstream.

A plasmid alone wouldn't stimulate the immune system to make antibodies. So if the researchers could detect antibodies, Dave thought, that must mean that the oncogene had induced host cells to manufacture its protein. And if this was happening, surely some of the protein was being transported to the cell's surface in a way that stimulates not just antibodies, which are the main actors in humoral immunity, but also the cellular arm of the immune system. And that interested Dave a great deal, because he was pretty sure that both types of immunity would be needed to protect people against AIDS.

Plasmids, for those cancer researchers and most other molecular biologists, were nothing more than convenient handles for picking up DNA and moving it from one place to another. But Dave was struck by a different idea. "I thought that what was a laboratory tool in these oncology experiments could be adapted for use as a vaccine. You just had to figure out how to do that."

Koprowski thought the concept of a DNA vaccine was wonderfully exciting and new. He was also impressed that Weiner, who had become an assistant professor only a few months earlier, already had experience presenting research to biotech and pharmaceutical companies. Dave had been the designated hitter for his lab chief on a couple of occasions, which is not an opportunity given to many postdocs. Over cognac and cigars, Koprowski offered Dave an appointment at the Wistar. Koprowski would work out the financial details with Penn, and Dave's lab would stay where it was. But he would also have an office at the Wistar, and the sign on the door would read "Director of Biotechnology." All this was tremendously flattering to David Weiner, a young man from Bensonhurst who slips back into Brooklynese when it suits him and who makes self-deprecating references to his roots when he worries about misusing a word or a fork. He said yes to Koprowski's offer.

As much as Dave relished his new ties to the Wistar, his real work was going on across the street in Room 573 of the Maloney Building, one of the oldest parts of Penn's hospital complex. Dave and another recently promoted assistant professor had moved into this lab suite in late 1988. Deserted for years, it was a jumble of antiquated glassware and cork-stopped bottles of mercury and other poisons. Bay by bay and bench by bench, the two young academics sorted and packed toxic reagents and radioactive materials according to instructions provided by the university's hazardous waste experts. Unwilling to expose their students or lab technicians to the detritus of a less-cautious era, they did everything themselves—down to the scrubbing and painting. They also set up containment spaces where Dave and his staff could safely handle HIV, which they were already inserting into bacterial plasmids.

Although the lab was much improved, on blustery winter days snow blew in through the ill-fitting casement windows, and in high summer, rivulets of water leaked onto the floor from overtaxed air-conditioning units. Just outside the hollow sliding door to Dave's office was a table where students and technicians crowded to eat lunch and talk, elbowing aside stacks of journals and books. Funky though it was, this was Dave's first lab of his own and he liked it.

●

The pranksters who wrote *Naked Came the Stranger*, like other writers, knew that the urge to edit a manuscript is powerful. Whether we are rereading our own words or those of someone else, we cannot resist feeling that a few small changes will make the work ever so much more powerful and effective.

Molecular biologists are no different. They tinker with the raw material of nature and edit their own inventions. For genetic engineers, the first draft comes in the form of plasmids—small, flexible rings of DNA that float around in a bacterium, carrying bits of genetic information that are copied independently of the blueprint carried in the organism's large central chromosome. Sometimes during conjugation, which is the bacteria's version of sex, these little loops of DNA are passed back and forth like gifts, transferring useful bits of code from one creature to the next. Some plasmids carry traits that make the bugs resistant to antibiotics; others tell how to make toxins that can destroy enemies. That is what plasmids do in the wild, before humans lay hands on them. This innate capacity of plasmids to move genetic material from point A to point B, and deliver it intact, makes them wildly attractive and utterly indispensable to molecular biologists. Pieces of DNA are hard to hold on to, and plasmids are a way of carrying them around in a reproducible form and inserting them in the right place. Being human, of course, biologists cannot resist the impulse to edit and rewrite what nature has supplied. And once a plasmid has been altered by one user, others can't keep their hands off it.

When Nancy Haigwood made her vector for expressing gp120 in Chinese hamster ovary cells, for example, she started with the plasmid's basics. She kept the "on switch" that enables the plasmid to replicate itself, over and over, as little circles inside bacteria. And she retained a gene for antibiotic resistance, because this would later help her distinguish CHO cells that had taken up the plasmid from those which did not. Then she began adding on.

She inserted the gene for gp120 because her central mission was to make lots of this protein in CHO cells. And because she wanted the gp120 signal to be loud and clear, she stuck in a eukaryotic promoter—a piece of DNA that would drive the expression of gp120 (or any other gene that followed it) specifically in mammalian cells. This effectively turned up the volume on gp120, so that the hamster cells responded by making more of it. Nancy used a promoter that originated in cytomegalovirus, referred to in medicine as CMV, a virus that multiplies easily in people and other animals. And because the promoter is always "on," she also inserted a termination code at the end of the gp120 signal, to tell the CHO cell to stop copying at that point.

In 1989, these elements added up to the best mammalian cell expression vector that anyone had ever seen. Officially, it was burdened by the designation pCMV6a gp120-SF2; unofficially, it was simply called 6a. Stick this baby in a cell and it would gush gp120. But even 6a was a work in progress, tinkered with over the years by every gene jockey who touched it, always in the interest of "optimizing the vector." A similar process took place in Dave Weiner's lab at Penn, where another of nature's rough drafts was revised time and time again, all in hopes of making a DNA vaccine against AIDS. An unintended consequence of all this editing and revision would be that as the years passed, it would become harder to determine who really owned any of these vectors. Ultimately, this uncertainty might lead to a latter-day version of the protracted dispute over whether American scientist Bob Gallo or French researcher Luc Montagnier first discovered the AIDS virus.

●

Once it became apparent that Chiron was not going to join forces with Vical, no matter how promising Gary's results were with the gp120 plasmid in mice, Phil Felgner began promoting the idea of naked DNA to any pharmaceutical company, bigger biotech, or venture-capital outfit that would listen. "The broad concept was that we had a new approach to gene therapy, but the near-term opportunity was this vaccine. So any company that we went to had to be interested in developing vaccines, and there weren't that many," Phil remembers.

In the first months of 1990, Phil and Gary put on suits and ties and flew to Switzerland to stage their dog-and-pony show for executives at Ciba-Geigy and Sandoz. They went to Indianapolis to talk with Eli Lilly, and to Massachusetts to meet with Amgen and Genetics Institute. Their efforts were crucial to Vical, which was trying to reinvent itself as a gene-therapy and vaccine company. By now it was obvious that the original business plan, which focused on liposome-encased AIDS drugs, was simply not going to work. Although injectable treatments had sounded good to Vical's founders, it was now clear that AIDS patients had no interest in shots when competing drugs were available as pills. Vical's original investors balked at coughing up more money, and bottom-feeding venture capitalists were beginning to circle the wounded company.

It was a tough time for scientists in a biotech that still had only about two dozen employees. Research staff were asked to work on everything at once because Vical needed to keep all its options open. There were no products or royalties bringing in money, and rumors flew about the company's precarious financial situation. Employees worried that the investors would walk away before the next paycheck cleared the bank.

In the spring of 1990, having been turned down by the other vaccine makers, Phil and Gary arrived at the Merck Research Laboratories in West Point, Pennsylvania. Beautifully situated in farm country outside Philadelphia, this research and manufacturing facility is bigger than many college campuses, with eighty buildings located on 400 acres of fenced and secured land. With some 7,000 employees, it dominates the nearby small town and its environs. Merck has the largest in-house research operation of any U.S. pharmaceutical company, but Phil was not impressed. He'd been to grander companies in Europe, after all, and had come away with nothing.

Still, Phil remained stubbornly optimistic as he and Gary were ushered into a conference room where three people were waiting. The most famous and imposing figure was seventy-one-year-old Maurice Hilleman, a lanky giant well over six feet tall, with piercing eyes and strong features, dressed in his customary three-piece suit. For twenty-seven years,

Hilleman headed Virus and Cell Biology at Merck, and although he had stepped down in 1984, the world-famous vaccinologist still headed Merck's charitable foundation and was an influential consultant to his old department. Hilleman's reputation was intimidating: He was universally recognized as having developed and brought to market more vaccines than anyone else. Not only that, but in person he was quick to deflate foolishness with his precise and profane wit.

Flanking Hilleman were two scientists in their early thirties, rising stars who had recently been promoted to the level of director. At Merck this is roughly the same as being an associate professor at a university; they had survived the first cut and their prospects were good. Emilio Emini, a stocky New Yorker with a thick thatch of black hair and a beard covering his throat as well as his chin, had earned a Ph.D. in microbiology at Cornell ten years earlier. His interest in vaccines had attracted him to Merck, but in 1990, the company gave him the opportunity to prove himself as head of HIV Biology and Immunology.

Instead of vaccines, Emini now worked on Merck's highest-profile AIDS project, an all-out effort to develop a new type of drug called a protease inhibitor. HIV-specific protease is an enzyme that baby viruses, or virions, need to package themselves so they can slip out of an infected cell and into the bloodstream, where they colonize and destroy other cells. Many scientists thought a drug that could block protease would not only outperform AZT and other treatments but would also have fewer side effects. Merck and other big companies were racing to have the first protease inhibitor on the market.

Margaret Liu, one year younger than Emini and a relative newcomer to Merck, was a Harvard-trained physician who looked at vaccines not as a virus expert might, but as an immunologist would. Her main goal was figuring out how vaccines could be used to summon the cellular immune system to the body's defense. A Colorado native, she was a slim Chinese-American woman with a firm handshake, an upright carriage, and no shortage of political savvy or ambition. At Merck, Margaret had recently been put in charge of immunology research for the powerful Virus and Cell Biology Department. In her new role, she traveled around, scouting biotech companies for promising ideas about how vaccines might generate killer T cell activity as well as antibodies. This strategy was a departure from Merck's do-it-yourself tradition, which holds that Merck makes its own discoveries instead of acquiring them from others. But innovation is where you find it, in Margaret's view, and she reported to a new vice president for research who was of the same mind.

●

The human body, like a big city, can be a rowdy and dangerous place. Some of its troubles are home grown, such as inherited disorders or normal cells that turn cancerous. But maladies as serious as AIDS or as trivial as a temporary stomach upset are generally the mischief of viruses or bacteria that roll into town from someplace else. These are the outside agitators that vaccines must prepare the immune system to overcome.

Just as cities need both street cops and detectives, the body has two types of protective immune response: humoral and cellular. The humoral response—named for the medieval term "humors," which referred to blood and other body fluids—sends specialized cells throughout the body to battle intruders. In this arm of the immune system, B lymphocytes manufacture antibodies that prowl the bloodstream and the spaces between cells. Like alert patrolmen on a familiar beat, antibodies are prepared to challenge dangerous-looking strangers. Vaccines against poliovirus, measles, and other microbes work by teaching the street cop the profile of a specific microbial wise guy. The job of memory B cells, which are stored in the lymph nodes, is never to forget the face of a villain they've tangled with in the past.

Although antibodies have a fighting chance against viruses that are out in the open, their reach doesn't extend to viruses that have sought shelter within the body's own cells. This is where the cellular response comes in. This arm of the immune system employs the special skills of T cells, the main actors of the cellular response. Like detectives going through garbage cans for evidence of foul play or contraband, T cells scrutinize the exterior of other cells looking for viral antigens, which are clues that a pathogen—a disease-causing microbe—is hidden inside.

Criminals invariably leave behind traces that can link them to a crime, when analyzed by a good detective: fingerprints, fibers, hair, DNA. So, too, do viruses, leaving debris on the outer surface of cells in the form of antigens. Made up of fragments from the virus and the injured cell, antigens are processed and sorted for disposal inside the cell. Just as we separate garbage from recyclables, the cell sorts trash before hauling it out. There are two routes to the curb, both of which involve specialized MHC molecules. MHC class I molecules attach to viral antigens, which makes them visible to cytotoxic T lymphocytes, also called CTLs or killer T cells. Once these CTLs know to look for an invader, they hunt down and kill every infected cell they can find—like detectives on a life-or-death mission. Copies of CTLs are archived and can be reactivated if the same antigen ever returns.

In the second disposal mechanism, MHC class II molecules grab the viral antigens and display them in a way that is recognizable to helper T cells. Having recognized the antigens, the helper Ts don't attack the virus directly. Instead, like a cop calling for backups, helper Ts sound a general alarm that boosts production of both antibodies and killer T cells.

Helper T cells have gained a sad notoriety in the age of AIDS. HIV uses CD4 receptors on the surface of helper T cells to penetrate and destroy them. As an AIDS patient's level of these CD4 cells falls, his or her immune system fails and the body becomes vulnerable to microbes that a healthy immune system would swiftly overpower.

Once it became clear that HIV obliterates CD4s—the very cells that would ordinarily coordinate defensive responses against an invading microbe—researchers became increasingly certain that a very special vaccine would be needed to defeat this virus. They disagreed, however, about what it should do. Many scientists believed a vaccine would have to elicit both antibodies and T cells to ward off HIV; others thought programming antibodies before the body's initial encounter with the virus would do the trick. In the absence of convincing evidence for either side, this argument was to drag on for years. As a consequence, some companies pursued vaccines that would activate the humoral arm of the immune system, unleashing antibody street cops to battle the virus. Meanwhile, other vaccine developers focused on generating CTL responses. And there was no way to know which strategy, if either, was the right one.

●

Although many vaccines elicit antibodies against specific pathogens, such as polio or measles, in 1990 scientists did not have a safe and sure method for getting T cells involved in self-defense. This troubled them, because most viral infections are intracellular. And clearly HIV is a virus that penetrates human cells quickly and efficiently with devastating results. In Margaret Liu's words, "The Holy Grail for immunologists was getting a CTL response." And not just a cellular response that could be measured in the laboratory, which is relatively easy, but one strong enough to fight off an attacker in the real world. Margaret wanted to know how a vaccine could use MHC class I molecules to display proteins in a way that would program killer T cells to attack a specific pathogen before the body actually encountered it.

And so she listened attentively as Phil and Gary described what happened when they injected a plasmid containing an HIV gene into mice. "When Vical showed these data indicating that you could have the gene taken up and have the protein produced within the cell, we said 'Wow. This is endogenous [in the cell] production. Let's see if we can use it to make CTL responses,'" Margaret said of her first encounter with naked DNA.

Phil and Gary were exhausted from repeating their story to groups of pharmaceutical company executives who just didn't get it. But their meeting with Merck was clearly different. "Margaret Liu obviously saw the potential of the thing," Gary said. But Emilio Emini, who had just been put in charge of developing a protease inhibitor to treat AIDS, was far less receptive. Although the Vical team correctly surmised that Emini would not be enthusiastic about any new undertaking that might divert resources from his drug project, they did not know that he also had his own reasons for being pessimistic about the prospects for an AIDS vaccine.

In the mid-1980s, Emini had been quite disappointed by a couple of HIV vaccine ideas that had turned out to be hopeless dead-ends. "What I did, personally, was I gave up. Gave out. And temporarily put the vaccine stuff aside," Emini said years later. In 1990, when Phil and Gary were doing their sales pitch, Emini had hitched his wagon to a winner and it was a protease inhibitor, not a vaccine.

By all accounts, it was the enthusiasm of Maurice Hilleman, Merck's grand old man of vaccinology, that tipped the balance in Vical's favor.

Phil Felgner says, "If he had been against it, we definitely would not have gone ahead, that's for sure. But he was really keen on it, and that's what it took at Merck vaccines at the time."

Six months after this initial meeting, Merck and Vical worked out an agreement to keep Vical afloat. Vical scientists taught Margaret and her team their protocol for immunizing mice, and together the two companies carried out a "proof of principle" experiment. HIV wasn't used because it makes no sense to challenge mice with this virus, since they resist infection with it. So the scientists put influenza genes into the plasmid, immunized groups of mice, analyzed their cellular and humoral responses, and finally challenged them with a whopping dose of flu virus. If immunized mice outlived ones that had not been given vaccine, then there would be reason to hope that naked DNA might hold promise as a vaccine for people.

Merck paid the bill for this research. So long as the initial experiments worked well and Vical met certain deadlines, the giant company agreed to license Vical's DNA technology to make vaccines against flu, HIV, and several other infectious diseases. "They had an option to pull out," Phil said, "Every year we had to perform in order for them to renew." In his view, the best part about the Merck deal wasn't the money, although that was certainly no small thing, but rather Merck's endorsement of a technology that lesser companies—and some greater ones in Europe—had scorned.

●

It was lunchtime, but on the first floor of Building 16, Margaret Liu closed the door to her office, clamped a set of headphones over her ears, and began to play from a score propped on the music stand. Her fingers galloped across the keys of the electric piano, which had been customized so that their action duplicated the feel of a concert instrument. Margaret was squeezing in some practice so that she would be ready to play for rehearsals with the Bala Cynwyd Symphony.

Ever since Margaret was a youngster growing up in Colorado, science and music have been her passions. After graduating from Colorado College, where she earned honors in chemistry, she enrolled in a Paris conservatory and earned a *diplôme* in piano. She became fluent in Chopin and in French, then went to Boston to attend medical school at Harvard. Her curriculum vitae glittered with awards and fellowships and prestigious appointments.

Margaret came to Merck in June 1988 via a worn path already traveled by the president of Merck & Co., the president of Merck Research Laboratories, the manager who recruited her, and scores of other Merck scientists. It leads from Harvard Medical School to Massachusetts General Hospital to America's most-admired drugmaker. Her husband, a Harvard-trained cardiologist, followed the same road to Merck.

Early 1991 was an extremely stressful time for Margaret, who had bet her rising career on naked DNA. Out in San Diego, Phil could relax after Merck had bought into the idea; here in West Point, the tense times were just beginning. Upstairs, in her laboratory on the third floor of Building 16, she and her colleagues were using Vical's plasmids and procedures to retrace every step the California scientists had already taken. And they were being ribbed for doing it.

Skeptical colleagues jokingly referred to naked DNA as "cold fusion," likening it to the discredited idea of creating atomic power in a mason jar. They poked their heads into Margaret's lab to ask, "How's the weird science doing?" Margaret's colleagues totally dismissed the idea that genetic material from a virus could be deliberately inserted into mammalian cells, then direct production of a viral protein that would stimulate a protective immune response.

Although scientists are supposed to make decisions based on objective data, old paradigms die hard. Margaret herself was skeptical about viral DNA being taken up by muscle cells and churning out enough protein to be clinically useful. But "either there's something here or these guys have made a mistake. And if there's something here, we don't want to miss out on it," she said.

It took most of 1991 to run the proof of principle experiment using flu. "One reason it took so long was that we were on different coasts," Gary Rhodes says. "It's much easier to show somebody how to do it than to describe how to do it." Vical sent people to tutor Margaret and her crew in mouse immunization, and that summer Margaret and two of her lab people traveled to Vical for more training. Margaret was thirty-three years old and pregnant with her first child, and while she was in San Diego, she collected some hand-me-down baby clothes from her sister. When her son was born, she took two weeks off from work.

Despite Margaret's growing administrative responsibilities at Merck, she also spent time in the lab injecting naked DNA into mice. Bench work would be too lowly an activity for most scientists at her level. But Margaret was a typical Type A personality and believed that the only way to be sure of something is to learn how to do it yourself. Because she had been trained in the procedure, Margaret would know whether the mouse work had been properly carried out by others.

No matter who conducted these experiments, each required nearly three months to yield results. Each mouse typically got two shots, and immune responses took several weeks to build up after each inoculation. Several additional weeks were spent observing mice that had been challenged with a huge dose of flu virus. By late summer, Gary knew he had successfully protected mice against flu. But he had to keep quiet about the results until Margaret's lab reached the same conclusion. By January 1992, both teams had demonstrated that naked DNA worked as a flu vaccine, at least in mice. Whether the same approach could be used for HIV remained to be seen.

At about the same time, Emilio Emini and other Merck scientists synthesized a series of protease inhibitors they began exploring as treatments for AIDS. Other major companies were also racing to make such drugs. Although the first four compounds were considered failures, the one they dubbed indinavir, eventually sold as Crixivan, would turn out to be a blockbuster. It entered clinical trials in 1993, and its climb toward the pantheon of history's most lucrative drugs consumed resources that might otherwise have been shared with Margaret's vaccine-development efforts. Ironically, a product that aimed to prevent AIDS in millions of people took a backseat to a drug that would treat the disease in thousands.

●

Meanwhile, on the Penn campus, Dave Weiner was paging through the March 23, 1990, issue of *Science,* when he ran across an article titled "Direct Gene Transfer into Mouse Muscle In Vivo." The first author was

Jon Wolff, at the University of Wisconsin, and the senior author was Philip L. Felgner of Vical, a biotech company that Dave had never heard of. Dave read this without knowing that only one week earlier Phil had been just a few miles away, making his pitch to Merck Research Labs in West Point.

Dave zeroed in on the observation that there was something special about muscle tissue. In Wolff and Felgner's experiments, plasmids generated more protein when injected into muscle than into the skin, bloodstream, or elsewhere. Throughout 1989, Dave and his lab workers had been putting HIV and various marker genes into plasmids and injecting them "all over the place" in mice, just as Wolff had earlier done. And Dave saw levels of protein expression that were all over the map, leaving him clueless about what the optimum injection site might be.

After reading the Vical paper, Dave decided to do more injections into muscle. About the same time, he noticed that marker genes appeared to express better in immature muscle cells. Remembering that biology professors use a dab of local anesthetic to trigger division in muscle cells, so students could see cell division in action, he guessed that this might also boost the uptake of plasmids—and thus the production of protein—in these cells. Dave soon found that exposing muscle cells to bupivacaine, a common local anesthetic, improved protein expression and made results more consistent within groups of mice. This was the discovery that Penn's intellectual property attorneys soon moved to protect. They applied for a patent on the use of DNA as a vaccine, with its delivery enhanced by the use of bupivacaine or other local anesthetics.

Dave was encouraged enough to begin talking about his findings with more people, both at Penn and at outside scientific conferences. "Whoever I spoke with on the HIV front said, 'It's very cute, but without a company you can't go anywhere.' So I was interested in finding somebody who could manufacture and test it," he said.

Hilary Koprowski, his mentor at the Wistar Institute, was eager to help. When venture capitalists came sniffing around the Wistar for new technology, Koprowski made sure that Dave—in his capacity as the institute's director of biotechnology—made presentations to them. Dave is a tightly knit fellow with a springy step, who looks a bit like a prematurely graying version of Robin Williams. He's got a dry delivery and a nice sense of humor, and Koprowski no doubt thought that Dave would make a good impression.

Some of the Wistar's visitors struck Dave as quick-buck artists, people who didn't know much about science and who would be impatient and difficult to work with. When he had a chance to interact with potential investors who knew a bit about experimental AIDS vaccines, many of them thought that Chiron and Genentech and a handful of other companies were right to focus on antibodies. They didn't see the need for a vaccine that brought cellular immunity into play.

One of these Wistar business lunches finally paid off, however, because it led to a meeting between Dave and an executive at Centocor who was spinning off a new company. He needed exciting technology to spark this new enterprise, which would be called Apollon, and DNA vaccines caught his fancy. It didn't hurt that Koprowski had been involved in the founding of Centocor and had strong ties with the top brass.

By January 1992, the University of Pennsylvania and Apollon had reached an initial agreement about Dave's DNA vaccines, although it would take longer to nail down the details of licensing the technology. "The agreement was that I was free and clear to work with them, and they were free and clear to move forward," Dave says. Apollon started in one wing of a Centocor building in suburban Malvern, Pennsylvania, but soon moved to Great Valley Corporate Center, a nearby office park filled mostly with computer start-ups. It was nothing fancy, but there was plenty of free parking.

From the start, Dave got along well with the executives at Apollon and their financial backers. "I can be frank with them. I can say 'I did this experiment and it didn't work.'" Dave feels more comfortable with this attitude than with investors "who only want to hear that you've cured cancer and are ready to go on to the next thing."

Although Dave now had the backing of a small biotech company, he lacked the imprimatur of the National Institutes of Health, the world's largest public underwriter of biomedical research. Repeatedly his grant proposals for DNA vaccine experiments were rejected by NIH study sections, committees of scientists who are called together to judge the work of their peers. He fared no better with the editors of major scientific journals, and at meetings people didn't hesitate to tell him that his approach couldn't possibly work. Dave was frequently warned that the FDA would never approve clinical trials, because they would be afraid that naked DNA would be taken up by human cells and copied with every cell division.

Despite a barrage of negative messages about his vaccine concept and his own worth as a scientist, Dave persisted. In 1992, with backing from Apollon, he began testing DNA vaccines in monkeys. He was running well behind a half-dozen companies whose HIV vaccines were already in human trials. Koprowski cheered Dave at every step of the way, giving this young assistant professor more confidence than he could have mustered on his own. Koprowski's advice was to go for it, and "if you fall on your face, who cares?" Dave sometimes worried overmuch about what others thought, and Koprowski's "damn the torpedoes" attitude helped keep him going.

●

During the 1980s and early 1990s, a migratory flock of vaccine researchers, public-health officials, and pharmaceutical-company executives returned every September to Cold Spring Harbor Laboratory on the North Shore of Long Island. Invited lecturers discussed various issues in vaccine science during working hours, after which convivial cocktail parties gave way to long, talky dinners. Participants renewed old friendships and perhaps met a few new people before heading uphill from the dining hall in the darkness, like tired campers, to sleep in rustic cabins or modern dormitories.

In 1992, however, something unprecedented happened in the cool, blue-and-green atmosphere of Grace Auditorium, Cold Spring Harbor's elegant main stage. For the first time, a major scientific conference devoted a session to research on naked DNA immunization. Although most of the old vaccine hands in the room either didn't know or didn't particularly care that this was a first, the four speakers and a handful of their coworkers were unbelievably keyed up.

For Dave Weiner, DNA vaccines "came together in the public eye" on this particular September day. Dave described mouse experiments using HIV genes and oncogenes. Margaret Liu and Harriet Robinson, a researcher at the University of Massachusetts, talked separately about their work with influenza and marker genes. Gary Rhodes told how in his lab DNA immunization had protected mice against flu.

Margaret Liu remembers this meeting as "an incredibly affirming experience" and says that until it happened, "we were considered to be out on the fringes of science." Dave felt tremendous relief that the audience listened calmly, unlike his experiences at other meetings, where "people would laugh at us, or abuse us publicly for our presentations." He winced at the memory of a 1991 talk, at which "a very eminent person from Columbia stood up and said, 'Dave, you're always doing these exciting things, but you know this really doesn't work this way.'"

Phil Felgner, who was not up on stage, watched the audience carefully. "I sensed that the bulk of the participants were preoccupied with other things," he recalls. "At that point they weren't really persuaded that this was a legitimate vaccine [technology]." Skepticism would have been overt if all the DNA vaccine findings had come from a single company or institution. That four groups had independently reached similar results added tremendous credibility to the DNA concept, as did the good name of Merck—a leading vaccine maker for nearly a century.

The people in the auditorium would have been surprised to learn how independent these researchers really were. "We had never before been in a room and heard everybody speak," Margaret remembers. Although she had talked to Harriet Robinson on the phone and was collaborating with Vical, she had never met Dave Weiner and knew nothing about his experiments—even though their two labs were no more than thirty minutes apart by car. "To find out that there were other groups doing this was really remarkable," Margaret said.

Dave Weiner was exhilarated. "It feels so much better to know that other people can get the same results! And I think the audience must have felt that. It was harder to say that his stuff is no good, or Harriet's is no good, or that Merck is just trying to make money, because none of us worked together but there we were."

When the official session ended, the pioneers of naked DNA strolled down the road to Blackford Hall, the laboratory's original 1907 dormitory and dining hall. They split off from the official cocktail crowd and huddled in the pub in the basement, relieved that their talks were over, senses sharpened by a mix of camaraderie and wariness. They tried to get a handle on one another, to figure out who knew whom and who worked where. Looking around the scarred wooden table, they saw for the first time that the faces of their kindred spirits and their rivals were the same.

But there was someone missing from the group. Stephen Johnston, a researcher from Dallas, likely would have been invited if the meeting's organizers had known about his work in time. Johnston had just published a paper in the prestigious journal *Nature*, reporting that the gene gun, a device he invented for doing skin-deep injections, could be used to immunize animals with naked DNA. "I can't believe he had that paper come out; we just had a paper rejected by *Nature*," said one of the researchers. Another admitted that two major journals had just turned down his latest manuscript.

"All of us realized that we had to get our papers published," Dave says of that moment in the pub. "Johnston's publication made everyone realize that there was another lap around the track. This made it more real. We couldn't continue to just bang the pavement, we had to get our stuff out there."

●

Dave Weiner stood on the stage of a darkened hotel ballroom in Atlanta. Behind him was a large projection screen. He glanced briefly at the remote control on the podium, pushed the button, then turned to look at the screen and smiled. On the left side of the slide was a ribbon of yellow undulating from top to bottom. This, according to Dave Weiner's five-year-old daughter, Rebecca, was a little girl's arm. On the right side of the picture, Rebecca had drawn a syringe that resembled a fountain pen, filled with a vaccine represented by alternating stripes of pink, green, and black. She drew this during a visit to Dave's lab, Dave told the audience, and of course he asked what was in her vaccine.

"Dad, it has all of the good things that you need and none of the bad things that would hurt you," she told him. The crowd laughed appreciatively, no doubt glad for a bit of levity during the annual meeting of the American Society of Microbiology. Dave Weiner and Margaret Liu were cochairing this session, and sharing the podium were the other charter members of the DNA vaccine club: Phil Felgner, Harriet Robinson, and Stephen Johnston from Texas. It was May 1993, eight months after the landmark meeting at Cold Spring Harbor.

The intervening months had brought a flurry of publications. In the March 19, 1993, issue of *Science*, Merck and Vical reported that naked DNA immunizations not only stimulated a CTL response in mice but also protected them against challenge with huge doses of flu virus. The names of the Vical researchers who had demonstrated protection in 1991, and who had been impatient for Merck to concur that these results were real, were buried in a list of seventeen authors. Although this delay didn't make Margaret popular with her collaborators, she stood by her judgment. "We were concerned that other people would scoop us, but I felt that something that was such a radical departure needed to be very well documented. And that's why our paper got published in *Science* and not in some other journal," she said.

In April, Dave Weiner's latest report on his HIV experiments in mice appeared in the *Proceedings of the National Academy of Sciences*. Here he showed that a DNA vaccine could elicit both antibodies and, as he had originally hoped, killer T cells against HIV. This meant the body might have a fighting chance against virus hiding in cells, as well as virus circulating in the blood. Other researchers had also published papers about DNA vaccines during the months leading up to the microbiology meeting.

On the day of the session in Atlanta, the DNA gang was stunned. "It had been scheduled for a big room but there were people out in the corridors listening because they couldn't fit inside," Dave Weiner said. No longer were DNA vaccines a subject for ridicule, as they had been in the past, or a matter of polite interest as they had been at Cold Spring Harbor. After the session, Harriet Robinson marveled aloud, "It has clearly changed. This was a very big event." And she was right. It would not be long before DNA vaccines, once shunned by high-profile scientists in government and academia, would be lionized as biotechnology's best hope against AIDS.

4

WHERE THE LIVE THINGS ARE

IN ADDITION TO THE THOUSANDS of species on this earth that are big enough to see, our world teems with more than 30,000 distinct types of viruses. The great majority of these submicroscopic creatures live quietly in the cells of a susceptible animal or plant, attracting little attention because they don't cause disease or prevent crops from growing. A few, however, have become notorious. These are the mass murderers of the virus world, perpetrators of Ebola, HIV, and other scourges. A select few of these villains have been domesticated and converted into heroes: These are the weakened, or attenuated, strains of virus that have been used to immunize millions against diseases such as smallpox, polio, and measles.

Despite their abundance, viruses were discovered less than 100 years ago. In 1915, when scientists had devised filters fine enough to trap bacteria they could see under the microscope, they found that invisible disease-producing agents were still getting through. Researchers called these gate-crashers "filterable viruses"—*virus* being a Latin word meaning "slime" or "poison." Later, when scientists developed techniques for identifying the chemical hallmarks of genetic material, they discovered that all these filterable agents harbored bits of DNA or RNA. For a time, viruses were thought to be plain and simple pieces of genetic material—equivalent to the plasmids now being used in DNA vaccines.

When electron microscopes burst on the scene in the 1940s, this idea was quickly discarded. Finally able to examine viruses in more detail, researchers were astonished to find that some looked like soccer balls, some like fishing worms, and some like the outline of a stop sign. Although scientists had been right in thinking that all viruses had a soft center of RNA or DNA, they had not guessed that it would be wrapped in a protein coat. This protective nucleocapsid, as it is officially known, keeps the genetic core from being damaged as the virus journeys from cell to cell, from one host to another. Some viruses, like HIV, have an additional outer layer called an envelope. Once a virus gets inside a cell, it throws off its overcoat and sets about reprogramming the cell's machinery to make more of itself.

Figuring out how each type of virus gets into a cell, hijacks normal cellular mechanisms, and sends forth its progeny is an endless source of fascination for the virologists who pursue it. From a public-health point of view, the rationale for studying medically significant viruses is to figure out how to prevent and treat infection. For most virologists, these are good things but not really the point.

Virologists love viruses for their own little selves. Many say a professor or lab chief introduced them to the world of viruses early in their scientific training, where they were unexpectedly captivated by what they found. Decades later, many are still working on the same individual or group of viruses that caught their youthful fancy. Some say that they can't walk away because there are still too many unsolved mysteries; others simply believe that their virus is cooler than the rest.

As anyone who has ever been in love knows, as time passes the desire to change the beloved becomes irresistible. In the old days, virologists changed their viruses like Mendel altered his peas, selecting and breeding for characteristics that were useful or interesting. It was a long and messy process. Molecular biology revolutionized this in the 1970s. Suddenly a virus was less like a hardbound book and more like a three-ring binder: The power to cut and paste genes enabled virologists to remove pages of genetic information and replace them with others. The implications for vaccine research were tremendous.

●

"Docs Discover Miracle Vaccine" was the huge page-one banner on the *New York Post* for October 18, 1983. As soon as the paper hit the streets that afternoon, a PR flack for the New York State Department of Health hustled some copies into a dark and smoky Irish pub in midtown. He marched over to a crowded table and held up the paper for all to see— including the "docs" pictured on the front page. Forty-year-old Enzo Paoletti and thirty-four-year-old Dennis Panicali were really not physicians at all, but research virologists employed by the state health department up in Albany. They were as stunned to see themselves on the tabloid as they would have been to find their faces engraved on dollar bills.

Notoriety was new to these men, whose natural habitat was a laboratory. Only a few hours earlier, they had been the main attraction at a packed press conference held at the World Trade Center, where the state health department had its Manhattan beachhead. On the front table, clusters of microphones bristled like giant black sea urchins, and the room was hot with television lights. Although the reporters had never seen these researchers before, most of them recognized State Commissioner of Health David Axelrod, the blunt fireplug of a man with them.

Axelrod told the reporters that these exciting new vaccines were the fruits of New York state's long-term investment in basic biomedical research, an expensive endeavor that he had backed while critics dismissed it as folly. Not only did these vaccines have the potential to protect the public against infectious diseases, Axelrod said, but they would bring needed revenue to the state treasury. The health department had already set up a company that stood ready to commercialize these products; they were just waiting for venture capital. When funding fell into place, Axelrod predicted that clinical trials of the new vaccines could start within three years.

When Enzo took over the microphones, he told how he and Dennis had inserted genetic material from herpes simplex, hepatitis B, and influenza into a type of vaccinia virus that had long been used as a smallpox vaccine. His thick russet hair shining in the camera lights, Enzo told how each of these new vaccines had stimulated immune responses in small animals and in one experiment had protected mice against a dose of herpes virus that should have killed them.

Reporters leaned in to hear his soft deep voice as he described even

more astonishing possibilities, such as a single shot that could protect
against three different diseases—or maybe even more. All in a product
that could be manufactured for thirty-five cents a dose, shipped to parts
of the world where there are no refrigerators, and administered with a
pinprick instead of an injection. No wonder the *Post* dubbed it a "miracle
vaccine." The *Daily News* picked up on the idea that this might be a way
of protecting against sexually transmitted herpes simplex. At this point,
most heterosexuals—still sure that straight people didn't get AIDS—
thought herpes was the worst thing that could happen to them in bed.

Dennis Panicali kept his mouth shut during the press conference.
Although he and Enzo had worked together on the vaccine idea for five
years, and although they were coinventors on patent applications for this
hot new technology, Dennis had moved out of Enzo's lab and into a space
of his own about six months earlier. The press event was only a few days
away when Dennis got wind of it. It had been set up by Axelrod's office,
apparently with lots of help from Enzo. Dennis insisted that he should be
there, and soon the rest of the lab—the people who'd done the grunt
work—were also offered a free bus trip to Manhattan for the day.

Listening to Enzo field questions, Dennis thought his former boss
sounded way too optimistic about speedy development of a herpes vaccine. Maybe five years, Dennis thought, or maybe ten. But to suggest that
clinical trials could begin in three years? That sort of claim was embarrassing.

Once they got to the Irish bar, where more reporters were brought in
by the state PR guys, Dennis was a good soldier. He talked with the writers, explaining the technology and being sure to thank Dr. Axelrod and
the state for supporting their research. Dennis and Enzo both spent time
with a *New York Times* writer, who the next day described the two as "part
of a new generation of laboratory scientists who are unlocking the genetic
secrets of cell biology." The Irish bar he upgraded to "a restaurant in Manhattan," a gentrification that amused both the scientists.

As it happened, the press conference took place on a slow news day, and
it was covered by all the major dailies, the wire services, and national and
local TV and radio outlets. "Everybody has their fifteen minutes, but this
was seventeen minutes of fame," Enzo would say later, with just a touch of
bitterness about the events that followed.

•

Dennis was twenty-eight years old when he came to Enzo's lab in 1977 as a postdoctoral fellow. A Connecticut Yankee, he'd been in graduate school at the Medical College of Georgia, which had a terrific cell and molecular biology program but was otherwise a hot, flat, dusty, and boring place to be. It was hard to believe that the lush fairways of the Augusta National were in the same city. Dennis was itching to escape Georgia and return to New England with his wife and two young sons, but after shopping around for a postdoc position he found that Albany, New York, was as close as he could come. As it turned out, he and his family loved it there.

In the lab, both Enzo and Dennis were fascinated by one of the largest and most medically significant viruses of all time—vaccinia, a descendant of the cowpox that Edward Jenner had used as a smallpox vaccine back in 1796. After 200 years of being used and manipulated by humans, the virus had changed in much the way a long-domesticated animal might. From wolf to golden retriever, from tiger to tabby. As a result, no one has seen a wild vaccinia in many years, and a large assortment of cultivated strains are used for vaccines and research.

While studying the genetic structure of a common laboratory strain, Enzo and Dennis noticed that it came in two versions—long and short—and that the latter was missing a big chunk of its DNA. Yet this deletion didn't seem to have any functional impact, and the short and long forms grew equally well in cell cultures. It was as though pages were missing from the virus's genetic binder but it didn't matter. This observation, Dennis later recalled, pointed them in a whole new direction: "If there are nonessential regions, and pieces can come out, then why can't we put something else in? With that, we decided that maybe we could use the poxviruses as a vector, as a delivery system for other genes."

When they had this revelation, back in late 1979, the two young researchers weren't thinking about using these vectors to immunize people against disease. They had no contact with the part of the health department that handled immunization and other routine public health measures; rather, they dwelled exclusively in the world of basic science. Only in retrospect would they see this as the first of many, many steps toward what the tabloids would eventually call a "miracle vaccine."

Enzo had fallen under the spell of vaccinia in 1966, shortly after he graduated from Canisius College, a small Jesuit school in Buffalo. Not knowing what he really wanted to do, except that he was drawn to the medical sciences, he got a job as a lab technician with a scientist who worked on vaccinia. Enzo hadn't been certain that he would go to graduate school before he crossed paths with the virus; afterward, he enrolled in a Ph.D. program at the State University of New York at Buffalo.

When Enzo and Dennis first had the idea of inserting foreign DNA into vaccinia, they headed for the library. The first step before careering off on something new is to search the scientific literature to see if someone else has already figured out how to do what you want to do or whether others have already tried and failed. In this case, they found that no one had taken the first step of moving DNA from one strain of vaccinia to another—much less trying to splice foreign, or heterologous, DNA into vaccinia. With no precedents to follow, they would have to break the trail on their own.

At about this time, Enzo went to visit his father, who was hospitalized in Buffalo. The Paoletti family is from one of Tuscany's ancient and beautiful hill towns, and Enzo's parents emigrated to Buffalo when he was a small boy. His Tuscan heritage shows in Enzo's face, with its chiseled features and warm dark eyes. After years in upstate New York, his manner smacks of Clint Eastwood in a Sergio Leone western. Enzo wears jeans and has a close-cropped beard, and when he squints through the smoke of his cigarette, it is as easy to imagine him lounging in an American pool hall as in a Tuscan piazza.

Enzo's mother, being Italian, made a big dinner for her visiting son. And late night found him sitting at his parents' kitchen table, just talking, perhaps with wine and cigarettes, with his brother-in-law. This man was not a scientist, but he had heard the buzz words: molecular revolution, gene splicing, genetic engineering, the whole hopeful new vocabulary of biology in the late 1970s. So, he asked Enzo, what is all this stuff good for? That's what he wanted to know.

"Vaccines," Enzo said without skipping a beat. And so the two of them talked about how recombinant DNA techniques might open the door to better and safer vaccines. When his father was out of danger, Enzo drove back to Albany on the New York State Thruway, a road not known for its scenic beauty. "It dawned on me during that trip that everything that I had been telling my brother-in-law about vaccines, one way of doing that could be through vaccinia virus," Enzo recalled twenty years later. He thought about this for the rest of the drive.

Back at the lab, he and Dennis realized that they faced some tough and very basic questions. They had not yet inserted a piece of foreign DNA into a vaccinia virus. If that could be accomplished, would the foreign DNA be expressed—along with the normal vaccinia DNA—in an infected cell? And, on a purely practical level, how would they know? They needed a way to detect whether the DNA was in place and what it was doing. If they got this far, then they'd have to see whether a souped-up version of a vaccinia could stimulate immune responses in animals.

Enzo and Dennis were excited and eager to get started on this project, but they were thwarted by some new regulatory barriers. Only six years had passed since the Boyer-Cohen experiment made recombinant DNA technology the hottest tool in all of biology. As exciting as genetic engineering was, some people feared that it would spawn dangerous, mutant organisms that would overrun the world. To reduce the odds of this happening, the National Institutes of Health set up guidelines and a review process for proposed genetic engineering experiments. This in itself was not a problem. The difficulty was that while some states were relying on the NIH guidelines, New York wanted to debate and develop its own. As a result, the vaccinia project was on hold for an entire year while the state compiled a rule book that ended up being nearly identical to the federal version.

●

When Julia Child set out to make the art of French cooking accessible to her fellow Americans, she reassured readers, "Sauces are the splendor and glory of French cooking, yet there is nothing secret or mysterious about making them." They fall into only half a dozen groups, she said, and each sauce in a group is made in the same general way. Every silky béchamel and velouté, for example, owes its texture to a roux—a simple mixture of flour and butter, cooked slowly together before any liquid is added. In molecular biology, plasmids are as basic and indispensable as a roux.

Plasmids occur naturally in bacteria, where they ferry genes among organisms. They are ubiquitous in laboratories because they serve as specialized tongs that researchers use to grip a specific bit of DNA and transfer it safely from one place to another. When Enzo and Dennis set out to make a live-vector herpes vaccine, for example, their first step was to make a plasmid that held a herpes gene. They also inserted pieces of vaccinia DNA that would steer this gene to a place in the vaccinia genome where it would blend in and be copied along with the viral DNA.

The vaccinia, at this stage of the game, was as plain as a cup of milk sitting on the kitchen counter. Only when it was put into the pot, in this case a culture dish filled with live animal cells, did it start turning into a live-vector vaccine. The gene-carrying plasmids and the basic vaccinia virus were dumped into the culture dish. Both penetrated the cells, and once inside, the vaccinia exposed its soft DNA core and set about copying itself. As this happened, the plasmids slid into the vaccinia's genetic code and inserted the herpes gene.

Not all these attempts at genetic recombination would succeed: Some strains of vaccinia could be fooled into copying the herpes gene along with their own DNA; others could not. In time, scientists figured out how to include markers in their plasmids, so that they could harvest only viruses that had accepted the foreign gene.

When a team of researchers successfully inserted their first gene into a live virus, it was as though they had mastered Julia Child's basic white-sauce recipe. Just as a cook can easily turn a white sauce into a Mornay by adding grated cheese, genetic engineers began adding a variety of disease genes to their basic vaccinia vectors.

●

Once the bureaucratic hurdles were behind them, Enzo and Dennis made dizzying progress on recombinant vaccinia vectors during the three years leading up to the press conference in New York. Their complementary skills made them excellent partners at this stage, with Enzo having more vaccinia expertise and Dennis being more facile with DNA cloning and sequencing. It was a time, Dennis would later recall, when there seemed to be no limits on what they could do. "We designed experiments, asking 'What if?' And they all worked. It was a matter of just doing it. There were tricks of the trade and breakthroughs and techniques that had to be developed, but everything came together."

In 1980, their experiments showed that a marker gene could easily be spliced into the vaccinia virus and delivered to cells in culture, which in turn expressed the protein it encoded. The first medically significant gene they inserted was from herpes, which they picked for two reasons. In addition to its status as the sexually transmitted disease of the moment, herpes was a sensible choice because other researchers had already cloned genes and shown that the disease could be emulated in mice. Elated when vaccinia willingly took up the herpes gene, Enzo and Dennis rounded up hepatitis B and influenza genes and went to work on those.

Enzo was sure that he and Dennis had discovered a new way to make vaccines. Their starting point was a vaccinia strain that had a long track record as an effective vaccine against smallpox, which had just been eradicated worldwide. They had made genetic modifications aimed at making this strain even safer than it already was, and they were retooling it to stimulate immune responses against other infectious diseases. It was like hiring an old friend in a new job. As wonderful as this concept seemed to Enzo, he knew that not even the best idea will move forward without corporate backing. Fortunately, this was not the first time that scientists on the health-department payroll had made a discovery with strong commercial potential. Years earlier, two New York health-department scientists had come up with the world's first antifungal cream, called Nystatin, and the state had licensed the rights to a major pharmaceutical company for development and marketing. This was clearly a precedent.

Unfortunately, the Wadsworth Center for Laboratories and Research, where Enzo and Dennis worked, was not a hotbed of entrepreneurial thinking in 1981. Frustrated by his bosses' ho-hum, "don't-bother-us" response to the vaccine idea, Enzo decided to tug on the old school tie that connected him with David Axelrod, the state's powerful, highly regarded health commissioner. The two had met a decade earlier at the National Institutes of Health, when Enzo went there as a postdoc in virology.

Although Axelrod was eight years older than Enzo and was already a Harvard-trained physician with impressive research credentials, the two hit it off. Both were the sons of immigrants, one Italian and the other Polish. Both grew up in cities outside the mainstream, Enzo in Buffalo and Axelrod in Great Barrington, Massachusetts. Both were smart and outspoken and interested in viruses. Equally important, neither ever wasted time pussyfooting around a subject or sparing anyone's feelings.

Axelrod left the NIH first, going to Albany to head New York state's laboratory and research operations. After Enzo completed three years of postdoctoral training at the NIH, Axelrod recruited him for the state labs. Axelrod was later promoted from laboratory head to commissioner of health, which elevated him from the subterranean hive of labs under the government mall to the fourteenth floor of the state office tower. Frustration propelled Enzo up this same trajectory during the summer of 1981. "I went to see David Axelrod alone, and I sat down with him in his office and I don't think it took more than thirty seconds for him to grasp not only the science but also the potential for biotechnology." The two met several more times to talk about how the state might commercialize the new vaccine technology in a more beneficial way than it had Nystatin, which had done very well for the drug company that licensed it but paid little to the state.

Ultimately, Enzo remembers, "Axelrod left it up to me. He said, 'What do you want to do with this?' And I said, 'Oh, I think I'd like to start a biotech company.' And he said, 'So go for it.'" Within a few months, health-department administrators had completed the legal paperwork needed to create Virogenetics Corporation. They were off and running. "On Christmas Eve, 1981, Dennis and I were in New York City, where we put our signatures on the first patent application," Enzo said. Biotechnology was new and happening mainly on the West Coast, so finding a New York patent attorney who knew anything about genetic engineering had been tough. But find one they did, and the patent application he prepared claimed, among other things, that genes selected from other organisms could be inserted into vaccinia and expressed, and that this technology would be useful for making vaccines.

Back in their underground lab in Albany, Enzo dreamed big dreams and worked incessantly. In 1982 and 1983, he and Dennis published a quick succession of papers showing that a series of vaccinia vectors could separately express genes from herpes, influenza, and hepatitis B viruses. By 1985, they had reported on their first "polyvalent" vector, a vaccine that delivered genes from three viruses at once. Although these accomplishments created quite a buzz in the scientific world, stimulating more and more laboratories to jump on the vaccinia bandwagon and make recombinant vectors of their own, all was not well in Albany.

For one thing, Virogenetics was going nowhere fast. "We had all sorts of offers during that time," Enzo said with a cynical laugh, "like $50 and a carton of cigarettes." In the lab, he and Dennis constantly postponed important experiments because they didn't have the people and resources to do them. There was a tremendous backlog of work needed to make the vectors as safe and as effective as possible. The longer they got by on a shoestring, the more sour the mood became.

Enzo felt especially ill-used by Bernie Moss, his former lab chief and mentor at the NIH. He had told Moss about the recombinant vaccinia concept when he and Dennis first began working on it. Moss had subsequently put his lab to work on vaccinia-based vaccines, and when Moss's team published articles, Enzo felt that they gave short shrift to the groundwork that he and Dennis had laid. Envy may also have been a factor: Moss was a world-famous virologist, and as an intramural scientist at the NIH, his resources dwarfed those of the Albany team. "Once he got his hands in a technology, he could work it much faster than we could, and that was part of what was bothering Enzo, and what pushed him to overreact, in terms of making sure that people knew that he, Enzo Paoletti, had done it," Dennis would later reflect.

Like a married couple who argue more when they're worried about how to pay their bills, Dennis and Enzo's partnership gradually fell apart during these lean times. Enzo did not think that Dennis was as passionately committed to the vaccine project as he should have been, while Dennis felt that Enzo was trying to claim all the credit for himself. Dennis moved into a lab of his own about six months before the 1983 press conference in New York.

In the wake of the press conference and their seventeen minutes of fame, Enzo and Dennis put aside their differences, donned suits and ties, and hit the road. Much as the developers of the naked DNA vaccine would later do, Enzo and Dennis took their scientific dog-and-pony show to venture capital groups, private investors, and major pharmaceutical companies in the United States, Switzerland, and France.

One of many negotiations in late 1984 was with Luc Montagnier, the French codiscoverer of the AIDS virus. During several meetings in New York City, Enzo and Dennis talked with him about teaming up to make a vaccine against AIDS. Montagnier's lab at the Pasteur Institute had cloned genes from HIV, which the Albany team wanted to test in a vaccinia vector. But the talks fizzled out. "It wasn't that they didn't want to deal with Americans, it was that they wanted the vaccine to be a French effort," Enzo said. At the time, he could not have foreseen what a prominent role he would later play in French efforts to make an AIDS vaccine.

In March 1985, after five years in the state lab, Dennis Panicali left Albany and joined a biotech company in Cambridge, Massachusetts. Enzo stayed where he was. In September, Enzo got a lot of press coverage when *Science* published his article on splicing genes from hepatitis, herpes, and influenza into a single vaccinia vector. When he talked with reporters about these accomplishments, Enzo always mentioned that Virogenetics, the company set up to commercialize this and other vaccines, "remains undercapitalized." That was an understatement.

●

Shiu-Lok Hu came from Hong Kong to the University of California-Berkeley in the fall of 1967, when Governor Ronald Reagan ordered helicopters to spray student antiwar protesters with tear gas. "It was an exciting time and I learned a lot, not necessarily in the classroom," Shiu-Lok said in his slightly British accent. Despite all the upheaval during his undergraduate years, he wrote a senior thesis about bacteria and graduated with great distinction in biochemistry.

Shiu-Lok left Berkeley for graduate school at the University of Wisconsin in Madison. "I thought it would be in the middle of the country and things would quiet down a little. But soon after I moved there, they bombed the math center. I like a liberal environment, and I certainly found it," he said wryly. It was in Madison that he was seduced by viruses—specifically the very tiny ones, called phages, that infect bacteria. In his postdoc years, Shiu-Lok pursued these creatures at Cold Spring Harbor Laboratory on Long Island, where phage biology got its start.

From there he signed on with a biotech company in Minnesota, which was okay for a few years, but not great. Shiu-Lok was ecstatic when an offer from a Seattle start-up enabled him to return to the West Coast. Oncogen was a spin-off of Genetic Systems Corporation, which was competing with Chiron and a host of other companies to develop lab tests that could be used to diagnose AIDS and screen donor blood for HIV. Oncogen, Shiu-Lok's new employer, was supposed to come up with novel ways of diagnosing and treating cancer.

When Shiu-Lok reported for work in the spring of 1985, however, Oncogen's laboratories hadn't yet been completed. Rather than simply sit in his new office, admiring the spectacular view of Puget Sound, he began casting about for something meaningful to do. Elsewhere in the building, he met the Genetic Systems group working on AIDS diagnostic tests. They had just received, from the Pasteur Institute in Paris, the very HIV genes that Enzo Paoletti had tried and failed to obtain from Luc Montagnier. In addition to clones of the genes, they had gotten all the genetic information and laboratory supplies needed to work with them.

Shiu-Lok was prepared to make the most of this unexpected opportunity. In Minnesota, articles by researchers including Enzo and Bernie Moss had inspired him to tinker with vaccinia vectors on his own. Although he made vectors mostly as experimental vaccines for veterinary diseases, he had inserted into vaccinia bits of an African virus that can cause fever and bleeding in humans. Now, in Seattle, he had reason to see if he could do the same with the French gene for gp160, the full-length HIV envelope protein.

Although Shiu-Lok believed a vaccinia capable of smuggling the gp160 gene into human cells might have great potential as a vaccine, that was not the official reason for his new project. The Genetic Systems team working on an HIV blood test needed large quantities of gp160 protein for their experiments. Shiu-Lok was helping them by making a vaccinia vector that could induce mammalian cells to churn out lots of envelope protein. The desire to make a vaccine, however, was what really drove him.

Unfortunately, Shiu-Lok's vaccine dreams were not part of Oncogen's business plan, and Oncogen paid his salary. It was also a small company that had to answer to several much bigger masters. Originally launched as a partnership of Genetic Systems and Syntex, a California drugmaker, Oncogen soon picked up additional backing from industry powerhouse Bristol-Myers Co. Innovative cancer tests and treatments were the money magnet for these stakeholders, not vaccines for infectious diseases. Still, Oncogen's top executives were intrigued by Shiu-Lok's efforts to make a vaccinia-based AIDS vaccine, and they agreed that he could pursue it— so long as he worked on cancer vaccines at the same time.

In the roller-coaster world of biotech in the 1980s, the scientific mission and the control of a company were subject to change without notice. In October 1985, Bristol-Myers beat out Syntex to acquire Genetic Systems and Oncogen. The two biotechs had been founded by Bob Nowinski, a University of Washington professor turned entrepreneur. Although Nowinski was widely criticized for shunning Syntex at the last minute in favor of Bristol-Myers, Shiu-Lok cared less about the business side of the deal than about the future of his vaccine.

Soon after the sale, when a Bristol-Myers executive told *Business Week* that Oncogen's AIDS vaccine "shows promise," it seemed as though Shiu-Lok's HIV project was on firm enough ground. Still, corporate leaders sent mixed messages: "Some were supportive, some tolerant, some opposed," he later recalled. Within a month, however, Shiu-Lok had enough support to start testing the new HIV vaccine in monkeys.

●

The Rain City Grill was a name known to foodies everywhere, whether or not they'd ever been to Seattle. In the fashionably funky and oh-so-gay Capital Hill section of the city, the chefs made exuberant use of the Pacific Northwest's abundant seafood, seasonal vegetables, and increasingly respected wines. The decor winked at the conventions of fine dining, with colorful parasols hanging overhead and sheets of butcher paper on the tables. Travelers whose appetites had been whetted by *Gourmet* and the travel section of the *New York Times* competed for tables with well-heeled locals celebrating special occasions.

One summer night in 1987, four people dining together at the Rain City Grill planned the world's first respectable clinical trial of a recombinant vaccinia vaccine against AIDS. They knew that in 1986 a French scientist had been criticized for an unsanctioned African experiment of a vaccinia-based AIDS vaccine, and what they had in mind would be nothing like that. They were determined to do an experiment that would be above reproach. Shiu-Lok Hu, who had designed the vaccine now called HIVAC, was of course there. With him were his boss and a colleague from Bristol-Myers Squibb Pharmaceutical Research Institute—which had swallowed up what had earlier been Oncogen's research division. The fourth member of the group was Lawrence Corey, a forty-year-old professor of laboratory medicine and microbiology at the University of Washington, who had been recruited to head the clinical study.

The table was charged with optimism and excitement. And no wonder: Shiu-Lok's monkey experiments had showed that the animals mounted T cell responses to HIVAC. This raised hopes that in humans it could stimulate a cellular immune response that might protect against HIV. He published a preliminary report of this work in the April 10 issue of *Nature*, alongside an article by Bernie Moss saying that he also had inserted the HIV envelope gene into vaccinia. A page-one story in the *New York Times* lauded both teams for "remodeling the most successful of all vaccines" and said that Shiu-Lok's monkey experiment could mean that an AIDS vaccine would be available before the 1980s were over. Back in Albany, Enzo Paoletti read these articles and knew that Shiu-Lok had made a landmark accomplishment in their field. Clearly, Shiu-Lok was now the front-runner in the race for an AIDS vaccine.

It is not unusual for basic scientists like Enzo and Shiu-Lok to finish their careers without ever having one of their discoveries make it from the laboratory to the clinic. Even those who have this satisfaction seldom take so many steps into the unknown—all at once—as Shiu-Lok and his team were prepared to do. No matter how many millions of people had been immunized with vaccinia, the fact remained that not a single person had ever been deliberately exposed to a poxvirus that had been genetically altered in a laboratory. Nor had healthy volunteers ever agreed to immunization with a live vector that carried a piece of the deadly AIDS virus. A trial that involved these "firsts" would have to be very carefully conceived and impeccably implemented, that was for sure.

Because Bristol-Myers Squibb was going to pay for a Phase I study of

HIVAC, the researchers would not have to appeal to the National Institutes of Health for funding. Still, a historic trial like this would inevitably be conducted in a fishbowl. One way to minimize embarrassing gaffes was to have strong leadership, which explained why Larry Corey had come to dinner at the Rain City Grill. Corey had successfully led a large, multisite study showing that an antiviral drug, acyclovir, could be used to treat genital herpes. He had published in the major clinical journals, spoken at important scientific meetings, and handled reporters' questions about this unpleasant, sexually transmitted virus. Corey's brilliant accomplishments, untarnished by any sign of self-doubt, led the University of Washington to name him a full professor at the tender age of thirty-seven.

As a result of all this, Corey possessed what he later called "the hubris of success." As the evening at the Rain City Grill proceeded, Corey pushed dishes aside and used the crayons—which were part of the table set-up—to sketch a trial design on the butcher paper. The collaborators wanted the study to include people who had been vaccinated against smallpox and those who had not. This was important because previously immunized volunteers might unleash antibodies that would kill the vaccinia messenger before it had a chance to deliver its HIV message. The group also decided to administer a standard smallpox vaccine to half the volunteers, so that their immune responses could be compared with the people who received HIVAC. Otherwise, researchers wouldn't really know how much of the overall immune response was to vaccinia and how much to the HIV envelope that it carried.

The trial could go forward only with the blessing of the Food and Drug Administration. The FDA's primary concern, as always, would be the safety of the volunteers and everyone around them. Like a standard smallpox immunization, HIVAC was going to be administered intradermally—scratched into the surface of the skin instead of injected into underlying muscle tissue. Vaccinia typically causes a small pustule to form at the immunization site, and standard practice is to cover this so virus won't be spread through casual contact. Although this would be even more of an issue for a vaccinia carrying a piece of HIV, Corey had an idea. When he treated babies with herpes infections, he sometimes used a special dressing that kept virus from leaking out. This same dressing could be used to cover immunization sites. And to make doubly sure that the vaccine trial was not seen as a threat to public safety, the scientists agreed that the first immunizations should be conducted in an isolation unit.

In the wake of this enjoyable and productive evening, the notes on the butcher paper—which Corey took with him at the end of the meal—were transformed into Investigational New Drug submissions for the FDA. Meetings in Washington followed, details were hashed out, and on November 25, 1987, the FDA approved the first human trial of a live recombinant viral vaccine.

Four months later, on March 25, 1988, the first volunteers were immunized in a quarantine ward that had been specially constructed on an upper floor of Pacific Medical Center, Seattle's public health service hospital. Several worked at the hospital or in research labs, the others were gay or bisexual men who had responded to advertisements or articles about the experiment. There was quite a bit of excitement and media hoopla, as the investigators had predicted, but no real problems.

The launch day was an emotional roller-coaster ride for Shiu-Lok. On the one hand, it was exhilarating to think that a vaccine against AIDS might be "on the horizon" and that he had invented it. Yet he was nagged by the thought that maybe he had missed something, and somehow the vaccine might hurt people. Everything he had seen in monkeys told him it was perfectly safe, but monkeys were not humans, and the animal experiment had not lasted long enough to rule out the possibility that some ugly surprise might crop up decades later. Shiu-Lok also worried that individual volunteers could be harmed in more immediate, if milder, ways. They might be stigmatized as homosexuals or intravenous drug users, simply because they signed up. And those who received HIVAC, instead of the smallpox vaccine alone, would very likely test positive on HIV blood tests. Those tests measure antibodies to several HIV proteins—including the viral envelope that the researchers hoped vaccinees would respond to.

Private worries did not spoil the upbeat mood of the volunteers and staff at PacMed, as the hospital is known in Seattle. As befits a trial that was conceived in a gourmet restaurant, the volunteers feasted on splendid meals from Gretchen's, one of the city's most upscale caterers. As the principal investigator, Larry Corey joked that "my job on this trial was to pick up the food and pick up the videos. The community was really supportive, and the trial went amazingly well." After the first six or eight patients were immunized and the researchers could show that HIV was not oozing from their immunization sites, the FDA allowed Corey to begin vaccinating people and sending them home. Volunteers no longer needed to put their lives on hold in order to participate, and by late July, twenty-five people had been immunized

●

Vaccinia had become the workhorse of designer vaccines. For one thing, scientists had a long history with this descendant of Jenner's cowpox virus: After two centuries in captivity, vaccinia had been tamed and—with the advent of recombinant DNA technology—taught new tricks. But this did not mean that vaccinia was completely trustworthy. Occasionally, a circus tiger unexpectedly slashes the trainer who's worked with the big cat for years. And occasionally, vaccinia-based vaccines wound, or even kill, people they are supposed to protect.

Although complications from vaccinia are rare, coupling this virus with HIV, which was 100-percent fatal, was a scary proposition. What if immunization somehow did cause HIV infection? Even if this occurred in only one person, it would be disastrous.

Maybe there were other roads that would lead to Rome—vectors that were safer than vaccinia but could still deliver the goods. One possibility was to create a viral mutant so dilute that it could not cause disease, hoping that it would still be powerful enough to stimulate an immune response. Another option was to use a virus that could not reproduce in human cells.

●

Even though Shiu-Lok Hu had surged ahead in the race to test vaccinia-based vaccines in humans, Enzo Paoletti had not been standing still. On the contrary, he had spent more than a year flying back and forth to France, promoting his vaccinia vectors to Charles Mérieux, head of

Institut Mérieux and a major figure in the vaccine world for more than fifty years. This venerable business, founded by Mérieux's father and now partly owned by the state-controlled company Rhône-Poulenc, was the kind of investor that Enzo and David Axelrod had been pining for since 1981. They wanted Virogenetics to have an experienced partner with vaccine expertise and a proven commitment to public health. They also wanted Virogenetics to make money.

Enzo's courtship of Charles Mérieux bore fruit in February 1986, when Institut Mérieux purchased 51 percent of Virogenetics for $4 million, spread over three years. The remainder of the company was held by a nonprofit administrative entity set up by the state health department. The ambitious vaccine that put antigens for herpes, hepatitis, and flu into a single vaccinia vector was the lead product in the agreement, but Mérieux also purchased access to other technologies that Enzo's lab might develop. A contract between the company and the state health department would fund vaccine research in Enzo's lab for the next three years. If Mérieux liked what it saw at the end of that time, the company would buy another 29 percent of Virogenetics and move the company into its own space, outside the health department.

The deal's immediate impact on Enzo was that he had more staff, equipment, and supplies than ever before. Virogenetics' research team grew from eleven to twenty, although that number included several people based in France. One of Enzo's key hires was a former graduate student of his, an easygoing young man named James Tartaglia. Jim had decamped to New Jersey for his postdoc and now returned to the state lab with considerable expertise in virology, immunology, and genetic engineering.

As a graduate student, Jim had witnessed the fireworks between Enzo and Dennis, and he knew that Enzo's ferocious intensity could make him a difficult guy to put up with. It takes two to make a fight, though, and Jim knew he was a patient man who did not fly off the handle easily. Besides, he had tremendous respect for Enzo as a scientist. "He would always drive you to the next step, always asking questions that made you have to extend yourself. In that way, he was very good," Jim said.

Shortly before Jim's return, Enzo had begun thinking about making live-vector vaccines out of something other than vaccinia. Although vaccinia had been his virus for many years, he realized that the same vaccine strains that defeated smallpox also caused complications in a few people. For example, a plug of tissue at the vaccination site might die and rot away, leaving an unsightly pit, in those with unhealthy immune systems. Or vaccinia pustules might spread over the body of a person with a skin condition such as eczema. In a few unlucky souls, vaccine strains have even caused encephalitis, an inflammation of the brain. Now that Shiu-Lok's HIV trial was underway in Seattle, people were beginning to spin doomsday scenarios about what might happen if people with undetected HIV infection were injected with a vaccinia-based vaccine.

Enzo wondered whether a better alternative might be fowlpox, the best-studied member of the avipox family. As the name suggests, viruses in this family cause diseases in birds. Fowlpox appealed to Enzo for two reasons. Veterinarian friends told him that animal vaccines are a huge and lucrative market, and Enzo thought that fowlpox might be versatile enough to deliver genes from other viruses. If this was true, it could be used to immunize poultry against various diseases. The second possibility was even more compelling: Fowlpox might be a safer way to make human vaccines. Because the bird virus cannot replicate in human cells, there would never be enough of it in the body to cause nasty side effects like skin lesions or encephalitis. The looming unknown was whether fowlpox could express spliced-in genes at a level high enough to stimulate a protective immune response in humans.

With new money from Institut Mérieux, Enzo could afford to put some of his people to work on these questions. One of his postdocs inserted genes into fowlpox and measured their expression levels in bird and mammal cells. She also sorted through other types of avipox, looking for ones that might be even better vectors than fowlpox. One of the most promising was a vaccine strain of canarypox that was already being used to immunize canaries.

When his lab tested this canarypox as an expression vector, Enzo was "pleasantly surprised" to find that "it was about ten times more efficacious than the fowlpox in inducing an immune response." Clearly it was worth pursuing, and in early 1987, canarypox joined vaccinia as the top priorities for Virogenetics. Jim Tartaglia focused on manipulating the genomes of both viruses, seeking ways to build a safer vaccinia and a more expressive bird virus. As it turned out, Virogenetics was going to need avipox vectors sooner rather than later.

In 1988, a World Health Organization report on smallpox eradication, coupled with increasingly dismal statistics about the spread of HIV, made researchers worry that safety concerns would block approval of vaccinia vectors for human use. The report said that of 14 million people immunized during the campaign to wipe out smallpox, there had been 8,000 complications, 153 of them severe. WHO also estimated that there were already 7 million HIV-infected people in the world, most of them in countries where blood tests for AIDS simply weren't available. If these people were immunized with vaccinia-based vaccines, a shot that was supposed to keep them healthy could make them very sick, and possibly even kill them. The cardinal rule of vaccinology is that immunization should be as risk-free as possible. So when major companies like Institut Mérieux and Bristol-Myers Squibb considered what could go wrong, and what their liability would be if vaccinia vectors did more harm than good, they became very nervous indeed.

In this tense atmosphere, Enzo's first articles about avipox vectors made a huge splash. When he and Dennis Panicali had published their vaccinia vectors nine years earlier, they added a novel twist to old strains of vaccinia. Avipox was different. "Here was something that was totally new, and therefore more exciting," Enzo said. Institut Mérieux was extremely interested in canarypox, not just for AIDS, but as a vector that might be used for other vaccines as well. A virus that could not reproduce in human cells was bound to be safer—and more easily approved by government agencies—than a replicating virus like vaccinia.

In 1989, when Enzo's accomplishments with avipox created a stir, Pasteur Mérieux Serums & Vaccines—which Institut Mérieux had formed by joining forces with the Pasteur Institute—was lagging behind their competitors in the race to develop an HIV vaccine. One of their responses was to license a protein subunit vaccine, similar to the ones being developed by Chiron and Genentech, from a little French biotech company called TransGene. The other was to authorize Virogenetics to work on live-vector vaccines for HIV. Enzo had been wanting to tackle this since 1984, when his attempted collaboration with Luc Montagnier fell flat. Now he seized the opportunity, obtaining HIV genes that had been cloned in Bob Gallo's lab at the National Cancer Institute. Enzo's lab set to work immediately, and soon they inserted the HIV envelope gene into both vaccinia and canarypox.

Just as Enzo had fixed his sights on the world's highest-profile disease, his elbow was jostled by New York's state comptroller. In an audit released just in time for Christmas of 1989, the comptroller charged that the health department had "given away" the rights to the vaccine technology and that various state employees—including Enzo and his old friend David Axelrod, the health commissioner—had conflict-of-interest problems because they simultaneously held positions at Virogenetics and the state. The comptroller claimed it was wrong for Axelrod and two other state officials to sit on the company's board of directors; Axelrod faced him down, while the other two resigned from the board. The comptroller was scandalized that Enzo's contributions to Virogenetics had been rewarded with equity and a few thousand dollars of extra pay, and he claimed that greed would impair Enzo's scientific judgment. Little did he know that whereas MBAs measure success in dollars and cents, Ph.D.s are more fixated on solving a scientific problem ahead of their rivals. It isn't that scientists are averse to getting rich, of course, and biotechnology turned many of them into multimillionaires. It's just that, in this crowd, ego is commonly a more powerful motivator than money.

When the state's inquiry was completed, both Axelrod and Enzo were cleared of any wrongdoing. Eventually it became apparent that the comptroller's motives may have been none too pure, as he was a Republican and a sworn enemy of Mario Cuomo, the state's popular Democratic governor. Regardless of subtext, the audit was a distraction Enzo could have lived without.

Corporate politics were also becoming more ornate. After a long bidding war with other companies, Pasteur Mérieux boosted its presence in North America by acquiring Canada's biggest vaccine maker, Connaught BioSciences. Although Connaught's HIV work wasn't the reason Pasteur Mérieux bought the company, three types of experimental AIDS vaccines were being developed in its Toronto laboratories. Now Pasteur Mérieux Connaught (PMC), as the entity was called, held four cards instead of one. Enzo and his colleagues didn't know which one the company would choose to play, but they worried that Virogenetics' AIDS vaccine might be left on the table while others got into the game.

Still, it was clear that PMC had not lost interest in Virogenetics. In 1989, the French company increased its stake in Virogenetics to 80 percent and rented office and laboratory space for it at Rensselaer Technology Park, in suburban Troy, New York. Enzo resigned his state job in January 1990 to become research director for Virogenetics, Jim Tartaglia moved over as assistant director, and many of the junior scientists and technicians followed. The main focus was on canarypox vectors, which they had named ALVAC (a contraction of "Albany vaccines"). In the lab, they inserted genes from HIV, herpes, rabies, flu, and several animal viruses into ALVAC vectors.

State Health Commissioner David Axelrod was the chairman of Virogenetics' board, having shaken off the state comptroller's attempt to unseat him. Axelrod had developed an excellent rapport with Alain Mérieux, Charles's son and the man who ultimately made the big decisions. Although PMC had an expanding web of relationships with entities great and small and executives jostled one another for position, Axelrod looked out for the interests of Virogenetics.

On February 25, 1991, Enzo and Jim boarded an Albany-to-Washington flight and discovered that, quite by chance, David Axelrod was also on board. They exchanged pleasantries, and in Washington went their separate ways: Axelrod headed for a health policy conference at the General Accounting Office; the two scientists went to meet with the FDA.

The next morning in Albany, Jim was stunned to read in the newspaper that the fifty-six-year-old Axelrod had suffered a massive stroke during his conference the previous afternoon. Now he was in the intensive care unit at George Washington University Hospital. A few weeks later, Axelrod was transferred to a hospital in Albany, and in mid-April, Governor Cuomo announced that he would not be returning to his job as health commissioner. In fact, Axelrod died three years later without regaining consciousness.

The loss of Axelrod hit Enzo hard. Axelrod had been the bulldog on the Virogenetics board when it came to looking out for the interests of the state. Not only that, but he looked after the interests of his old friend and colleague as well. If Enzo ruffled feathers by blowing off suggestions from PMC executives, or even walking out of meetings with them, then Axelrod smoothed it over. Without Axelrod on duty, Enzo worried that PMC would push Virogenetics off to one side, like Cinderella in the chimney corner. Enzo felt that for the corporate executives in France, "Virogenetics was not their most important fish."

And that was true, because PMC had dozens of experimental vaccine programs underway at once. All were under the control of infectious disease expert Stanley Plotkin, an American vaccinologist who joined the company in 1990 as its medical and scientific director. Author of major vaccinology textbooks, inventor of the rubella vaccine, and for decades a department head and distinguished physician-researcher at Children's Hospital of Philadelphia, Plotkin was a towering figure in vaccine research.

Plotkin saw AIDS as a complex infection that was not likely to be fought off by either arm of the immune system acting alone. He wanted Virogenetics to keep improving its canarypox vector for HIV, which seemed likely to stimulate cellular immune responses, while other company researchers worked on subunit vaccines designed to elicit antibodies. It was crucial, Plotkin felt, not to put "all our eggs in one basket."

In 1990, Plotkin assigned a newly hired physician to set up human vaccine trials in France and in the United States. Jean-Louis Excler, like Plotkin himself, was originally trained as a pediatrician. He had been working in Burundi when the AIDS epidemic surfaced in Africa in the early 1980s. "When you see every day, children dying of measles, or tetanus, or whooping cough, and of course of AIDS, you think, 'If I could do something upstream, that would be more beneficial,'" reflects Excler, a soft-spoken man with wavy black hair and limpid spaniel-like eyes. His growing interest in public health led Excler to leave Burundi for the Central African Republic, where he ran a World Health Organization program that immunized children against the common killers that he had come to know all too well.

When Excler decided to return with his family to France, he felt fortunate to land a job with PMC's medical department and to work for someone as distinguished as Plotkin. Being assigned to HIV vaccine work was the icing on the cake, a lucky break that he attributes to his experience with AIDS in Africa and his command of English. Soon, Excler and Plotkin were traveling regularly to Bethesda, seeking NIH support for clinical trials of the canarypox vaccine for HIV.

●

It was 105 degrees Fahrenheit in Maryland on July 14, 1988. The entire East Coast had gone limp in the rank, sweaty grip of a heat wave that showed no signs of letting go. It was late afternoon when Nancy Davis pulled off the highway and rolled to a stop beside the pumps at a gas station. Nancy and her traveling companion, Loretta Willis, had set out nearly six hours earlier from Ralcigh, where Nancy was a virologist and Loretta a lab tech at North Carolina State University, familiarly called NC State. They were driving a ponderous brown four-door Chevy, circa 1977, that had been passed down to Nancy by her husband, Steve. It wasn't the greatest car in the world, but its trunk was big enough to hold all the coolers and boxes of laboratory supplies that their mission required.

The station attendant apparently figured that two ladies in an eleven-year-old car needed help, so he pumped gas while they paced stiffly on the hot, soft asphalt, trying to shake out the kinks that come from sitting too long. They were wearing rumpled shorts and T-shirts, and it would be fair to say that neither was having a good hair day. Just making conversation, the young man drawled, "Sooo, what are you up to?"

"We're army scientists," said Nancy. She and Loretta cracked up, giddy with heat and disbelief that, at least for the moment, this was true.

"Right," smirked the gas jockey, who knew when his leg was being pulled.

As strange as the idea seemed to them, Nancy and Loretta were on their way to the U.S. Army Medical Research Institute of Infectious Diseases, or USAMRIID, headquartered at Fort Detrich, Maryland. Nancy was a forty-two-year-old child of the 1960s, born and educated in California, a self-described bleeding-heart liberal who until recently had had no dealings at all with anything military. Nine months earlier, however, the U.S. Army had made a major research grant to the NC State University laboratory where Nancy and Loretta worked. The head of the lab, virologist Robert Johnston, had come up with a plan for making a vaccine to protect soldiers against Venezuelan equine encephalitis, a tropical disease usually called VEE. U.S. military personnel are sometimes sent to South America, where epidemics of this mosquito-borne fever have been known to strike as many as 100,000 people at a time. Although VEE kills only about 1 percent of its victims, it can easily incapacitate a local population or an army. Bob was the one who typically thought up new projects like this; Nancy excelled at making those visions real.

The rest of the drive to Fort Detrich was a fetid crawl on an interstate clogged with commuters heading home from Washington to the Maryland suburbs. The base itself is about forty miles from the city, a sprawling installation with hundreds of buildings spread out over many acres. It was nearly dark when they reached the security gate and were met by their army collaborator, Jonathan Smith. He led them to a long, low building filled with containment suites, or BL-3 labs, where dangerous microbes can safely be handled. They had driven all this way because they didn't have a BL-3 lab at NC State. Two summers earlier, Bob Johnston had come to this same building to take the first steps toward a VEE vaccine. Now Nancy and Loretta had to assemble the first real version of the vaccine over the next two weeks. They had a long list of experiments to do, and Bob would be coming soon to lend a hand.

Jonathan helped the two women empty the Chevy's trunk of Styrofoam coolers and cardboard boxes filled with precious supplies for their experiments. Their budget was so tight that Nancy had carefully measured out plasmids, restriction enzymes, and all the other solutions and reagents that she expected to need. "We weren't rich enough for me to take whole tubes," she would later say.

By 10:00 p.m., they were ready to get started. In one of the isolation suites, Nancy and Loretta put on gowns, masks, booties, and gloves, and then pulled two tiny tubes from the cooler. In each were cloned halves of a weakened VEE virus that it had taken them two years to develop at NC State. Digging into their supplies, Nancy and Loretta combined the half-clones in a single tube, along with a buffer solution and an enzyme called ligase. Left to work overnight, the ligase would stitch the cloned halves together into a whole VEE that—if everything worked right—would be a vaccine against this disease. Although they were permitted to handle the two pieces separately at NC State, regulations dictated that the two could be combined only in a BL-3 facility. Once the mixture was nestled into a warm-water bath, the tired and sweaty army scientists went to Jonathan's house, where they were staying. It was still hot, despite the lateness of the hour, when they cracked open cold beers.

Fort Detrich was already parched and shimmering in the heat wave when they arrived the next morning. Inside the containment building, Nancy and Loretta saw gowned and gloved workmen frantically transferring biological specimens from broken-down freezers into replacements. The huge air-conditioning units on the building's roof were failing, and in the labs the big freezers filled with biological specimens were overheating and crashing every day. Some of these samples probably don't exist anywhere else in the world, Nancy thought. Working in such a place was not unlike being an unknown artist who was suddenly given a painting studio at the Louvre. She was a bit awestruck at first.

The more familiar Nancy and Loretta became with USAMRIID, the less like a museum it became. They quickly discovered that the place was not only as hot as a frontier town, but also as lively with gossip. They had come on the scene just as military vaccine researchers, like their civilian counterparts, were questioning the safety of vaccinia vectors they had embraced a few years before. Fort Detrich scientists had worked with Shiu-Lok to insert the HIV envelope gene into vaccinia. On their own, the military researchers had spliced genes from VEE and other exotic pathogens into vaccinia vectors, hoping to make vaccines that would protect soldiers, sailors, and airmen sent to the far corners of the earth. But many of these vectors, including the one bearing VEE, elicited disappointing immune responses. And the military researchers had a sinking feeling that vaccinia-based products might not be safe enough to use.

As a result, Fort Detrich scientists were curious about whether the visitors from North Carolina had anything that might replace vaccinia. Nancy remembers walking down a corridor and overhearing one stranger say to another, "Johnston, he's making a clone," which in this case was labspeak for an attenuated VEE. It was a creepy feeling to know that people who didn't recognize them in the mess hall were intensely interested in what they were doing. In the privacy of the BL-3 lab, Nancy and Loretta put the stitched-together VEE into the workhorse laboratory bacterium, *E. coli*, which would copy the viral DNA as it divided. They put the clones into culture dishes where skin cells from chicken embryos, called chick embryo fibroblasts, were growing in a thin, cloudy layer that adhered to the dish. They settled the dishes in a closed, climate-controlled incubator where they would remain for several days. At the end of this time, they hoped to see that the attenuated VEE virus had thrived—making more of itself inside some of the fibroblasts and killing its host cells as it multiplied. If there were no dead cells, however, this would mean that the halves of their clone—two years in the making—did not add up to a whole.

Soon after the cultures were sequestered in the incubator, Nancy made a terrible discovery. She was doing a routine analysis of the clones, which involved using enzymes as a kind of molecular scissors to snip them into predictable lengths. She knew what these lengths should be from earlier studies of the two partial clones, done in the lab at NC State. But when she chopped up what was supposed to be the full-length clone, the pieces were the wrong sizes. It appeared that a big chunk of genetic material was missing. Nancy was devastated by the thought that the clone was not viable, that it would not grow in the chick cells, and that she had failed while all the virologists at Fort Detrich were watching.

By this time, Bob Johnston had arrived, which gave the North Carolina team even more visibility among the local scientists. Many recognized Bob from his previous visits. He is a tall, lanky Texan with broad shoulders, a droopy mustache, and a kind of cowboy slouch. He and Jonathan Smith got their Ph.D.s together at the University of Texas, where Bob first began to study alphaviruses—the family that includes VEE. During the summer of 1986, Bob spent two months in the BL-3 building at Fort Detrich. That's when he selectively snipped out genes to create mutant strains of VEE that he hoped would be less virulent than the original: too weak to cause disease but able to stir up a protective immune response. It had taken two years of additional experimentation at NC State to sort through all these mutants and come up with the vaccine strain that Nancy and Loretta had just assembled. Now he was in the lab with them day and night, grinding out experiments while waiting for the cell cultures to come out of the incubator.

With his booming baritone voice and confident manner, Bob doesn't come across as a guy who is afraid of much. But he didn't want to be the first to find out whether two years of hard work had been wasted. So, at

11:00 P.M. on the night of July 20, he took the tissue cultures out of the incubator and handed them to Nancy. "You look at them first," he said. The NC State trio was alone in the BL-3 suite, garbed in their blue scrub suits.

When Nancy slipped the dishes under the microscope, she saw spots where the chick cells had "rounded up" and pulled loose from the dish. This meant that they were dead because rapidly multiplying VEE had killed them. After that it was bedlam in the lab—three people in identical scrubs jumping up and down, hugging and screaming. They phoned Jonathan Smith at home and woke him up with the good news. Despite the missing chunk of viral DNA, the clone was alive and growing. Now they could start testing it in animals to see what immune responses it stimulated, which was the next step in their mission for the U.S. Army. The military wanted a vaccine against VEE and, by damn, the virologists from North Carolina were determined to make one.

●

Meanwhile, the testing of HIVAC, Shiu-Lok Hu's vaccinia-based AIDS vaccine, was about to spread beyond Seattle. About the time that Larry Corey finished immunizing volunteers in the Phase I study sponsored by Bristol-Myers Squibb, the federal government decided to pull together a network of university-based clinics where experimental AIDS vaccines could be tested. Corey's group at the University of Washington was funded as one of five units in the AIDS Vaccine Evaluation Group, or AVEG. The idea was that companies would be more motivated to do costly preclinical development if they knew the government would pay for clinical trials.

Before the first government-backed study of HIVAC could begin, unsettling news began emerging from laboratories at Bristol-Myers and the University of Washington. Vaccinated volunteers didn't appear to be making neutralizing antibodies against much of anything; sometimes their antibodies killed tame, lab-adapted strains in the test tube, sometimes not. And the antibodies were useless against fresh HIV samples from AIDS patients, the so-called primary isolates. On a brighter note, HIVAC did stimulate production of killer T cells, or CTLs, against HIV.

When Shiu-Lok saw these data, he thought of a prime-and-boost regimen that he had tried in monkeys. When he gave a live-virus vaccine followed by a protein subunit boost, the monkeys generated antibodies and
CTLs. On the strength of this result, he and the clinical researchers got
FDA approval to prime volunteers with one or two doses of HIVAC, then
boost with one or more doses of gp160, a protein subunit vaccine made
by MicroGeneSys, a small Connecticut biotech company. They hoped
that this one-two punch would mobilize both the cellular and humoral
arms of the immune system against HIV.

In November 1988, recruitment for the prime-boost study began in
Seattle and four other AVEG sites. AVEG sought young volunteers who
had come along after the United States stopped vaccinating all children
for smallpox, because Corey's initial study at PacMed indicated that these
"vaccinia-naive" individuals responded better to HIVAC than those who
had gotten the immunizations. Sixteen months later, the NIH launched a
second study of HIVAC with a gp160 boost, this time signing up volunteers who had been exposed to smallpox vaccine in childhood.

Even as these studies moved forward, Bristol-Myers was reconsidering
its involvement with AIDS vaccines. As the 1990s began, more and more
articles cautioned that vaccinia vectors might be hazardous to people
whose immune systems had been damaged by HIV. Pharmaceutical
companies had already spent millions of dollars defending themselves
against lawsuits alleging that childhood vaccines were harmful, and they
were not eager to expose themselves on another flank.

Not only that, but the immunology data from the prime-boost studies
were discouraging. "It went pretty well, until we hit the early roadblock,
which was that vaccinia vectors only worked in vaccinia-naive people.
And then it became harder and harder to demonstrate good CTL activity," Larry Corey recalled. In the laboratory, immunologists could see that
more CTLs were activated in immunized people, but they could not tell
whether these cells were stimulated by vaccinia or by the HIV antigens it
carried. The tests were difficult to perform, and there was no way to vali-
date their results.

Although Shiu-Lok can't pinpoint an exact date when Bristol-Myers
decided to "pull the plug" on the vaccine work, funding for the clinical
studies was phased out during 1991 and 1992. In June 1991, AVEG agreed

to assume responsibility for the volunteers originally immunized at PacMed and to continue studying them at government expense. "After 1992, we basically gave up clinical development of AIDS vaccine," Shiu-Lok said.

Although he had officially dropped out of the competition to develop a vaccine that would protect healthy people against HIV, Shiu-Lok could not walk away from something that meant so much to him. NIH grant money was still flowing into his lab at the University of Washington, where he did monkey experiments as a member of the research faculty. With Bristol-Myers's permission, he continued to carry out animal studies that he hoped would help show the way to a successful AIDS vaccine.

●

In the 1980s, when Bob Johnston and Nancy Davis first cloned a weakened VEE virus that they hoped to use as a preventive vaccine against VEE itself, the idea of working on an HIV vaccine had not crossed their minds. So far as they could see, the only connection between HIV and VEE was that both viruses archive their genetic code as RNA instead of DNA. The North Carolina scientists defined themselves as alphavirus researchers; although AIDS was obviously a tremendous public-health problem, it seemed to have nothing to do with them.

But in 1992, just as Shiu-Lok withdrew from the HIV vaccine field, Nancy and Bob considered throwing their hats into the ring. One reason was that alphavirus experts at Washington University had spliced foreign genes into a virus much like VEE, had incubated the altered virus with mammal cells, and had detected expression of the added genes in the cells. This was the first hint that alphaviruses, like vaccinia, might be capable of delivering genes from unrelated viruses into human cells. Bob put this news together with some of his own observations about VEE's activity in animals and saw two more reasons why VEE might be a good way to present HIV antigens to the immune system.

Both these reasons had to do with location, which is just as important in immune protection as it is in real estate. When VEE enters the body, it heads straight for the lymph nodes. Here, the two arms of the immune system first recognize foreign antigens and begin programming B cells to make antibodies, which nab free virus in the bloodstream, and T cells, which hunt down and destroy infected cells. In addition to VEE's affinity for the lymph nodes, Bob also saw that it apparently stimulates immune responses in mucosal surfaces, such as the vagina and rectal lining. Since HIV infects most of its victims through sexual contact, this was another point in VEE's favor as a possible vaccine vector.

Bob and Nancy also had other, more visceral reasons for wanting to make a vaccine against AIDS. Several years earlier, they had left NC State and moved to the University of North Carolina in nearby Chapel Hill. Now, instead of being in a pure research setting, their lab was part of a medical-school complex where many of the state's AIDS patients came seeking state-of-the-art medical care. "We were in the middle of all this HIV research, and we were looking at VEE as a vaccine vector. People were starting to talk to us about HIV," Bob recalled.

Nancy remembers an occasion early in 1993 when Ron Swanstrom, a retrovirologist who had been working on HIV since the early days of the epidemic, was hanging out in Bob's tiny office, which barely accommodates two people amid teetering stacks of journals and books. Nancy was lounging against the door jamb, listening to Ron as he tried to entice Bob into working on an HIV vaccine. "You know, if you think your vector is going to be a good vaccine vector, you're almost obligated to try it for HIV," he told them.

The more Bob and Nancy considered this, the more they agreed with Ron. It would have been different if the protein subunit vaccines made by Chiron and Genentech or Shiu-Lok's vaccinia-based product were yielding good results in clinical trials. But none of these looked very promising to Bob and Nancy. The other highly touted concept at the time was immunizing people with an attenuated strain of HIV itself, and the two North Carolina virologists thought that sounded far too risky. In this context, it made sense to try to make an HIV vaccine using VEE. Having resolved to try this, they also knew they would have to work overtime to convince others that a vector with the word "encephalitis" in its name was safe.

In April 1993, Bob applied for funding from a special National Institutes of Health program intended to stimulate HIV vaccine research. Although the request was quickly turned down, they began work on an HIV vector anyway. Ron Swanstrom nudged them forward by giving

Nancy plasmids into which he had inserted genes for several different pieces of HIV. On May 17, Nancy tried for the first time to insert the gene for HIV gp120 into their VEE vector. They were in a hurry to prove they could do this so they could use the results of the experiment to bolster another grant application to NIH. Despite long hours staring through the microscope, desperately seeking signs that VEE-infected cells were making gp120, they saw nothing.

It is a fact of laboratory life, however, that dozens—sometimes hundreds—of experiments fail before the first one works. So instead of giving up, Nancy put the Yorkshire lad on the case. Ian Caley was an apple-cheeked Brit who had come to UNC for the summer from the University of Bath, where he was working on a Ph.D. He had a deft touch with gene splicing, and he got the experiment to work before returning to England. Ian showed that gp120 could be inserted into the lab's favorite VEE vector, delivered into animal cells, and the HIV envelope protein expressed. Nancy, meanwhile, had been equally successful with a series of experiments using genes from influenza. Instead of making Julia Child's basic white sauce every day, a world of other possibilities was opening up: VEE looked like a versatile tool for making vaccines against at least several important diseases.

About this time, Bob's team hooked up with Philip Johnson, a researcher at Children's Hospital in Columbus, Ohio, who was using simian immunodeficiency virus, or SIV, as a model for HIV in humans. Eager to give the VEE vector a try, Johnson sent SIV genes to North Carolina. Ron Swanstrom spliced them into plasmids, and Nancy's team used the plasmids to insert them into their top-of-the-line VEE vector. The SIV-bearing VEE went back to Columbus, where Johnson began testing it in macaques.

Funding was a constant problem during this time. Although the military continued to back development of a live attenuated vaccine against VEE itself, and the NIH was underwriting basic studies of the VEE virus, Bob and Nancy had yet to win a single grant for vaccines against HIV, flu, or any other disease. It seemed to Bob, who was responsible for raising money, that it was the kiss of death to put the word "vaccine" in an NIH grant.

In October 1993, Bob read in the newspaper that the U.S. military had just gotten an extra $20 million to spend on HIV vaccine research. Congress had originally earmarked this money for a specific clinical trial, but after that plan was derailed by controversy, the army gained control of its use. "When I saw that news report, I said, 'I wonder what they're going to do with that money?'" The plan, Bob soon learned, was to distribute it to researchers with novel ideas about AIDS vaccines. This was great news but no solution to the immediate funding needs of the lab, because proposals weren't due for nearly six months.

When they weren't obsessing about money, Bob and Nancy were caucusing with Jonathan Smith, their Fort Detrich collaborator, about how they could make the safest VEE vector imaginable. At UNC, Bob and Nancy had been adding HIV or flu genes to a genetically complete, but weakened, strain of VEE. The theoretical drawback of this strategy was that although this strain was attenuated, it might make so many copies of itself that an immunized person would get sick. Even the remote possibility of such a thing could keep the Food and Drug Administration from approving it for human testing.

At Fort Detrich, Jonathan had been working on a different approach. He first removed the genes that code for VEE's nucleocapsid, the protein coat that protects the virus's RNA core as it moves from cell to cell, or from one person to the next. In their place, he inserted the foreign genes that he wanted the vector to deliver. Once the altered virus got inside the host cell, the added gene and the virus's remaining genetic material would be copied. But—and here's where Jonathan's vector differed from the UNC version—the virus could not replicate because it lacked the genetic instructions for making its protective outer coat. In technical terms, this was a "propagation-incompetent vector particle," called a "replicon" for short.

As appealing as the replicon looked in terms of safety, the scientists did not know whether a nonreplicating vector could generate enough foreign antigen to stimulate an immune response. Enzo Paoletti and the Virogenetics team had faced the same uncertainty with canarypox, which also can't reproduce in host cells, and only after many costly experiments had they decided that it was worth pursuing as a vaccine.

As strapped for funding as they were in early 1994, Bob and Nancy knew it was important to keep working on both kinds of vectors. Until they answered some basic scientific questions about safety and potency, it would make no sense to pick one and drop the other. Still, how were they going to pay for all this research? As Enzo and many other scientists had done before them, Bob and Nancy realized that they needed corporate support to keep the ball rolling.

Unfortunately, North Carolina universities had been slower to jump on the technology transfer bandwagon than institutions in California and the Northeast. Lacking a licensing office of its own, UNC had gone in with two other schools to start one. The head of this fledgling outfit helped Bob and Nancy apply for a patent on their original VEE vector and began promoting the idea to Merck, Chiron, and other companies that were active in vaccine research and development. Although they were prepared to trade their blue jeans for business clothes and fly off to deliver their spiel in the fancy conference rooms of the pharmaceutical industry, that didn't happen. There were no takers.

●

Up in Albany, the early 1990s were an intensely frustrating time for Enzo Paoletti. With Axelrod out of the picture, it seemed to Enzo that no one was in a hurry to move his AIDS vaccine into human trials. The chain reaction of mergers, acquisitions, and reorganizations that had turned Institut Mérieux into Pasteur Mérieux Connaught had made it the world's largest vaccine company. His view was that Virogenetics was small, distant from France, and lost in the corporate shuffle.

Stanley Plotkin, who was in charge of vaccine research for PMC, realized that the HIV vaccine project was moving slowly. Part of the problem rested with the NIH, which was struggling to set up an orderly process for selecting experimental vaccines and launching them in clinical trials. But he also acknowledged that the company didn't move as fast as it might have on the HIV vaccine.

One cause for delay was a battle between Enzo and PMC over how the prototype HIV vaccine, known as ALVAC vCP125, should be manufactured for clinical trials. Because they would be injected into healthy volunteers, and not animals, these batches had to comply with Good Manufacturing Practices established by the Food and Drug Administration. Pasteur Mérieux Connaught had GMP plants in France and in Swiftwater, Pennsylvania. Virogenetics had no such facility, but the company did have the experience—even the art—that Enzo said was required to produce the vaccine.

Canarypox grows best in chick embryo fibroblasts, skin cells that thrive only when they have a surface to adhere to. They are cultivated in roller bottles, which resemble large soft drink bottles lying on their side, and much care is required to keep cells happy in this system. Because the yield of vaccine from each bottle is low even when everything works fine, Enzo insisted that Virogenetics was best equipped to grow the large batches needed for clinical trials. PMC said no: The company refused to build a multimillion dollar GMP facility in Albany when they already owned others.

Instead, PMC executives pressured Enzo to find ways to make production more efficient, so that the yield would be higher. Although he came up with minor technical improvements, Enzo claimed the process was essentially sound. He maintained that production was being slowed by a PMC manufacturing team that didn't know much about canarypox and wasn't working hard enough to grow it.

By the time vCP125 entered Phase I trials in the spring of 1993, relations between Enzo and PMC were less than warm. NIH officials and the PMC clinical team, Plotkin and Excler, had agreed to test canarypox in a prime-boost strategy modeled on Shiu-Lok Hu's pioneering work with vaccinia and a protein subunit boost. They wanted this because in animal experiments, canarypox, like vaccinia, appeared to stimulate a cellular immune response but no antibodies. Plotkin and the NIH wanted to see both types of immunity, and the NIH persuaded Chiron to supply its gp120 as the booster for canarypox.

Enzo groused that antibodies are what "old timers" expect, because this is the type of immune response stimulated by classic vaccines. His view was that "antibodies are irrelevant" and that his product should be tested without any kind of boost.

As the clinical trials went forward, blood samples were drawn from volunteers and sent to two laboratories for analysis. One was the central immunology laboratory for all NIH-sponsored trials of AIDS vaccines, located at Duke University in Durham, North Carolina. Its official role is to independently measure immune responses to all the vaccine candidates in human trials. Samples were also shipped to a French lab that PMC hired to do immunology studies on its behalf. Both confirmed that the canarypox vaccine appeared to be quite safe—that wasn't in dispute. But they differed dramatically over its capacity for stimulating an immune response. The Duke laboratory found that volunteers had T cell activity against HIV, which is a promising sign. But the French lab showed absolutely no immune response to vCP125.

Enzo was beside himself at the French findings, and protested to PMC that this could be possible only if the lab had tested samples from people who hadn't actually been injected with his vaccine. He insisted that some of the samples be sent to Duke for retesting, and he was not surprised that the Duke lab found positive immunologic results. When the French lab did the tests again, this time their results squared with those from Duke. Plotkin attributed the discrepancies to technical glitches, which plagued both labs from time to time and are to be expected when complex immune assays are performed.

Not surprisingly, Enzo took a less benign view. While the testing problems were being resolved, Enzo imagined that the executives at PMC who didn't like him were gossiping that the HIV vaccine didn't work, that the poxvirus technology was a failure, and that "we don't need Enzo anymore."

5

TROUBLE IN THE IVORY TOWER

A HOLLYWOOD MOVIE ABOUT the early days of public health in America would be an action flick, with health officers as real-life heroes risking their own skins in the fight against pestilence. The pioneering scientists of the 1800s were trained in controlling infectious diseases, but they also faced physical challenges that today's public-health officers can scarcely imagine: slogging through swamps to capture mosquitoes, braving tenements to interview the stricken and their families, patiently tracking down leads that only sometimes paid off. They were a band of hands-on adventurers who were nearly always "in the field."

That image of nineteenth-century public-health officers is in stark contrast to U.S. Public Health Service officers of today. Now most USPHS personnel inhabit offices where they administer, delegate, and enforce the official policy du jour. Few engage in fieldwork or come face-to-face with lethal disease. Hands-on research has given way to database management, and risk is something to be assessed with a questionnaire, not taken personally.

Nowhere is this change more apparent than at the National Institutes of Health.

●

Before any kind of vaccine can be given to millions of healthy people, first it must travel a long and costly road that drug developers call "the pipeline." The journey begins when a scientist like Kathy Steimer or Phil Berman makes a vaccine in the laboratory, where it is tested, often for five years or longer, in test tubes and animals. If it appears safe and stimulates a desirable immune response, the candidate vaccine's owner asks the Food and Drug Administration, the FDA, for permission to mount a Phase I study in a few dozen volunteers. If the vaccine continues to appear safe and if it stimulates the immune system in positive ways, it will gradually move into larger Phase II and Phase III human trials. And this is where money and control become issues.

Each stage of testing costs more than the last, and the government almost always organizes and pays for the Phase III study. This final phase is designed to test the efficacy of a vaccine, which means how well it protects against disease. A Phase III study usually requires collaboration among medical centers in different cities, where many thousands of volunteers will be enrolled at a cost of millions of dollars. But experimental AIDS vaccines needed government help earlier in the development process. This was an entirely new disease, there were no established animal models for studying it, and it was unknown what type of immune response would protect against infection. Uncertainty was the order of the day.

Although top executives at a biotech might have been willing to wager $100 million on a vaccine, which is about what it costs to make one and shepherd it through the preclinical stages, or even into a Phase I trial, they weren't willing to bet an additional $100 million or so on further testing. That would be hard to justify to investors, who could easily see that drugs cost less to develop than vaccines and would earn more. So the young scientists who invented the first generation of HIV vaccines saw the money and know-how of the National Institutes of Health as essential to the future of their products.

After several years of work in their own labs, Kathy, Phil, and their counterparts at a handful of other biotechs began making pilgrimages to the NIH in Bethesda, Maryland. Although biologists of their generation had benefited greatly from NIH largesse as grad students or postdocs, few of them had ever negotiated with NIH bureaucrats, hammered out a major grant proposal, or won a big-dollar award. The nitty-gritty of getting funded had mostly been handled by their mentors and lab chiefs. Now these young scientists were lab chiefs themselves, eager to test their vaccines in people and acutely aware that doing so would require support from the NIH. The FDA would license these products for sale only if the clinical trials complied with formal scientific and ethical standards, and if all the paperwork was done exactly right. Few young biotechs knew how to navigate this part of the development pipeline, and without help, their vaccine might languish in a laboratory refrigerator. If the NIH stepped in and conducted the trials, on the other hand, it would be possible to find out whether these products could help stop AIDS.

Nothing in their formal training prepares young researchers for the NIH, which is intimidating and mysterious in much the same way as the Internal Revenue Service. It is a massive institution, with thousands of staffers plugged into an organizational chart that is constantly changing, and it has rigid customs and peculiar jargon that are tough for outsiders to grasp. More important, it deals in money and power, verities of postwar science. When the makers of the first HIV vaccines began to knock on the NIH's door in the late 1980s, the Institutes were being buffeted by an un-precedented tsunami of AIDS activism. On public television the the NIH was hailed as the "jewel in the crown" of federal research; in the streets it was accused of murdering people with AIDS—Dr. Jekyll one day, Mr. Hyde the next.

●

In 1987, U.S. government support for biomedical research turned 100 years old. To mark this event, PBS stations aired a series called *The Health Century,* which vied with *Cheers* and *St. Elsewhere* for viewers' attention. In 1887, the forerunner of the NIH was a Staten Island hospital devoted to the control of epidemics, home base for mustachioed health officers, jaunty in khaki and puttees, who fanned out across the country to battle typhoid, plague, yellow fever, and other scourges. A few years later this program relocated to Washington, went through several name changes, and was staffed by a growing band of U.S. Public Health Service officers imbued with the pragmatic, can-do spirit of their predecessors. Their mission expanded to chronic as well as infectious diseases, and the National Institute of Health was officially created within the USPHS in 1930. In 1937, it became the Institutes, with an *s* on the end, when Congress set up the National Cancer Institute (NCI). Over the years, more disease-specific facilities would spring up when powerful people, usually members of Congress, were afflicted by a particular malady.

The real impact of the NCI legislation was not that it cured anyone of cancer, but that one of its provisions revolutionized the funding of American science. Before 1937, the entire USPHS budget was spent on research conducted in its own laboratories, by its own scientists. This new law empowered the USPHS, for the first time, to make research grants to scientists at universities and other outside institutions. Although this extramural program started small, eventually its budget would dwarf that of the intramural research programs. It also put top-ranked scientists at NIH in a position to shape the direction and pace of biomedical research in the United States—and beyond.

The NIH assumed the appearance of landed gentry in 1938, when private donors gave a lovely, rolling forty-five-acre estate in suburban Bethesda to its parent agency, the USPHS. Despite its genteel new home, in reality the NIH was not yet rich, not with a $2.8 million budget that was small potatoes compared with $26.3 million for the Department of Agriculture. World War II changed all this: When mass-produced malaria drugs and penicillin became crucial to the war effort, their manufacture was swiftly accomplished by lavishing massive amounts of government funding on a consortium of independent research institutions.

Once the war was won, policy makers thought that the same strategy could be used to solve other major medical problems if the NIH had enough money and manpower. Viewers of the PBS series saw how a dynamo named James Shannon, a hotshot kidney doctor from New York, came on board first as research director for the new Heart Institute, and then in 1955 as director of the whole shebang. When Shannon took over, the NIH budget was $100 million; when he retired in 1968, it had surpassed $1 billion.

When Shannon taught medical students, he never hesitated to say outright that something was a stupid idea. He was smart and blunt and determined to change the character of NIH by changing who worked there. Shannon disdained the muscular microbe hunters who excelled at slogging through swamps and imposing quarantines. Instead, he demanded that civil-service rules be abandoned so that he could recruit people from the nation's top universities and hospitals.

Shannon's goal was to create an NIH peopled with modern scientists, medical doctors with an interest in what he called "the quantitative approach to serious biological problems with application in medicine." The genial rough riders were replaced by battalions of physician-scientists with Ivy League degrees and clinical training at the nation's elite hospitals. The only thing they shared with their predecessors was that almost all were white and male. Shannon and the high-minded men he recruited were confident that they practiced "good science," and they weren't at all shy about saying what this meant or about enshrining their opinions as the core values of NIH. That others might disagree simply didn't matter.

When virologist Robert Gallo came to NIH in 1965, Shannon's hiring policies had been in place for sixteen years and he had been NIH director for a decade. In Gallo's autobiographical book *Virus Hunting*, he says that at this point "spending time at NIH was virtually a prerequisite to academic medicine." Young men who served a tour of duty in Bethesda could expect to have great careers and someday to head departments at top medical schools. Joining the public-health officer program at NIH had another advantage as well: It was a shelter from the Vietnam-era draft, a respectable alternative to military service.

Although Shannon talked about the importance of bench-to-bedside research—laboratory experiments that will help doctors prevent or relieve human suffering—he also set in motion a snob factor that bestowed second-class citizenship on such pragmatic work. Gallo recalls that during his early years at NIH, research with direct implications for patient care was considered "empirical, not very intellectual, and often rather crude." Basic science, the attempt to unravel the inner workings of biology without regard for the practical implications of one's work, was the highest calling and the greatest challenge for intramural scientists. Outside researchers who fed off NIH also understood that the most prestigious and well-funded labs specialized in amassing knowledge for its own sake. For the most part, high-profile academic researchers were content to let drug companies translate basic science into products that would prevent or treat disease. After all, the researchers were engaged in science, not commerce.

Unprecedented wealth and authority came to the NIH when the War on Cancer was launched by Congress in 1971. The National Cancer Institute's budget went from $190 million in 1970 to $815 million in 1977, thanks to legislation that was meant to develop a host of new therapies for cancer patients, and the other parts of the NIH grew as well. Although Nobel laureate David Baltimore and other prominent scientists testified before Congress against the cancer initiative, fearing that channeling so many resources into a specific disease would shortchange basic science, half of this tremendous windfall was spent on exactly the kind of rarefied projects favored by Baltimore and other academics. This happened because clever scientists quickly realized that almost any grant proposal could get funded if it contained a reference, no matter how strained, to cancer.

Although the War on Cancer did not yield the cures that members of Congress had hoped for, it revolutionized the life sciences by giving rise to molecular biology. Most of the knowledge and tools that scientists now use to pick apart the inner workings of health and disease—including AIDS—were made possible by the tremendous increase in NIH funding during the 1970s and 1980s. And although unplanned, the War on Cancer actually gave birth to the biotechnology industry as well.

The 1987 PBS series on the NIH was exciting, full of cliff-hangers and triumphs. AIDS was portrayed as the latest tough problem that brilliant, hardworking NIH scientists were working to solve. It showed immunologist Anthony Fauci, director of the National Institute of Allergy and Infectious Diseases (NIAID), reminiscing about the fateful day in 1982 when he decided to dedicate his own laboratory to the study of AIDS. Bob Gallo's discovery of HIV was spotlighted as an exemplary use of the new molecular biology. The NIH was ready for AIDS, the filmmakers concluded, and was attacking it as vigorously as the dashing, khaki-clad scientists had attacked epidemics 100 years ago.

●

An entirely different view of the government's readiness for the AIDS epidemic showed up on television news broadcasts on June 1, 1987. Hundreds of gay activists from around the country blockaded the White House driveway, chanting "Shame! Shame!" and carrying placards excoriating President Reagan, the NIH, and the FDA for failing to mount an all-out effort against AIDS. More than 36,000 Americans had been diagnosed with the disease, more than 20,000 had died, and the CDC estimated that close to half a million were infected with HIV. Activists insisted that the government wasn't spending enough on the discovery of new treatments, the NIH wasn't pushing hard enough to test new medicines, and the plodding machinery of the FDA was delaying the release of drugs that might help people with AIDS.

Many of the protesters wore stark black T-shirts bearing the slogan "Silence = Death" and "ACT UP" in bright pink letters. "Dr. Fauci You Are Killing Us!" read one of the posters waving above the crowd. "NIH = Not Interested in Homosexuals" said another.

The TV footage looked much the same as the antiwar protests of the 1960s, where the White House was a backdrop for earlier groups of scruffy young people who marched and chanted because they were angry with their government. Until the camera shifted to the mass of blue-uniformed police who were preparing to move in and reopen the driveway. Bulky and anonymous in their helmets and thick carapace of gear, each officer tore open a sealed package of bright yellow, elbow-length rubber gloves, the kind found in millions of kitchens, and pulled them on. Then they waded into the crowd and dragged the protesters, most of whom went peacefully, into waiting paddy wagons.

News of the rubber gloves electrified participants in the Third International Conference on AIDS, which had just begun that June day in 1987 at the Washington Hilton. Physicians who'd been struggling to have their patients treated like other sick people, instead of shunned as carriers of vile contagion, were outraged. Only twenty-four hours earlier, some of the most prominent AIDS doctors had been at a black-tie fund-raiser in Georgetown where President Reagan gave his first speech on AIDS, six years after the epidemic was officially identified. Like most Reagan speeches, it was light on content, urging compassion and lauding the nobility of volunteer efforts to help people with AIDS. Doctors and researchers were disappointed but not surprised that the president launched no new government initiatives and failed to mention that most of the people who had died—and most of the volunteers who had helped them—were gay. Now the bright yellow gloves made it clear that these street protesters were seen as vectors of disease who should not be touched unless precautions were taken.

No matter how inadequate the government's efforts seemed to the activists in the streets, no matter how out of touch the president seemed, the fact was that Congress increased NIH's budget for AIDS each year. Most of this money went to NIAID, which made Anthony S. "Tony" Fauci's Institute the biggest spender in global AIDS research. Not only did NIAID's grant-making clout directly affect what was going on in the nation's laboratories, but Fauci was now ubiquitous in the media. He had become the Reagan administration's point man on the epidemic, the government's cool, authoritative voice on scientific and public-health questions. On a table just inside the press room at the Washington Hilton, NIH flacks had stacked eight-by-ten glossies of the handsome, dark-haired Fauci next to the programs and scientific abstracts for the international AIDS conference.

The activists in the streets feared they might die before effective AIDS treatments were developed, and the burned-out doctors who had not cured a single AIDS patient during the six years since the epidemic surfaced were equally pessimistic. At the conference, a parade of epidemiologists showed tables and graphs demonstrating that AIDS had spread from its splash point in urban gay communities and was now rippling fast through the social pond in ever-widening circles. AIDS was the leading cause of death for women aged twenty-five to thirty-four in New York City, U.S. prisons were crowded with HIV-infected inmates, and blood transfusions still weren't as safe as public officials had hoped. And although U.S. activists were mainly focused on America, the World Health Organization estimated that an astonishing 5 million people were already infected with HIV in Africa and other parts of the developing world.

Not all the news at the 1987 conference was bad, however. The general gloom was pierced by early reports that the drug AZT, or azidothimidine, interfered with HIV's growth in human cells and that some patients who took the drug lived longer than expected, even though many suffered terrible side effects. The tremendous buzz about AZT, and about the need to quickly find other, less toxic treatments, largely overshadowed news about vaccines or other means of prevention.

During one session, an intense, dark-haired Frenchman with bushy black eyebrows described a vaccine he had made by inserting the gene for HIV gp160 into a harmless vaccinia, the same virus that had long been used to inoculate against smallpox. Daniel Zagury, a physician and researcher at the Université Pierre et Marie Curie in Paris, read his presentation in slow, heavily accented English. He told how in November 1986, he had conducted the first human trial of an experimental HIV vaccine. Following an old tradition of physician self-experimentation, Zagury first immunized himself. When there were no ill effects, he took some of his new vaccine to Zaire, where eighteen children, the youngest two years old and the oldest eighteen, were inoculated with the permission of Zairean government officials. Unfortunately for Zagury and his collaborators, including the NIH's famous Bob Gallo, the parents of these children were not asked to consent to the experiment. This omission violated international covenants governing research on human subjects, which were regarded as sacred in the wake of the Nazi abuses during World War II.

Instead of making history, Zagury's experiment was an embarrassment to science. A scandal had broken out back in February 1987, when the *New York Times* published an article critical of the study. After making his presentation at the International AIDS Conference, Zagury failed to show up for a scheduled press conference. Reporters grumbled and went on to other things, secure in the knowledge that there was no imperative to cover what little news there was about HIV vaccines. There were no crowds of healthy people outside the White House or the Washington Hilton, demanding that science find a way to protect them against AIDS.

●

By the time of the tumultuous 1987 AIDS conference, NIH had grown to a 318-acre establishment with more than sixty buildings. Few of the Institute's thousands of employees worked on anything related to AIDS. Tony Fauci's laboratory at NIAID studied "host factors," characteristics of the human immune system that influence its interactions with viral invaders like HIV. Over at the National Cancer Institute, Bob Gallo had a large group working on HIV itself. But they were exceptions among the intramural researchers. On the extramural side of NIH's operations, about twenty physicians and Ph.D.s worked for the AIDS program within NIAID, administering grants and contracts to outside researchers. Fauci had set up this program in 1984, shortly after he became director of NIAID and Gallo was heralded as the discoverer of the AIDS virus.

When AIDS surfaced in the early 1980s, the Centers for Disease Control was the lead public-health agency on the new disease. The CDC, headquartered in Atlanta, had counted the bodies, figured out that sex, dirty needles, and blood transfusions were the major ways that people became infected, and realized that containing the epidemic was going to be a formidable task. Most of the "good science" crowd at NIH, the intellectual descendants of former director James Shannon, saw AIDS as a public-health problem that held little interest for them.

But the NIH elite sat up and took notice after Gallo and Luc Montagnier, his rival in Paris, discovered in late 1983 that the disease was caused by a bizarre retrovirus whose behavior was entirely new to scientists. This virus broke all the rules: It invaded the cells of the immune system itself, causing myriad signs and symptoms before eventually killing its host. The discovery was wildly provocative to scientists able to sniff out the next big thing before others are onto it. At NIH, Fauci and Gallo were among the first intramural researchers to see that AIDS, like cancer in the 1970s, could be the raw material of a new empire. There were discoveries—and careers—to be made.

Part of Fauci's portfolio was NIAID's new extramural AIDS program, which had the makeshift look of a hastily assembled political campaign office. It was housed not on the main NIH campus but in an ugly office park a few miles north in Rockville, Maryland, where about two dozen employees worked in cubicles and rudimentary offices. Vaccines were such a small part of this new operation that the whole vaccine staff could have driven to the meeting at the Washington Hilton in a Toyota Corolla. And if they had made this trip together, the long slender hands of Wayne Koff would have gripped the steering wheel.

Wayne Koff was a tall man of thirty-four with a lean and hungry mind and looks to match. He had a long, narrow face made less severe by his curly brown hair and his ready laugh. Wayne came to NIH from Texas, where he had earned a Ph.D. in microbiology and immunology at Baylor College of Medicine and then studied influenza virus. As a postdoc he realized that he had no intention of devoting his entire life to the analysis of a single gene, as many molecular biologists did at that time. Instead, Wayne yearned to tackle a major medical problem, something that would change the world.

In March 1986, he began an elite, twelve-month internship program at the NIH, with the aim of deciding what his focus should be. Wayne rotated through various disease-specific institutes in Bethesda and got an overt taste of politics in the White House and Congress. Put simply, he saw that it was not scientists but politicians who called the shots. A research program got funding if enough pols thought that a "yes" vote would guarantee reelection, pay off a political debt, or get them appointed to a high-profile congressional committee. Wayne was attracted to Alzheimer's disease, which he believed was going to be so lavishly funded that NIH staffers would have unusual opportunities to think big and be creative.

But meanwhile, a National Academy of Sciences report on the challenges facing AIDS research had generated a lot of buzz, and clearly AIDS would be a promising arena for an ambitious young man with a background in infectious-disease research. "I had absolutely no interest in being a prototypical project officer, who sees all of the grants but really doesn't have a say in where the field is going," Wayne recalled a decade later. Avoiding dead-end bureaucratic dullness was much on his mind when, at the end of his internship, Wayne had job opportunities in burgeoning NIH programs on AIDS and Alzheimer's. In the end, he ruled out the latter because "frankly, I didn't know a helluva lot about brain research." The upshot was that Wayne Koff became NIH's first project officer for AIDS vaccines in March 1987, just three months before the police pulled on their rubber gloves outside the White House.

●

"It took a while to get organized," Wayne said of the early HIV vaccine program. "I had never made a vaccine and I hadn't come out of industry.

So I said, 'Let's get some opinions.'" This meant calling in vaccinologists from pharmaceutical companies and universities, because few people at NIH knew anything about making vaccines. If intramural scientists thought of vaccines at all, they saw them as an engineering job, holding about as much interest for them as telescope construction holds for a cosmologist.

One of the first people that Wayne turned to for advice was Mary Lou Clements, a dark-haired, blue-eyed Texan who knew all the players in the larger world of vaccines. As a young public-health physician at the Centers for Disease Control, Mary Lou had worked on the global eradication of smallpox. In India, one of her CDC colleagues during that effort had been Don Francis, who in 1987 was rapidly becoming a household name thanks to Randy Shilts's heroic portrayal of him in *And the Band Played On*.

Mary Lou designed and ran clinical trials for vaccines against rotaviruses, hepatitis B, and other diseases at Johns Hopkins University in Baltimore, where she founded a special center for immunization research. She rounded up the nation's leading vaccinologists—most of whom worked for large companies—for small, informal brainstorming sessions that helped Wayne chart a course for NIAID's new HIV vaccine effort.

For starters, Wayne needed scientific program officers. He quickly hired one basic immunologist, one virologist, one expert on animal experiments, one expert on adjuvants (substances added to vaccines to enhance their effectiveness), and a physician who had worked on clinical trials for CDC. The group had two initial goals: to strengthen the vaccine development pipeline and make sure there would be products ready to test, and to devise a long-term funding scheme that would enable vaccine developers to spend more time working and less time applying for federal grants.

Wayne's vaccine team was ferociously busy and suffused with optimism, even though the new AIDS program was rocked by frequent reorganizations, changes of command, and periodic firestorms of bad publicity about NIH's shortcomings in developing new AIDS treatments. AZT had been approved at this point, and activists claimed that Tony Fauci was not doing enough to move other, possibly better, drugs forward.

In 1988, the AIDS program was elevated to the status of a division, thereafter known as DAIDS, and Wayne was promoted to branch chief for vaccine research and development. Blessedly ignored by AIDS activists, Wayne and his colleagues met quietly with more than a dozen companies working on experimental vaccines. They set about "building a machine" that could weed out inferior products and propel the best ones all the way through the pipeline and into human trials. They cobbled together and funded a network of primate researchers, for example, to carry out pre-clinical studies of experimental vaccines made by academic scientists or small biotechs.

Knowing that NIH already paid a network of university-based researchers to test vaccines against other diseases, Wayne's crew persuaded these researchers to also become the AIDS Vaccine Evaluation Group, or AVEG. "The clinical area was straightforward: give the units some money and get them ready to run AIDS vaccine trials," Wayne later recalled. Mary Lou Clements, head of immunization research at Johns Hopkins, and other AVEG investigators put their heads together with Wayne's team to develop "protocols," detailed plans for every conceivable aspect of future clinical trials. The protocols spelled out what a study might hope to accomplish, such as demonstrating that the product was safe and that it elicited antibodies against an HIV surface protein, and how these goals would be measured. AVEG members began to debate the social and ethical aspects of HIV vaccine trials. Topics ranged from which volunteers would be accepted to what would happen when immunization caused people to test positive for HIV, even though they weren't really infected.

●

Laboratory testing was an even more complex and difficult issue. The new vaccine branch had to determine not only what should be tested and how, but also who should carry out the lab work and how the data should be stored and analyzed. The logistics alone were staggering. Over the course of one year, a small Phase I study, which must demonstrate that a vaccine stimulates immune responses without disrupting any normal physiologic function, might call for thousands of individual lab tests on blood collected from a small number of volunteers. Most of these assays had nothing to do with the product's intended effect, but they were needed to make sure that the vaccine was safe. Once it was clear that immunization had no impact on most of these measurements, the number of tests per volunteer would drop sharply in larger, later trials. Nevertheless, a Phase III study with 10,000 volunteers could require hundreds of thousands of lab tests over three or four years.

Towering uncertainties were involved in clinical testing. First off, scientists did not know exactly what the immune system would have to learn from a vaccine in order to win an encounter with HIV. If the virus had just entered the body, would antibodies—the roving street cops of humoral immunity—be able to overpower it? Or must a vaccine also alert the detective squad, the killer T cells of the cellular immune system, so that they could find and destroy HIV that had sneaked into human cells? The only way to define a protective response would be to develop a battery of laboratory tests that could monitor antibody and cellular immune responses to immunization, and later to HIV encountered by vaccinated individuals. Although this sounds relatively straightforward, in fact it would prove hellishly difficult.

Wayne hired immunologist Bonnie Mathieson, who had been studying the basic biology of T cells at NIH and elsewhere for more than a dozen years. Bonnie had tenure as an intramural researcher at NIH, she had authored more than 100 scientific articles, and she was expected to bring much-needed expertise in cellular immunology to Wayne's new group. Bonnie was forty-three, a rumpled woman with disheveled hair and glasses that slip down her nose. She has bright, darting eyes, and when she talks with fellow scientists, she asks rapid-fire questions about their work, rattles off the details of other studies, speculates about what it all means, and proposes which questions should be tackled next. For all this, she is not an impatient person. Rather, Bonnie is like a beloved junior-high algebra teacher who keeps explaining the part that you don't understand, rewording the explanation until you finally get it.

When Bonnie came on board in early 1988, the modus operandi of the vaccine program was to "think up ideas and get them out on the street as fast as possible," in Wayne Koff's words. This was accomplished by announcing that money was available to fund investigations on certain topics, or by issuing requests for proposals, or RFPs, inviting researchers to compete for long-term contracts. One of these RFPs was for a core immunology laboratory for AVEG, which would be responsible for most of the lab work needed to evaluate vaccine trials.

Bonnie immediately caused a ruckus by insisting that the RFP was fatally flawed, because it focused almost entirely on antibody testing and pretty much ignored the need to measure cellular responses to immunization. New products like the live-vector and DNA vaccines were intended to elicit cellular protection, yet no reliable, universally accepted assays for T cell activity were available at this point. Bonnie believed that a core laboratory for AVEG could help speed the development of such tests but that this could be accomplished only by writing a new RFP and restarting the bidding process. To her, this made more sense than spending millions of dollars on a five-year contract that did only half the job. Bitter debates raged within NIAID, eventually reaching as far as Tony Fauci's office. In the end, a new RFP was sent out, and in 1990, a group at Duke University won the contract and became the core laboratory for AVEG. Over the coming years, the central immunology lab would become indispensable to the pursuit of an AIDS vaccine.

Although Bonnie prevailed on the laboratory issue, that often wasn't the case when the pragmatic goals of the vaccine branch conflicted with NIH's proud allegiance to basic science. Vaccine manufacture was a major sticking point. Wayne and his colleagues knew that many experimental AIDS vaccines were being invented in tiny companies and universities that had no way to make these substances in amounts large enough to test in chimpanzees, much less in human trials. Chiron and Genentech were exceptions, because they had GMP manufacturing facilities that complied with FDA standards. Smaller biotechs, however, did not.

Wayne wanted to enter into contracts for GMP manufacturing, so that when a new vaccine was far enough along, it would be produced in one of these facilities at NIH expense. He soon found, however, that his bosses at NIH disdained this sort of lowly product development work. NIH's leaders had great ego investment in basic research and were proud of the institution's track record with vaccine efficacy trials, but they seemed to have little interest in translating discoveries into products. Making things was the job of industry, not of the NIH.

●

In June 1989, the Fifth International Conference on AIDS in Montreal was knocked off the front page by the Tiananmen Square massacre in Beijing and the death of one of democracy's most caricatured enemies, the Ayatollah Khomeini. But for the 12,000 people who attended the AIDS conference, lack of media coverage didn't obscure the reality that this meeting was even more raucous than its predecessors, as some 300 activists stormed the stage minutes before Canada's prime minister was scheduled to appear.

The program officers from the vaccine branch at NIH were there, and dismal statistics washed over them at every session. In the United States, more than 97,000 people had been diagnosed with AIDS and more than 56,000 of them had died. Worldwide, more than 500,000 AIDS cases had been officially reported in 149 countries and somewhere between 5 and 20 million people were already infected with HIV. For the first time at one of these international meetings, crack cocaine use surfaced as a catastrophe in the making. Although the drug was smoked instead of injected, users appeared willing to perform any imaginable sexual act in exchange for crack. Clearly the need for a preventive vaccine was growing more urgent by the day.

At the conference, the vaccine that generated the most media coverage was Jonas Salk's product called Remune™, a whole-killed virus preparation being tested as a treatment for people who were already infected. Remune™ would do nothing to help the millions of healthy people who were unaware that a killer was stalking them.

Back in his office after the Montreal conference, Wayne found himself ruminating about the Human Genome Project, NIH's high-profile effort to lay bare the entire human genetic code. With Nobel laureate James Watson at the helm and millions of dollars invested in long-term contracts with leading research institutions, the project appeared destined for success. This kind of directed program might also work for AIDS vaccine development, Wayne thought, if only the top brass at NIH would back it.

Evaluating one vaccine candidate at a time was going to take forever. "My sense, beginning in 1989, was that we needed the ability to make products and to facilitate the making of products. We needed to get them through and tested and screened across the board, so at the end of the day we could say which were the best three or four approaches and could drive them into multiple efficacy trials," Wayne said.

In 1990, Tony Fauci called together a "committee of elders" to consider whether the NIH should invest in a long-term, directed program aimed at speeding development of a vaccine against AIDS. Maurice Hilleman, Merck's most famous vaccine developer of all time, was at the table. So was David Baltimore, the MIT professor and Nobel laureate who had chaired the National Academy of Sciences' 1986 appraisal of government AIDS research. Wayne, the youngest and lowest-ranking person in the room, described the kind of start-to-finish development effort he hoped to see.

Members of the committee chewed over Wayne's words, expressed their various points of view, and planted their feet firmly in mid-air. Instead of recommending that an all-out effort to make a vaccine be launched, they advised NIH to "proactively coordinate" AIDS vaccine research. Although he hadn't protested during the meeting, Maurice Hilleman later opined that this term was absent from the pages of the *Oxford English Dictionary* and that if the NIH wanted a directed program, it should simply build one. If not, it should avoid coining new verbiage.

If this blue-ribbon committee had urged Tony Fauci to throw his weight behind the pursuit of an AIDS vaccine and if he had been willing to invest his career in applied research instead of basic science, history might be different. A safe and effective HIV vaccine might be in use today. Or we might have mounted an effort of Manhattan Project proportions, only to find that the biological challenges remained insoluble. As it happened, the pace of HIV vaccine research remained the same. When Wayne Koff looked back on this 1990 meeting, years after he had left NIH, it struck him as a historic moment that did not announce itself loudly enough, a time when opportunity knocked but no one listened.

●

Kathy Steimer and Nancy Haigwood arrived in Washington on a muggy summer day in 1990, having flown in from San Francisco for a meeting with the DAIDS vaccine staff. Six years had passed since they had begun work on gp120 vaccines, and their project was now part of Chiron Biocine, a joint venture between Chiron and the giant drug maker Ciba-Geigy. In Geneva, Chiron's Swiss partner had already conducted a small trial showing that the vaccine was safe and stimulated an immune response. They were in Washington to talk about what happened next.

Although Kathy had definitely not dropped the reins on recombinant gp120, she'd cut back on her working hours since adopting a newborn baby girl back in March. As co-leader of the gp120 project, Nancy had taken over preparation of the Investigational New Drug application for the U.S. Food and Drug Administration. If the IND was approved, and Nancy and Kathy were confident that it would be, then the product could be tested in human volunteers.

Chiron had strong ties with the University of California-San Francisco. The company's top executives would pay for a small, short-term safety study—maybe a dozen or so volunteers—at UCSF. Such a study would be invaluable to Kathy, whose lab could use blood samples from this experiment to refine lab tests for measuring immune responses to the vaccine. Young biotechs like Chiron could afford small clinical trials; the problem was scaling up.

Kathy and Nancy had heard Wayne speak at scientific meetings, where he impressed listeners with tales of how hard it had been to line up volunteers for a vaccine trial NIAID initiated two years earlier, in February 1988. This study involved a therapeutic vaccine, not a preventive one, which should have simplified recruitment because sick people are generally more motivated than healthy ones to expose themselves to something that might be risky. Impecunious vaccine inventors were horrified when Wayne showed a slide depicting how a pool of 1,000 interested people ultimately shrank to 128 actual volunteers. It seemed that the more people learned about the uncertain effects of an experimental vaccine and about how many appointments they would have to keep at the research site, the less willing they were to sign up.

Only the NIH had the money and infrastructure needed for this kind of massive screening, which is why Kathy and Nancy had traveled from California to DAIDS headquarters in Rockville, Maryland. On the second floor of the Solar Building, a black-sheathed box in an office park, the two visitors were soon seated at a small conference table in Wayne's office. There was ample room for them and the entire HIV vaccine staff, all four or five of them. The two California blonds, tanned and colorfully dressed, contrasted with the office pallor of the NIH staff.

None of the waffling or infighting that had disturbed Wayne so deeply, causing him to question whether NIAID was genuinely committed to developing an AIDS vaccine, was revealed to the visiting scientists. Kathy and Nancy saw people much like themselves, scientists mostly in their thirties, who had come of age during the flowering of molecular biology and who believed that biotechnology could solve many of humanity's most vexing problems. The urgent need for an HIV vaccine was a no-brainer, as obvious as a shrieking siren. The issue was how to get one as soon as possible. Now that Chiron, Genentech, and another half-dozen companies had invented possible vaccines, their scientists came to Rockville wanting NIH to help march their products through the pre-clinical stages and into the new AVEG sites, where doctors would inject them into the arms of willing volunteers.

Sitting around in Wayne's office, Bonnie Mathieson and the other vaccine staff asked what they could do to help Kathy and Nancy. Sometimes Wayne's team served as matchmakers, putting together corporate and academic scientists who had been struggling in isolation to perfect the same difficult lab assay. Other times they arranged for NIH to provide reagents—raw materials used in laboratory tests—to researchers in the field. When expensive chimp or monkey studies were needed in the later stages of preclinical testing, these could be arranged through NIH's contracts with several primate research centers. In Chiron Biocine's case, NIH agreed to subsidize some primate experiments and some later clinical trials.

In the early years, a vaccine that had been approved for human testing by the FDA could get into an NIH-sponsored trial without much ceremony. It was pretty much a matter of whoever got a bathing suit on the fastest got first dibs on the diving board. Before Wayne was put in charge of the HIV vaccine program, for example, NIAID had decided that its maiden study, number 001, would be of the gp160 made by Phil Berman at Genentech. When this product failed to protect chimpanzees against HIV infection in a 1986 experiment, however, it got stuck in the locker room.

After 001 was scrapped, and the study designated 003 got off the ground before 002, NIAID decided that a more systematic approach was needed. So one of Wayne's assignments was to set up an AIDS vaccine selection committee, a group of about ten extramural scientists who would screen candidates for testing. They would review written materials about the vaccine, hear oral presentations by its sponsors, ask questions, and vote. Only products with IND approval would be considered, but this alone would not guarantee a government-funded study. The committee wanted to see evidence that the vaccine stimulated the immune system in ways that its members considered desirable.

By taking the authority for choosing vaccines away from government employees and handing it over to a select group of extramural scientists, NIAID was repeating a pattern that had already proved disastrous as a means for selecting AIDS treatments for human testing. In street demonstrations, press conferences, and magazine articles, high-profile AIDS activists accused NIAID of squandering $250 million on studies of old drugs that would never work and on new types of antivirals that originated in NIH's intramural laboratories. The choice of which drugs moved forward was purely political, they claimed. If a potentially useful therapy was "Not Invented Here," taunted the activists, then NIH was not interested in testing it. If the vaccine selection committee operated in the same way, then products would be chosen based on who made them, not on how promising they looked.

The vaccine selection committee was the first of many ad hoc committees, advisory panels, and groups of every stripe that NIH brought to bear on AIDS vaccine research between 1990 and 1993. Simple discussions in Wayne's office in Rockville, where decisions could be reached in an afternoon, were replaced with layers of committees, procedures, and approvals. Like barnacles that build up on a ship's hull and slow its progress, these bureaucratic accretions slowed the pace of vaccine development. The results were extremely frustrating to the biotech scientists, who were used to making their own decisions and fixing them if they were wrong. If something needed doing right way, they would pull an all-nighter. Accustomed to being as quick as racing sloops, the scientists found that trying to launch a vaccine trial with NIH was like trying to steer a ponderous tanker.

Biotech company scientists weren't the only ones who grew frustrated as a small and nimble HIV vaccine effort was weighed down by bureaucracy. Wayne and his team found it increasingly difficult to get anything done. Even though vaccines weren't a high-profile item, AIDS research was more highly politicized than anything else NIH was doing. In May 1990, for example, 1,000 AIDS activists from around the country stormed the Bethesda campus, occupying the DAIDS director's office and causing so much disruption that there were more than eighty arrests.

Under the circumstances, Wayne thought that the vaccine program would function better if it was relocated from DAIDS to the Microbiology and Infectious Disease Program. This program was developing vaccines against other infectious diseases, and the issues that Wayne's branch faced had more to do with vaccinology than with the rest of AIDS research. He had also found that it was difficult to hire people with vaccinology experience, because they were reluctant to work in the fishbowl that was DAIDS. None of this carried any weight with Wayne's bosses, and the HIV vaccine branch stayed where it was.

In 1992, Wayne Koff left NIH to work for United Biomedical, Inc., a small vaccine company on Long Island that had an HIV vaccine in the preclinical stages. His valedictory comments on the state of the NIH vaccine effort appeared in journal articles and letters written around the time of his departure. In one article, Wayne and two coauthors argued that the time had come for NIH to seriously consider a Phase III efficacy trial of the most promising candidate vaccines. They gave three reasons: a vaccine is the best and least expensive way to slow the epidemic, NIH could show the world that vaccines are an international priority, and the trial would help identify immune responses needed for protection, which would help scientists design better vaccines.

•

Although 1992 was not the best year of Wayne's life, it was an excellent time for Tony Fauci and some others in the AIDS establishment at NIH. Fauci realized a long-standing dream when he was elected to membership in the National Academy of Sciences, the most elite club in all of American science. This was heady stuff for an Italian-American from Brooklyn, where the family business was a corner grocery store. Small, trim, compulsively neat in appearance, Fauci was as focused as a laser. Except for two years as a resident at New York Hospital-Cornell Medical Center, NIH was the only place he had ever worked.

And work he did, incredibly long days, to good effect. In 1984, he became director of NIAID. He was forty-three years old. That same year, he married Christine Grady, an auburn-haired, high-strung nurse he had met on the AIDS ward at the NIH Clinical Center. By the time Fauci was tapped by the old boys at the National Academy, about $1 billion of the NIH's $10 billion budget was dedicated to AIDS research. As NIH's associate director for AIDS, Fauci advised NIH director Harold Varmus about how the AIDS money should be divvied up among the institutes specializing in cancer, mental health, drug abuse, and infectious disease—his own shop. About $450 million went to NIAID, where Fauci directly controlled its use. Eventually his sway over the budgets of rival institutes drew fire from AIDS activists, who protested that this was a conflict of interest, and later Fauci was briefly humbled when that broad advisory role was taken away from him. But that day had not yet arrived, and he was riding high in 1992.

And so was Margaret "Peggy" Johnston, although her place in the hierarchy was several rungs—and many millions of dollars—lower than Tony Fauci's. Like Fauci, Peggy had the makings of a career NIH administrator. Armed with a Ph.D. in immunology and a background in basic lab research and medical-school teaching, she signed on with the AIDS program in 1987, when it had a staff of about twenty. She was rapidly promoted from program officer to chief of the branch working on AIDS drugs and in 1993 became deputy director of DAIDS. At the same time, she was put in charge of all basic research and development programs, which encompassed both vaccines and treatments.

In early 1992, Peggy received the NIH Merit Award, which was presented to her by Tony Fauci at a ceremony on the Bethesda campus. In the grip-and-grin photos, it is difficult to tell whether the steelworker's daughter from Pittsburgh or the grocer's son from Brooklyn looks more pleased. Fauci's gold-rimmed aviators gleam in the photographer's flash; Peggy's dark wavy hair and dark eyes shine. He is in one of his trademark gray suits; she wears the kind of colorful silk dress favored by confident female executives.

But AIDS had a more personal dimension for Peggy than for most of the executive corps at NIH. At age forty-two, she'd been part of Washington's gay community for years, and while she didn't advertise that she shared a suburban home with her female partner, neither did she waste energy hiding it. There was little point since her boss, Jack Killen, was also gay. But Killen had taken some hard knocks as the organizer of the highly controversial network for testing AIDS drugs and now had withdrawn into a more bureaucratic, less program-oriented role.

Legend has it that gay men have held even higher positions at NIH, an institution generally more likely to promote men of any persuasion than women. Peggy was not held back by much of anything, however, and she apparently figured out what traits open the doors to the largely male upper tiers of NIH. She was cordial to everyone, but gave away little. She rarely exhibited an emotional response to a professional issue, building her arguments with the brick and mortar of data and detail. The end result looked like science, with no frivolous touches. Although James Shannon didn't hire many women in his time, he would probably have thought that Peggy Johnston was a good fit.

●

Another manifestation of NIH's "knowledge for its own sake" culture is the mechanism for deciding which extramural research projects will win government funding. "Study sections"—committees of outside scientists deputized to review grant applications—date back to the World War II era, when academic researchers were called in to decide which institutions should be included in the all-out effort to manufacture penicillin.

Study sections are made up of researchers with a certain type of expertise, such as viral pathogenesis or measurements of immune response. Ideally they are "true peers" of the grant applicants, who have carried out research projects comparable to the ones being voted on by the study section. Rarely is anyone invited to serve who is below the rank of associate professor, or the equivalent in the corporate world. When AIDS first appeared, naturally there were no study sections set up to handle it. Until these were created in the late 1980s, AIDS proposals were usually sent to groups devoted to the broader topics of virology or immunology.

A special office at NIH assigns each grant proposal to a study section and to a program within one of the institutes. This is an important decision, because one group of reviewers may be more sympathetic than another to a researcher's goals. The study sections rank proposals in the areas of content, facilities, and staffing. What really matters in the latter category is who the principal investigator is. Although science claims that only hard evidence matters, many study-section veterans admit that personalities and networking are as important in scientific careers as in law, real estate, or any other field. Many young Ph.D.s have seen proposals bearing their own name rudely turned down, only to be praised and fully funded when resubmitted with their major professor's name at the top. An experience like this sparked Kathy Steimer's decision to leave academia for industry.

None of this means that study sections reach decisions lightly. Each proposal is assigned to three reviewers, two of whom write detailed commentaries on the experimental design and one of whom takes a broader view. Reviewers may spend weeks critiquing stacks of material sent to them by NIH. Three times each year they gather for meetings in Bethesda, which takes time away from their own laboratory research, teaching, and other commitments. Study-section membership generally lasts at least two years, and the members' home institutions simply swallow the costs.

Study-section rosters are large, so that members can disqualify themselves from voting on research proposals where they have an obvious conflict of interest. A more subtle question is what happens when reviewers hold sway over a grant application that comes from a rival, or even an enemy. Ideally, being on a study section is a prestigious form of jury duty, in which people try to exercise the fairness they would expect if the tables were turned. But because there is no guarantee that the Golden Rule will prevail, scientists with a Hobbesian view of human nature sometimes importune NIH staff to keep their proposals out of the hands of obviously unfriendly reviewers.

The worst proposals sink like a stone in study section. Better ones are reviewed, summarized, scored, and returned to NIH staff for administrative review. At this stage the investigator's proposed budget may be accepted or modified as program officers see fit. The proposals are then subjected to a Rube Goldberg sort of calculation that determines what proportion of the highest-ranking proposals will actually be funded— usually not more than one in four. Proposals below that "payline," as it is called, are turned down. In an especially competitive year or in one where the budget for a particular type of research can't accommodate many new projects, it is possible to have a high score and still come away empty-handed.

Most HIV vaccine proposals never reached this bittersweet stage. The quest for a preventive vaccine is the kind of "high risk, high payoff" research that study sections often disdain—unless the principal investigator is a giant in his or her field, someone they all know and respect. The inventors of the early AIDS vaccines, working at small biotechs or on the ground floor of academia, definitely did not fit this mold. Nor were the sections enthusiastic about projects where the "Eureka!" moment had already occurred. NIH's view was that companies, not the government, should fund the scut work required to gain approval for human trials.

NIH program officers routinely attend study sections to hear the debate about grant proposals assigned to them. Later, they'll be able to help investigators revise their applications if they want to try again. More often than not, DAIDS vaccine staff would leave these meetings in despair. Again and again, they saw vaccine-related proposals assigned low scores because they were judged too applied, too pragmatic, and not as interesting as more basic scientific questions. In fiscal year 1993, when federal AIDS spending topped the $1 billion mark, only 7.9 percent of that money went for vaccine research. It wasn't until FY 1998, in fact, that it crept over the 10-percent line.

●

"I turned on the television and there was AIDS. I opened the newspaper and it was AIDS again. I thought to myself, if I'm ever going to do anything important in this life, this is it." The year was 1989, and Patricia Fast was about to enter private practice as a pediatrician in the Washington suburbs. She had started her professional career with a Ph.D. in immunology but had changed courses and gone to medical school in her late thirties. She completed her clinical training in pediatrics at NIH, spent enough time in a molecular biology laboratory to realize that it wasn't for her, and decided to practice medicine.

But when a job opened up in Wayne Koff's vaccine program for a physician to coordinate clinical trials, Pat Fast jumped at it. She had a hand in launching every vaccine trial after the first two, which were underway when she arrived. She got AVEG up and running and helped organize the National Cooperative Vaccine Development Group, usually called the NCVDG, a mechanism for giving vaccine developers long-term funding. Kathy Steimer, for example, was the principal investigator on an NCVDG grant that put $1.3 million into Chiron's gp120 project between 1988 and 1994.

When Wayne resigned, Pat took over his job as chief of the vaccine branch and was soon named associate director of DAIDS for vaccine and prevention research. Although NIAID's system for deciding which vaccines to support had become increasingly ponderous, Pat's program began grinding out clinical trials. In 1992, it launched ten new Phase I trials and in 1993 initiated eight more of these small experiments. This doesn't mean there were eighteen separate vaccines involved, as many of these studies looked at the same products, varying the dosage or immunization schedule. Nevertheless, the vaccine development pipeline was bulging with promise.

The real highlight of Pat's first year on the job was the December 1992 launch of NIH's first Phase II vaccine trial. All five AVEG sites were involved in this landmark study, and more than 300 volunteers were being recruited in Baltimore, St. Louis, Nashville, Seattle, and Rochester, New York. Each volunteer would receive four injections of Chiron's gp120, Genentech's gp120, or an inactive substance. All would be repeatedly counseled to avoid unsafe sexual practices or drug use and would be warned that these experimental vaccines offered no guarantee of protection. The volunteers would agree to return for blood testing and other medical studies for either twelve or eighteen months, depending on what the investigators thought was needed.

It took twelve months for the AVEG sites to enroll 300 volunteers, and during that time NIH officials, company executives, and most reporters who covered the field assumed that a Phase III efficacy study was just over the horizon. In 1992, NIAID funded eight institutions, including Johns Hopkins and Case Western Reserve, to identify large high-risk populations in the United States and abroad and begin setting up the infrastructure—such as clinics, laboratories, and communications networks—needed for a Phase III trial that might enroll from 6,000 to 25,000 people.

In late 1993, NIAID requested bids from institutions to participate in HIVNET, the new HIV Network for Prevention Trials. By the end of the year, the government had signed multimillion-dollar contracts with research groups that would coordinate a network of sites. In early 1994, NIAID also contracted with a central laboratory and data-management facility. Many of the sites that had been studying high-risk groups, as well as other institutions, jumped at the chance to be part of a mammoth network of eight domestic and nine international sites. During the fiscal year when the big HIVNET contracts kicked in, NIH's budget for clinical trials for HIV vaccines more than doubled—from $20 to $42 million. The goal was to build a system big enough to determine, as soon as possible, whether any of the experimental products could actually stop—or even slow—the transmission of AIDS.[50]

As early as February 1993, DAIDS had drafted guidelines for what a vaccine would have to demonstrate before it could be selected for a Phase III trial. By April, Pat and her staff had come up with a protocol for an efficacy study that would run parallel tests of two candidate vaccines in groups of homosexual men, injecting drug users, and heterosexual partners of HIV-infected people. The unspoken assumption was that the candidates would be the gp120s made by Genentech and Chiron. But it was not a done deal: Internal documents show that NIAID was anxious about funding such a mammoth trial, which could easily cost $20 million annually and take four or five years.

In September, DAIDS showed outside researchers its guidelines for advancing vaccines into efficacy trials. The opening paragraph of the

DAIDS document states that because scientists don't know exactly what type of immune response the human body needs to protect against its first encounter with HIV, "it is impossible to develop rigid criteria for moving potential vaccine candidates into pivotal Phase III efficacy trials." And then the document reads as though the ghost of James Shannon guided the hand of Tony Fauci or one of his minions to write: "However, we do need data to judge whether a vaccine candidate has a reasonable expectation of being effective prior to entry into a pivotal efficacy trial."

This statement served notice that laboratory data are sacred, as they always have been in the traditional culture of NIH, even when there was no clear way to link them to what happens in the real world. If an efficacy study had been completed and scientists could compare immune responses of vaccinees who were protected with those who were not, then it might be possible to determine whether certain antibodies, certain T cell responses, or a mix of the two was needed to keep people safe from AIDS. For many scientists, the most important reason for doing an efficacy trial was exactly this—the opportunity to identify the immune correlates of protection. Street cops? Detectives? Both? That is what everyone wanted to know but no one could find out for sure, not until they had data from a big field trial.

In the absence of such data, top NIH officials apparently still hoped that laboratory observations could predict what sort of immune response would be needed to protect against HIV. If they asked the experimental HIV vaccines to jump just one more hurdle, perhaps it would be possible to pick a likely winner. The gp120 vaccines were meant to teach the immune system to make neutralizing antibodies, the roving street cops that recognize HIV bad guys and kill them. Faced with the prospect of a huge, expensive Phase III trial, NIH asked the vaccine makers to perform an additional set of neutralization tests. This wasn't a formal requirement for getting their products into an efficacy study, but clearly it was something NIH wanted to see.

The first neutralizing antibody assays were simple: Mix blood from a vaccinated person with a sample of one of the standard HIV strains—a virus like SF2, originally sequenced at Chiron, or the MN strain used by Phil Berman. These laboratory-adapted strains were easy to grow in immortalized cell lines and were always on hand in labs that worked with

HIV. The first test usually pitted vaccinee sera against the strain on which the vaccine had been based, so that Chiron's vaccine would have first squared off against SF2, and Genentech's against MN. If antibodies in the blood sample killed the virus in the tube, that was a good sign. The next step would be to mix vaccinee sera with samples of other lab-adapted strains, to see if broader, nonhomologous neutralization was possible.

In the early 1990s, however, scientists realized that primary isolates— HIV samples gathered from infected people and cultured in fresh blood cells—were harder to neutralize than lab-adapted strains of HIV. An early warning came from studies of Genentech's failed AIDS drug, soluble CD4. Although the drug had neutralized lab-adapted strains just fine, out in the world it proved powerless against the various strains of HIV that thrived in the bodies of AIDS patients. In this situation, it was apparent that success against lab-adapted HIV did not predict success against primary isolates.

No one knew whether the same disappointing pattern would hold true for vaccines. NIH administrators decided that before they made a decision about a Phase III trial, they wanted to know whether gp120 products induced antibodies that could kill primary isolates. Although this may sound like an easy question, in fact each team took a slightly different path to the answer. HIV primary isolates had to be grown in fresh human blood cells known as PBMCs, or peripheral blood mononuclear cells. These cells are infected with HIV and then bathed in chemicals and manipulated so they will divide. When they divide, they copy the virus's genetic code, so that new viral progeny can be produced. Exactly when the chemical growth prods should be added, and in what quantity, varied from lab to lab. Nor was there agreement on how a panel of primary isolates should be selected to do battle against vaccinee blood.

At Chiron, Kathy Steimer had been growing HIV in PBMCs since the early 1980s, so of course she developed her company's methods for measuring primary isolate neutralization. She worked to the point of exhaustion, doing experiments over and over again to make sure that they were right. No one was more shocked than Kathy when her new assays showed that blood from vaccinated volunteers did not kill any of the primary isolates in the panel she put together. Not 80 percent of them, not 50 percent, but zero. This did not conclusively prove that the vaccine was worthless, but it was not a good sign.

Bad news travels fast, and before long everyone in the field knew that Chiron's gp120 did not neutralize primary isolates. Genentech scientists soon weighed in with results of their assays, which were done a bit differently from Kathy's but arrived at essentially the same conclusion. Nor was it reassuring when the central immunology lab at Duke, which processed samples for all NIH-sponsored HIV vaccine trials, used slightly different methods to obtain similar results. No two labs did the assay the same way. None used the same array of primary isolates. All subjected the viral cultures to chemical torments that would never have occurred as it passed from one person to the next. Yet for anyone looking for a reason not to go forward with clinical trials, these results were convincing.

While the whole HIV research community buzzed over the primary isolate results, an internal document circulated within DAIDS. It was headed "Talking Points on HIV Vaccine Efficacy Trials for NCVDG, 1993, Meeting (or the Party Line Revisited)." The opening paragraph explained that its purpose was to encourage DAIDS staff to "speak with one voice" when asked about where preparation for large efficacy trials stood and how the decision to proceed would be made. It was organized in a question-and-answer format and emphasized throughout that scientific data would be the basis for decisions about future trials.

One of the questions was "What will be the process for evaluation of the scientific data?" In a draft dated October 19, 1993, the response was that the Vaccine Working Group, composed of "non-government and government scientists and community representatives" would judge when there were enough scientific data to justify advancing one or more vaccines into an efficacy trial. The VWG recommendation would be forwarded to the AIDS Research Advisory Committee (ARAC) and the AIDS Subcommittee of the NIAID Council, two broadly constituted advisory bodies, for a decision about whether such a trial was worth the money it would cost.

One week later, the sarcastic subhead about "the Party Line" had been deleted, and the verbiage about consensus and committee decisions had an entirely new first sentence: "The final decision and responsibility for stewardship of federal funds rests with NIAID." This was another way of saying that Tony Fauci would decide.

At the NCVDG meeting, Kathy Steimer presented her findings about the neutralization of primary isolates. There was much discussion about the difficulty of determining what these results would mean in a clinical situation, in part because a virus that is passed from person to person might not be as resistant to neutralization as primary isolates that have been manhandled in culture. Others argued that although the primary isolates might not have been grown in wholly natural circumstances, they were closer to the real world than lab-adapted strains that have lived for years in the same cell line.

In the wake of these discussions at the NCVDG meeting, Peggy Johnston and Tony Fauci made a wager. Peggy bet that Kathy's negative results were at least partly due to the assays themselves, and that they didn't necessarily mean that vaccinee blood was useless against primary isolates. Fauci bet that the assays were not flawed, and that the results meant exactly what they seemed to mean. Far from being trivial, this dispute would soon turn out to be the cosmic thumb on the balance scale.

6

SOLDIERS AT WAR

SEARCH YOUR MIND'S EYE for images of the brave citizen-soldiers of General Washington's Continental Army. In one familiar scene they huddle stoically against the hard-blown snows of Valley Forge; in another they strain at the oars in their commander's lee, struggling toward the far shore of the Delaware River. Harder to imagine is a homespun-clad medic inserting a needle into an angry smallpox lesion on one soldier's body, then using the pus-dipped instrument to score the unblemished skin of a healthy patriot. Yet that is what took place during the first mass immunization campaign in military history.

Like other educated people of his time, General Washington knew that this crude forerunner of the modern smallpox shot, called variolation, had been used for more than fifty years by the privileged classes in England. They had found that it triggered a mild, nonscarring form of smallpox and protected against full-blown disease. Although variolation killed one in 100 people, those odds beat having smallpox itself, which was fatal for one in four infected adults. As a commander in chief, General Washington needed to ensure that his soldiers were fit and ready to fight. And he worried not only about natural outbreaks of disease among the troops but also about biological warfare. He knew that the British had already used smallpox-contaminated blankets to neutralize hostile Indian tribes, and there was nothing to stop them from using the same horrible strategy against his army. No matter how disgusting variolation might seem, it was better than the alternatives.

More than two centuries later, preventive immunization is one of the mainstays of military medicine. All recruits are inoculated against the infectious diseases commonly encountered in the United States, as well as others that they would be exposed to only if they were deployed to such faraway places as Africa, Asia, or the Middle East. All told, they receive vaccines against nearly two dozen different pathogens. The rationale is that troops may be sent to any part of the globe on short notice and that combat is dangerous enough without also having to worry about attacks of yellow fever, Japanese encephalitis, or other exotic microbes.

The army is the lead agency for infectious-disease research, and this effort is headquartered at the Walter Reed Army Institute of Research This century-old institution, which has campuses in and around Washington, D.C., is universally referred to by its acronym, WRAIR (pronounced "rare"). It has more than 700 employees, many of them physicians and doctoral-level researchers trained at the nation's finest medical schools and universities. Although it resembles a mini-NIH, WRAIR keeps a much lower profile. If civilians know it exists at all, they generally confuse it with the famous Walter Reed Medical Center. WRAIR's main research interests are injury and disease prevention and treatment of combat casualties. One of the army's proudest—and least recognized—accomplishments is that it has developed a larger number of successful vaccines than any other medical institution.

When AIDS hit in the early 1980s, WRAIR scientists were as riveted by the new epidemic as their civilian counterparts. It was not immediately apparent to the Pentagon, however, that this killer of gay men and drug addicts was anything the army needed to bother about. Physicians at some of the military's leading hospitals, however, soon realized that uniforms did not protect soldiers against HIV. Once AIDS showed up on military bases at home and abroad, army doctors were duty-bound to care for these patients, as they would be for any other gravely ill soldiers. A few years into the epidemic, AIDS was added to the military research agenda after army researchers made key discoveries about heterosexual transmission and about the virus's gradual death march through the human body.

The armed services' battle against what might be called "straight AIDS" appealed to various members of Congress, who soon appropriated larger and larger sums for HIV research at WRAIR. In the military, as in civilian institutions, individual scientists who mounted the earliest assaults on HIV found that their careers accelerated. They were showered with fame and funding that would otherwise have come much later in life. Army researchers, who had previously gone about their work without much attention, were now thrust into the limelight along with Bob Gallo, Luc Montagnier, Tony Fauci, and other AIDS-research celebrities. As it turned out, this high-stakes game was not one that officers would always play like gentlemen.

●

Lieutenant Colonel Robert Redfield's army uniform made him stand out in the throng of university researchers, doctors from inner-city hospitals, and gay activists who flocked to Atlanta for the world's first International Congress on AIDS. Redfield was thirty-four years old and going bald on top, and his tunic fit snugly on his stocky frame. It was April 1985, and most epidemiological studies pointed to homosexual men, intravenous drug users, and hemophiliacs as the groups at highest risk for infection with HTLV-III, as the AIDS virus was called then. At a session on the closing day of the conference, Redfield stepped up to the microphone to deliver a presentation with an iconoclastic title: "Heterosexual Promiscuity: An Emerging Risk Factor for HTLV-III Disease?"

Bob Redfield was both a clinician and a researcher. As an infectious-disease doctor at Walter Reed Medical Center, he had been treating AIDS patients since 1983. As a virology researcher at WRAIR, he had also been collaborating with Robert Gallo at the National Cancer Institute. When Redfield combined what he learned from interviewing patients with results of blood tests run in Gallo's lab, he concluded that one-third of Walter Reed's AIDS patients were not gay, did not shoot drugs, and had not received blood transfusions or medicines derived from blood.

Instead, he said, they were heterosexual men who had sex with lots of different women and sometimes visited prostitutes.

Many in the audience did not want to believe Redfield's claims. Some scientists had garnered headlines by speculating that gay men got infected due to mysterious "co-factors" that were unique to the post-Stonewall, let's-get-it-on urban homosexual lifestyle. Maybe illicit drugs made these men vulnerable; maybe it was repeated exposure to nasty venereal diseases—those in the co-factor crowd weren't absolutely sure, but they thought there had to be something special about gay men. IV drug users also lived outlaw lives, far from what Reagan administration officials referred to as the "general population." And hemophiliacs, innocent victims of this terrible disease, were doomed because they'd been given clotting factors distilled from thousands of blood donations, some of which were bound to be contaminated with the AIDS virus.

As Redfield showed slides and described the data he'd collected, gay activists—and worldly wise reporters, as well—scoffed from their seats in the auditorium. Sure these guys are straight, they sneered. The U.S. military was famously homophobic, and everyone knew about closet gays and lesbians who had been outed and discharged from the military, stripped suddenly of reputation, career, income, and medical benefits. No sane soldier or sailor or airman would admit to an officer, even a physician, that he was gay. Far better to paint yourself as a real he-man who bedded thousands of women. Besides, it was unthinkable that plain old hetero sex could spread AIDS. If that were true, many thought, the disease would be more widespread.

Although it would later become obvious that heterosexual contact is responsible for more than 90 percent of AIDS cases in the world, Redfield was ahead of his time in 1985. One man who took his findings seriously, however, was a powerful army colonel named Edmund C. Tramont, the Pentagon's top adviser on infectious diseases and chief of Communicable Diseases and Immunology, the largest division at WRAIR. Whereas Redfield was somewhat abstracted and professorial in manner and always a tad rumpled in appearance, Tramont was a straight shooter who looked people in the eye and said exactly what was on his mind. He was a big man, with strong chiseled features and thick hair, and in uniform he looked like a model officer.

Tramont had no doubt that the AIDS virus was sexually transmitted, just like gonorrhea and syphilis and the other nasty infections that are as familiar to soldiers as bad rations. The difference was that AIDS appeared to be killing a high percentage of its victims, and Tramont knew that it might turn out to kill all of them, given enough time. And there was another worry: Carriers of the virus might appear perfectly well for years after infection, so that on the battlefield a healthy-looking soldier might spread the virus by bleeding on a compatriot or donating blood for an emergency transfusion. It was Tramont's job to make sure this didn't happen.

Some of the Walter Reed patients had been identified in a way that was especially troubling to Tramont, whose responsibilities included picking which preventive vaccines were administered to new recruits. A few inductees had narrowly escaped death after being immunized with vaccinia, the normally harmless virus used to protect against smallpox. Because their immune systems had been damaged by the AIDS virus, unknown to them or anyone else, a little jab of vaccinia sent them into a ghastly tailspin.

During 1985, Tramont and Redfield worked with the army's top brass to develop policies for dealing with soldiers who tested positive for the AIDS virus. Most of these people were discovered when they donated blood to a military blood bank or to civilian organizations that held blood drives on bases. Civilian blood bankers had balked at forwarding HIV results to military authorities, but they finally capitulated when the Defense Department assured them that test results would be used only for medical purposes and would not trigger disciplinary action.

Of the service branches, only the army really made good on this promise. Bob Redfield and Ed Tramont convinced their superiors that preserving the confidentiality of infected soldiers, and keeping them in the army with full medical benefits, gave military scientists a unique opportunity to chart the progression of the disease over time. Civilian researchers couldn't accomplish this, Redfield and Tramont told the generals, because out in the world, people who are diagnosed in the early stages often move, change doctors, or simply disappear before the disease runs its full clinical course. Soldiers, on the other hand, are assigned to specific jobs and locations, and their health-care and medical records are part of a national system. Military hospitals would also be in a position to make cutting-edge treatments available, as such drugs came on line, by conducting clinical trials in the same clinics the soldiers already visited.

Because top army officials agreed with this approach, Redfield was able to observe the natural history of AIDS in patients at Walter Reed. By following other chronic diseases in this manner, such as congestive heart failure, doctors have developed specific criteria for "staging" the disease. Patients are said to have stage 1, or stage 2 disease, depending on their symptoms and results of laboratory tests. These labels help doctors chart the progression of individual cases and enables them to put together groups of comparable patients for clinical trials. Redfield used long-term studies of military patients to develop the Walter Reed Staging Classification for HIV Infection, which was widely used after its publication in 1986.

Although the generals had agreed not to force infected soldiers out of the army, they wanted to shut the door against recruits who were harboring the virus. The creation of a national AIDS screening program was assigned to Lieutenant Colonel Donald S. Burke, a thirty-nine-year-old infectious-disease physician who had previously studied exotic viruses at an army laboratory in Bangkok. Born in a small town in Ohio and trained at Harvard Medical School, Burke at first had no yen to travel or any real interest in international health. In Thailand, however, he'd become fascinated by research on dengue, Japanese encephalitis, and other viruses that routinely killed children at the pediatric hospital across the street from the army facility.

At one point, recognizing that his laboratory skills weren't nearly as good as those of the doctoral-level virologists around him, Burke considered going back to graduate school. He dropped the idea, though, when a crusty general who'd been a mentor advised against it. "Why bother with a Ph.D.," the general said. "You're a doctor and you're smart enough to understand everything you need to understand. Besides," the sage concluded, "soon you'll be in a position where you won't be doing the lab work anyway." Burke forgot about grad school.

He stayed focused on laboratory work, however, and in 1984 returned to WRAIR to become chief of the Department of Virology, which was part of Ed Tramont's command. Burke was a man who had always yearned to be in charge of vast undertakings, and he jumped at the chance to organize a nationwide system for handling hundreds of thousands of young people who applied to join the army each year. Initial screening for HIV would be done with commercially available antibody tests, which were already being used by blood banks. These tests were simple and cheap, but sometimes their results were unclear. A different, more complicated test was required to figure out whether the person was really infected or not. After evaluating numerous tests and ways of using them, Burke devised a system that, in his words, "did not ruin people's lives with false positive results. It's better to miss a few positives than wrongly identify people who were really negative." This made sense at the time, when there were no effective AIDS treatments available and when being told you had the AIDS virus was tantamount to a death sentence.

Burke's HIV screening protocol was field tested at Fort Dix, New Jersey, before it was put into national use. The chief of preventive medicine at the army hospital there was Major John McNeil, a tall, dark string bean of a fellow who had just earned a Master's of Public Health degree at Harvard. John was thirty years old, an army brat whose mother—a nurse who retired as a major—outranked his father, an infantry lieutenant. The army had paid for John's medical education, and Fort Dix was his first posting as a medical officer.

Harsh experience had already convinced John that it made sense to screen healthy-looking young people for the AIDS virus. He had immunized a basic trainee with vaccinia, only to have the young man nearly die as a result. As an epidemiologist, John could see that a national screening program would give him an unprecedented opportunity to detect the previously silent spread of HIV among young Americans. On a more immediate level, John had to sit down and talk to individuals whose tests showed they were positive. In these situations, reassuring words were difficult to come by.

In October 1985, the Defense Department instituted mandatory testing for all civilian applicants for military service and all active-duty personnel. Hundreds of thousands of test results were channeled to WRAIR, in Washington, and to Great Lakes Naval Station, north of Chicago, where the recruiting command was headquartered. The Defense Department was reluctant to look too closely at this newly stockpiled information about recruits, because high rates of infection might reflect badly on young people seeking entrance to the military.

The prestigious Institute of Medicine, the best-known arm of the National Academy of Sciences, pressed the Defense Department to examine these swelling databases. Don Burke flew to Great Lakes in early 1986, during a cold and inhospitable season in the Midwest, to spend a weekend cloistered with results from the first 300,000 blood tests performed on would-be recruits.

"It just blew us away," Burke recalled years later. In some cities, 2 percent to 5 percent of young men tested positive for the AIDS virus. "Nobody had any idea at the time that this was anything other than a very rare disease," he said. "That was when we realized that a vaccine was going to be a crucial part of the effort, because the prevalences were much higher than anyone expected. Suddenly it went from being an abstraction, a small percentage of people, a marginalized gay population, to several percent of civilian applicants for military service."

Back at Walter Reed Medical Center, where he had little to offer the AIDS patients in his care, Bob Redfield agreed that a vaccine was sorely needed. He was eager to move ahead with this as soon as possible. Although he insisted that his ultimate purpose was a vaccine that could keep healthy soldiers safe from initial infection, Redfield believed he could approach that goal by studying "therapeutic" vaccination. This was not really vaccination in the classic sense, but a treatment that Redfield hoped would help his AIDS patients battle and perhaps even defeat HIV.

Like other doctors, Redfield had been taught in medical school that what happens in natural infection—the unplanned encounter of virus and host—demonstrates the capacity of the immune system to respond to a specific bug. For example, when the body is invaded by one of the hundreds of rhinovirus strains that causes the common cold, the immune system mounts a response that clears the virus in about one week. Once the cold is over, the person is forever protected against this particular cold virus—though not against its many relatives. That's how it seems to work for acute viral illness.

Viruses like hepatitis A or B, on the other hand, persist for years because the immune system cannot clear them on its own. But is that really the best that the body can do against a chronic infection? Redfield and a handful of others, including Jonas Salk and the French researcher Daniel Zagury, thought not. They believed it was theoretically possible that a vaccine, which stimulates immune response, might tip the scales so that the body could eliminate viruses that ordinarily linger for years, gradually killing their victims. In the case of AIDS, Redfield believed that the body's response to HIV could be broadened and improved by giving vaccines that mimicked proteins on the virus's protective envelope.

Many scientists found this idea ridiculous, because in their view, the last thing that AIDS patients needed was to be injected with a vaccine that mimicked HIV protein. These patients were swarming with viral proteins already, and eventually they all died. Redfield ignored these naysayers, because he was confident that the injection of genetically engineered immunogens would elicit different responses than sexual exposure to HIV itself. He felt completely justified in shaking off critics. Although his ideas about the heterosexual spread of HIV had initially been scoffed at, they were later confirmed by dozens of other studies. And his staging system for tracking the clinical course of AIDS was now widely used by physicians in civilian and military settings alike. "By that time, I had credibility and had done good work in the military," Redfield said later. "I could pursue these ideas."

When the annual federal spending bills were put together in late 1986, the Defense Department was surprised to discover that the Republican-controlled Congress had handed them $40 million for AIDS research. Some said this was a way for conservatives, who supported the army's aggressive HIV screening program, to do something positive for "the right kind of AIDS, the military kind." WRAIR took the bolus of new money and began contracting with a long list of HIV researchers, ranging from Gallo's lab at the National Cancer Institute to private companies, as a way to expand the scope of its work on virology and immunology.

Now that there was enough money to go around, vaccines were definitely on the agenda. Burke and Redfield were both enthusiastic about preventive vaccines, and no one was going to stop Redfield from exploring therapeutic vaccination as a means toward that end. There was a great deal to do in the laboratory and in the field before human trials could begin, but everyone on WRAIR's retrovirology team was hustling toward the same goal.

•

In March 1988, life was good for Major Deborah Birx. She had been in the army for eight years, which surprised her distinctly unmilitary family and friends, and had excelled as a researcher and clinician. Debbi had enlisted fresh out of medical school at Pennsylvania State University, so that she could train with her husband, a cardiologist who owed the army for putting him through med school. They both got postgraduate slots at Walter Reed Medical Center, and she had since completed her clinical training as an allergist and immunologist and turned into a crackerjack laboratory researcher. At age thirty, Debbi was assistant chief of the Allergy/Immunology Service at Walter Reed and ran her own lab, where she and three assistants had been studying Epstein-Barr virus, which causes nothing worse than mononucleosis in healthy people but wreaks havoc in patients with HIV-damaged immune systems.

Although Debbi was initially more interested in Epstein-Barr than in HIV, her work overlapped with Bob Redfield's. Both were trying to analyze the precise and insidious ways in which the AIDS virus affected helper T cells, killer T cells, and other players in cellular immunity. They had met at Walter Reed, and for two years Debbi had been collaborating with Redfield's lab on occasional projects.

Early 1988 brought ground-floor opportunities at WRAIR's Division of Retrovirology. Don Burke was the head of this high-powered new division, with two department chiefs under him. One handled retroviral diagnostics, and the other—Bob Redfield—had a broad mandate to perform retroviral research. There was ample money, and one of Redfield's top priorities was to test a vaccine in HIV-infected patients. He and Burke met with Jonas Salk, Phil Berman from Genentech, and other vaccine makers, checking out products they might want to test at Walter Reed. And Redfield was beefing up his own laboratory staff in a big way, gearing up for clinical trials, and, on occasion, alienating other army lab chiefs by luring away some of their best immunologists.

Now Redfield was courting Debbi Birx, who was not only a lab researcher but also a physician who could care for AIDS patients enrolled in the vaccine trials Redfield was planning. All Redfield could offer her at the outset, however, was a desk in a four-foot cubbyhole and a laboratory hood of her own. This wasn't even close to the resources Debbi had at Walter Reed, where she ran her own lab, supervised her own technicians and projects, and had an office door that closed. Debbi listened to Redfield's offer, but was pretty sure she'd say no. For the sake of politeness, she told Redfield that she'd think about it and let him know.

A few days later, Debbi and two fellow docs from Walter Reed boarded a flight from Washington to California's Orange County Airport, headed for a big clinical immunology conference in Anaheim. The flight was uneventful until Debbi started in on the fruit plate she'd requested for lunch. Within minutes she was flushed and sweating, her throat swelled shut, and she struggled to breathe as spasms gripped her bronchial tubes. Although nothing remotely like this had ever happened to her before, Debbi and her seatmates knew right away that she was in the throes of anaphylaxis—the most explosive and dangerous form of allergic reaction.

Without immediate intervention, her blood pressure would plummet, her heart would collapse, and Debbi would die—incontinent and twisted by convulsions—in the aisle of the plane. Fortunately, there were two preloaded syringes of epinephrine—the essential treatment for anaphylaxis—in the DC-10's first-aid kit. Her immunologist buddies injected the first vial and insisted that the plane be landed as quickly as possible. They were somewhere over Iowa, the closest suitable airport was in Omaha, and the pilot would have to dump fuel before they could get down safely. Debbi's struggle to breathe was so all-consuming that she was aware of little else, except the sense that it took forever to land. Her friends hung on to the second vial of epinephrine until the last possible minute, injecting it only when touchdown was imminent.

On the ground in Omaha, an ambulance rushed Debbi to Creighton University Hospital, where she was stabilized with drugs and intravenous fluids. Once the danger had passed, tests showed that paprika dusted on a scoop of cottage cheese was to blame for the near-fatal attack. Moreover, tests showed that Debbi had become horribly allergic not just to Hungary's favorite red pepper, but to all its kin. Mild or hot, large or small, red peppers would be lethal to her. Although red peppers might sound easy to avoid, in fact they are used in thousands of foodstuffs from nearly every cuisine. Never again would Debbi sit down to a restaurant meal; after this she would not eat anything unless she had prepared it herself or was absolutely, 100-percent certain that it contained no red pepper. Yogurt became her favorite appetizer, entree, and dessert.

As Debbi recovered from the anaphylaxis episode, she could not help thinking about a narrow escape from death she'd had five years earlier. In 1983, while giving birth to her elder daughter at Walter Reed, Debbi lost so much blood that the obstetrician ordered that she be transfused with four units. Only weeks before, Debbi had read a report saying that the new immunodeficiency disease, which had first surfaced among homosexual men, also appeared to be spread by blood transfusions. In the delivery room, "I was screaming at my husband, as they were hanging the units, 'Do not let them give me blood!'" Debbi passed out and her husband refused the transfusion. That afternoon, in the same hospital, a heart patient with her same blood type was given a transfusion during surgery. The blood later turned out to be contaminated with HIV.

Debbi had missed a fateful date with HIV in 1983, and now she'd survived the sudden treachery of her own immune system. Twice she had been saved, and for what? All of a sudden, for reasons she could not quite explain, it made sense to join Bob Redfield's possibly quixotic battle against AIDS. He thought that by manipulating the human immune system, he could save people from a disease that so far appeared to be 100-percent fatal. Not only that, but he believed that by analyzing how infected people responded to immunization, it would be possible to design a vaccine that would keep healthy people safe. These were big goals, maybe destined to be always out of reach, but definitely worth trying for.

By May 1988, Debbi was no longer commuting to the dignified old Walter Reed complex, in northwest Washington, but to a cookie-cutter office park just north of the Beltway in Rockville, Maryland. Her new cubby was on the upstairs floor of a two-story, red brick building at 13 Taft Court. Redfield's office was nearby, along with the lab where Debbi and the rest of his crew did their work. Don Burke had an office on the same floor, but his laboratory—staffed mostly by civilian scientists employed through a military research foundation—was at 1500 East Gude Drive. The two buildings faced each other across a blacktop parking area.

Debbi didn't really know Burke before she came to work for his division; she'd only seen him around Walter Reed. He was a lot more spit-shined than Redfield, more conventionally military in his upright bearing and his way of barking commands. Yet Don Burke and Bob Redfield seemed to her a good team, with different personalities and complementary strengths. "Bob was very big picture and Don was very good at the details and at implementation. They were good at throwing ideas back and forth and discussing each other's concepts," she later recalled.

While Debbi and the rest of Redfield's team worked to refine assays needed to measure patient responses to immunization, Redfield got clearance from the Food and Drug Administration and Walter Reed's institutional review board to test a product called gp160. Made by a Connecticut-based biotech company, MicroGeneSys, this vaccine was a genetically engineered version of HIV's entire surface protein—not the smaller piece known as gp120. This vaccine had entered the NIH pipeline about two years ahead of the gp120 products made by Chiron and Genentech, and a small NIH study had already shown that gp160 could safely be given to healthy, HIV-negative volunteers. In that NIH study it had not, however, generated antibodies that could neutralize HIV in test tubes. Many scientists took this to mean that the vaccine had little or no promise, but Redfield wasn't discouraged. He thought it might work differently in AIDS patients, who were already making some antibodies of their own against the virus.

On April 3, 1989, the first of thirty HIV-positive volunteers was injected with gp160 at Walter Reed. None of these volunteers had symptoms of AIDS, because their infections had been detected very early. Debbi and the other laboratory immunologists were looking for signs that blood from vaccinated people reacted differently, when mixed with HIV, than blood from patients injected with an inactive substance. The researchers hoped to see an increase in CD4 count, indicating that fewer helper T cells were being destroyed as HIV disease progresses, and an increase in the variety of T helper responses directed against HIV.

Six months into the trial, Redfield was invited to speak at a small NIH vaccine meeting held in Florida. Reporters, eager for anything new about vaccines, went into a feeding frenzy when he said that the vaccine appeared to have boosted immune function in eight patients over a five-month period. Most scientists would have hesitated to make any public pronouncements based such a small number of people and short study period; even fewer would have allowed themselves to be quoted in the corporate press release that MicroGeneSys issued the same day. Redfield did both, then clammed up when reporters at the meeting asked follow-up questions. When journalists phoned the company's voluble young chairman, Frank Volvovitz, he happily expanded on Redfield's remarks at the NIH meeting, saying that CD4 cell counts in the volunteers had either increased or remained stable, instead of falling as they usually do in people with HIV infection, and that Walter Reed would launch a larger clinical trial in early 1990.

This is not the kind of publicity that conservative, mainstream institutions like WRAIR want to see. Nor could Bob Redfield afford to become more famous than he already was, because whether he realized it or not, Don Burke's enthusiasm toward therapeutic vaccines was cooling faster than late November weather in Washington.

●

Redfield's Phase I trial marched on during 1990, eventually enrolling thirty HIV-infected volunteers. Debbi Birx was in the lab every day except Friday, when she put on her white coat and went to Walter Reed to see HIV patients—among them some of the gp160 participants. By now she was assistant chief of Redfield's department, which meant worrying about whether they were asking the right questions in the lab, as well as whether they had the right tools for answering them.

Busy as she was, Debbi heard rumors that serious rifts had opened between Redfield and Burke. Supposedly, they were fighting behind closed doors when they met to talk about which type of vaccine research the retrovirology division should put first—therapeutic or preventive? Other scientists who worked at WRAIR during this period had a darker view: "It was a war zone," one said. "They could barely speak a civil word to one another." "An ugly place to work," another recalled. The parking lot between the two buildings, one housing Redfield's lab and the other Burke's staff, became known as "the moat."

By November 1990, studies done by Debbi and her coworkers showed that patients immunized with gp160 churned out antibodies to parts of the HIV envelope protein that could not be detected in unvaccinated patients. Clearly, something was going on immunologically, and the researchers thought this was encouraging. But the vaccinated patients would have to be closely observed for a lot longer before the doctors could tell whether these responses could slow the progression of HIV disease or, better still, prevent full-blown AIDS.

Redfield was impatient to proceed with a Phase II trial that would be large enough—and last long enough—to determine whether gp160 immunization truly kept people healthier. The FDA and Walter Reed's review board approved his plans for a larger trial. Don Burke, on the other hand, was opposed.

"He thought I shouldn't do the trial unless we knew that it worked," Redfield recalled later. "And I said, 'Don, how can you do a trial and put people on placebo if you know it works?' If you know it works, you don't do a trial. You just stand up and say, 'I know it works.' But the truth is that we didn't know."

Redfield also took flak for collaborating with Frank Volvovitz and MicroGeneSys, viewed by many as shameless publicity hounds who would say anything to attract more investors. Although Redfield realized that MicroGeneSys had gone overboard in hyping preliminary results from the Phase I trial, after he gave the talk in Florida, he thought it would be "unethical" for him to refuse to work with the vaccine company simply because he didn't approve of everything they did. "We set criteria, and if the company met the criteria, we were moving forward," he said. "It wasn't a personality contest."

Although Burke and Redfield disagreed about the scientific merits of the larger study, Burke did not try to derail it. Redfield's trial had been funded by the army and approved by all the requisite authorities, which gave it considerable momentum. In November 1990, as soon as the Phase I study officially ended, Redfield and collaborators at army, navy, and air force hospitals around the country began enrolling the 300 volunteers required for the Phase II trial. It wasn't long before blood samples began pouring into Debbi Birx's lab, having been flown to Washington and driven to Rockville on the same day they were drawn. Debbi rarely went home before nine o'clock at night.

●

When Don Burke left Thailand in 1984, having worked there as an army virology researcher for six years, many doctors mistakenly believed that Asians were somehow genetically resistant to the AIDS virus. Bangkok's first AIDS case was identified only months after Burke left, however, in a Thai man who had lived in the United States with his male lover. More cases soon turned up among male sex workers, then female sex workers, and then intravenous drug users in Bangkok—no surprise in this crowded metropolis of nearly 10 million people, the country's biggest, wickedest city.

By 1989, Thailand's Ministry of Public Health, usually called the MOPH, was worried enough to set up a bare-bones HIV surveillance system in more than a dozen cities and towns in this country of 60 million people. The U.S. Centers for Disease Control helped devise methods for screening blood samples from commercial sex workers and IV drug users, who were known to be at high risk, and from soldiers. No HIV cases had yet turned up among Thai soldiers, but it made sense to think that infections might occur among young men who were probably away from home for the first time and who were no doubt sexually active.

Although Burke had revisited Thailand on numerous occasions since moving to the Washington area, those trips had nothing to do with AIDS. In December 1990, however, Burke went to Thailand's first major AIDS conference. Sponsored by Princess Chulabhorn, one of several science-minded members of the royal family, it attracted speakers from the NIH and from major universities in the United States and Europe. Although Burke's official purpose was to give a talk at the princess's conference, he spent most of his time not in fancy hotel ballrooms but in the utilitarian laboratories of the MOPH.

He had been called to the lab by Royal Thai Army authorities, who had discovered a skyrocketing number of HIV-positive soldiers through screening at army blood banks in northern Thailand. Like their U.S. counterparts, the Thai labs relied on antibody test kits for initial screening, but Burke knew that a more precise and labor-intensive assay was needed to rule out false-positive results. The test kits might be mistaking antibodies to malaria or some other tropical disease for antibodies to HIV, or the kits might simply be faulty. Burke asked to take some blood specimens to WRAIR for additional testing, and the colonel in charge of the Thai lab readily agreed.

Back in Rockville, Burke brought the soldiers' blood samples to a gifted civilian scientist named Francine McCutchan, who worked on his side of the moat at 1500 East Gude Drive. She was a molecular virologist who excelled at analyzing the genetic makeup of HIVs from different parts of the globe, then fitting them into different viral genotypes, or genetically defined strains. Each of these clades, or subtypes, is designated by a letter of the alphabet. Clade B typically causes AIDS in the United States and Western Europe. In Africa, AIDS is more likely due to subtypes A, C, or D.

McCutchan had earlier analyzed a batch of specimens from the Thai Red Cross in Bangkok. All were clade B, which Burke thought of as "the cosmopolitan strain" because it typically caused trouble in big cities around the world, where AIDS struck first among gay men and IV drug users. It did not take McCutchan long to figure out that the Thai soldiers were indeed infected with HIV, but not from subtype B. Once she had the genetic sequence for the new virus's "gag" gene, which codes for part of HIV's internal structure, she compared that string of genetic letters with the gag genes from all the known subtypes. The northern Thai HIV came closest to clade A, which is widely distributed in Central and West Africa. McCutchan classified it as an A strain at this point. Later, she would describe it as "Thai E," after discovering that its A-type innards were encased in an E-type envelope.

No one knew how a virus indigenous to Africa made its way to northern Thailand, or what conditions were allowing it to spread so rapidly among troops stationed around the ancient city of Chiang Mai. Don Burke made another trip to try to find out. In Bangkok, he met up with Arthur Brown, an army infectious-disease physician and epidemiologist who had been in Thailand for nine years, had a Thai wife, practiced Buddhism, and spoke the language fluently. Burke spoke some Thai as well, and together they took the one-hour commuter flight to Chiang Mai.

Thai Army authorities had asked the HIV-positive soldiers to report to an army hospital near the city for interviews with the visiting American officers. For these young men, the simple act of donating blood had thrust them into a nightmarish situation. One by one, they were ushered into a plainly furnished room to be interrogated by a towering pair of Americans who were said to be military officers but who were out of uniform. Burke was plain-spoken and barrel-chested, with thick, prematurely gray hair that would only be seen on a *farang*, as the Thais call foreigners. In contrast, Art Brown was soft-spoken and lean, barely stirring the air when he moved. For the soldiers it was like facing Lorne Greene and David Carradine.

Speaking in Thai, the two Americans quizzed the soldiers about their personal pleasures—about sex with women, sex with men, social diseases, and drugs. And the young men, who had been taught that men are free to do as they please, so long as they are discreet and do not bring shame on their families, answered. When the interviews were complete, Burke and Brown saw no evidence of IV drug use or homosexual behavior. It was obvious, however, that all the soldiers spent their off-duty hours in a certain Chiang Mai neighborhood. "What I learned was that they all frequented female prostitutes," Burke said. "Other than that, they were just a bunch of kids who were scared shitless."

In the wake of these interviews, it seemed clear that Thailand was gripped by two different HIV epidemics: in Bangkok and the South, cosmopolitan clade B was spreading among male homosexuals, commercial sex workers of both genders, and IV drug users. In the North, heterosexual contact was spreading an entirely different viral subtype at lightning speed.

Burke was fascinated by the coexistence of these two epidemics, and he began seriously considering Thailand as a place for testing preventive AIDS vaccines. One of the country's major advantages was that it already had an infrastructure for doing large clinical trials. For decades, vaccine development and testing had been strengths of AFRIMS, the Armed Forces Research Institute of the Medical Sciences in Bangkok. This is the largest of the U.S. Army's overseas biomedical research laboratories, and it is operated jointly by the U.S. and Royal Thai Armies, each with about 200 employees on site. When Burke was posted there from 1978 until 1984, he had laid the groundwork for a huge clinical trial of a Japanese encephalitis vaccine that had since proved protective. In late 1990, one AFRIMS team was coordinating a 40,000-person study of a hepatitis A vaccine, and Art Brown's group was working on a separate malaria vaccine trial. Burke figured that this research portfolio could stretch to accommodate HIV vaccines as well.

•

When John McNeil made his first trip to Thailand in April 1991, the commander of the American component at AFRIMS was friendly and polite to the newcomer who had been sent by Don Burke. John's mission, as Burke had explained it to him back in Rockville, was to establish scientific collaborations and set up studies that would enable WRAIR to determine whether experimental AIDS vaccines could be tested in a scientifically valid, cost-effective manner in Thailand. Beyond that, John was on his own.

The commander welcomed John, telling him he was free to meet with anyone in the U.S. or Thai components of AFRIMS. At the same time, the commander said, "You're here as an agent of a department back in the U.S., and if you can establish some studies that are collaborations between people in Thailand and in the States, that's fine. But I don't have anybody here who can work on HIV. And we don't have any capability to support an HIV effort." In other words, John recalled, the bottom line was "we're glad to have you here, just don't bother us."

John left the meeting thinking, "Wow. This is going to be a challenge."

In fact, everything about the new assignment in Thailand seemed a bit daunting on this, his first morning in Asia. John had left Fort Dix for WRAIR's Division of Preventive Medicine in 1986, lured by the promise of studying the spread of HIV on a scale that civilian epidemiologists could only dream of. Right away, he was named principal investigator on a study that tracked the occurrence of new HIV infections among the army's 770,000 active duty personnel. This effort stood out from a slew of others that could only tally AIDS cases, which reflected not today's infections but ones that had occurred as long as a decade earlier. The results of John's study appeared in the prestigious *New England Journal of Medicine*, and he soon published other noteworthy papers as well.

By early 1991, however, John wanted to do more than count infections, AIDS cases, and deaths. "I'm a preventive medicine officer, and our number-one tool to prevent infectious diseases is vaccines," he said. John yearned for a more active role in the HIV epidemic, and so he said yes when Don Burke offered him a chance to scout international sites for testing AIDS vaccines.

And so it happened that John, who grew up in a small North Carolina town and had no particular desire to explore Asia, whose only knowledge of Thailand came from Burke's reminiscences and what he read in guidebooks, made his first visit to the kingdom formerly known as Siam. After nearly twenty-four hours of folding his six-foot-plus frame into a series of coach seats, John arrived feeling as though he had been beaten with rubber hoses. Fortunately, an AFRIMS car and driver were waiting to take him to his hotel.

Everything about the trip from the airport to the city was cacophonous and strange, a jumble of modern construction and fierce congestion, with the gilded spires of Buddhist temples poking up in completely unexpected places. It was a relief when the car delivered the bone-weary John to the Siam City, a cool oasis of mirrors and teak, staffed entirely by people who were both extremely courteous and quite attractive. The air was scented softly with sandalwood, and he got a decent night's sleep before paying his first call at AFRIMS.

For several days, John trooped from meeting to meeting at AFRIMS, an unabashedly utilitarian complex of gray-streaked stucco buildings on the edge of a large medical area. In its immediate vicinity are a military hospital and pathology institute, several large academic hospitals run by Mahidol University, a Buddhist crematorium, and even a brig filled with Thai soldiers who'd lost their minds. John learned about the projects being juggled by American and Thai scientists and quickly came to realize that the U.S. component already had a packed research agenda. For one thing, the demands of running a hepatitis A vaccine trial with 40,000 participants were considerable.

Eventually, however, a Thai army epidemiologist named Narongrid Sirisopana sought John's advice about the *tahangain* surveillance program. *Tahangain* is what Thais call the twenty-one-year-olds who are conscripted into military service via a national lottery, which approximates a random sampling of men this age. The Royal Thai Army (RTA) began testing some of them for HIV antibodies in 1990, but the program was haphazard and not standardized in any meaningful way.

Dr. Narongrid wanted to improve the RTA's surveillance system, and John had experience with the U.S. Army's very exacting program for testing new recruits. It was a good match, even though there were cultural divides to be bridged. During their first serious technical meeting, Dr. Naongrid grabbed his head and said "Can we stop? My head is hurting from listening to English."

John made five more trips to Thailand during 1991, and the collaborators soon developed a coherent system for collecting blood, running tests in a centralized laboratory at the Thai Institute of Pathology, located next door to AFRIMS, and collecting basic personal information about the conscripts. The Thai army conscripted 120,000 *tahangain* each year and accurate information about HIV in such a large group would be helpful in deciding whether large HIV vaccine trials could be carried out in Thailand.

At first, John told Burke that he was commuting to Thailand only to help gather and analyze data that they could use to evaluate Thailand as a test site. He had not signed on, John insisted, for the far more complicated job of making trials happen. He was married, he had two small children back in the Washington suburbs, and he sensed that this assignment could morph into a huge, life-devouring project.

John's feelings changed, however, as he spent more time in Thailand. Epidemiologist that he was, the horror of the Thai AIDS epidemic first came to him from reading numbers on paper. What he saw was frightening, a situation far beyond anything documented in the United States. Among female sex workers in Chiang Mai, the rate of HIV infection went from 1 percent to 44 percent during one six-month period. Nationally, 15 percent of women in the sex industry were already infected. In northern Thailand, young men were five times more likely to be infected than their peers in the South.

The statistics were chilling enough, but the flesh-and-blood impact was worse. This hit John in November 1991, during a visit to a district hospital located in Lampang, a town in the mountains east of Chiang Mai. He was taken there by Dr. Chirasak Khamboonruang, the head of a major research institution in Chiang Mai University. Many Thai physicians were of Chinese descent and raised in Bangkok, but Dr. Chirasak was a Lanna Thai, raised in one of the nearby hill towns, and he was powerfully affected by what this new disease was doing to his homeland. He wanted John to see for himself.

"The male and female medicine wards, and the pediatric ward, were absolutely, totally full of AIDS patients," John said. "It absolutely blew me away, especially the pediatric wards. It was overwhelming. And I went into the labor and delivery suite, and several of the women who were in labor were HIV infected, and this was before there was any knowledge of how to intervene. The children had a very high likelihood of being infected." And from then on, John McNeil was determined that an AIDS vaccine would be developed for Thailand, as well as for the United States, and that he would have a hand in making this happen.

●

Meanwhile, back at WRAIR in Rockville, working conditions deteriorated after Ed Tramont left the army to work in the vaccine industry. Tramont was Burke's boss, and he had long-standing loyalties to Redfield as well. Without ever appearing to take sides with either man, he kept a lid on their disagreements and made sure that nobody let the air out of anybody else's tires. Redfield pursued therapeutic vaccines as a stepping stone toward preventive ones; Burke moved forward with efforts to test preventive vaccines in Thailand. The two approaches coexisted.

When Tramont left, Burke hung onto his role as chief of the Division of Retrovirology, but he also stepped into Tramont's spot as manager of HIV/AIDS research for the army and coordinator of tri-service research on controlling the epidemic. This made Burke literally his own boss. In the fall of 1991, when the budgets were passed, Congress allocated $100 million for AIDS research within the Defense Department. Some of the money went directly to navy and air force research efforts, but the largest share was under Don Burke's control.

Burke channeled much of the army's share into the Henry M. Jackson Foundation, a private nonprofit organization that hires civilian scientists for biomedical research projects run by the military. This is a mechanism for bringing in expertise that can't be found among active-duty personnel. Jackson-paid scientists like Francine McCutchan, for example, have been key players in army AIDS research. As the director of the Division of

Retrovirology, Burke contracted with the Jackson Foundation for the people and projects he wanted. Some of the money he used to renovate nearby 1600 East Gude Drive, a four-story building with three floors of offices and 40,000 square feet of new lab space on the top floor. As soon as the makeover was completed, Burke moved into a large office there. From the new lab, Burke could look across the moat to dumpy old 13 Taft Court, where Redfield, Debbi Birx, and the immunology lab remained.

"It was wonderful," Burke says of his situation in late 1991. "I got to call all the shots for the program. I had people who were very competent leaders and managers, but they didn't lay claim to the science." Burke moved quickly to reorganize research into "program areas." For the first time, he split research on therapeutic and preventive HIV vaccines, designating preventive vaccines as Program Area 1 and moving Redfield's therapeutic vaccine work to Program Area 4. It was obvious to everyone that the numbering system reflected Burke's scientific priorities.

During this period, Redfield recalls, "the personal relationship between Don Burke and I became very strained." The fundamental disagreement that had divided them for several years had not cooled: Redfield insisted that insights for designing better preventive vaccines would emerge from the study of therapeutic vaccines in HIV patients; Burke was certain that potentially protective vaccines should be tested in healthy volunteers, in real-world settings where the risk for exposure to HIV was high. Neither had ever conceded an inch in this standoff, but Tramont had made sure that both approaches stayed on the research agenda. Now Burke was the boss.

Redfield and his crew were buffeted by humiliations large and small. Although Burke did not interfere with the ongoing Phase II study of gp160, he decided that two small treatment trials in AIDS patients at Walter Reed should be halted earlier than expected. Redfield was distraught. He hated telling sixty people with advanced AIDS that they could not continue with a treatment that was safe and elicited immune responses, even though there was no guarantee that it would help in the long run.

Back at 13 Taft Court, the laboratory scientists felt like Cinderella in the chimney corner: Up-to-date telephones were snatched away and replaced with cranky old ones that didn't work, and when computers broke no one came to fix them.

On the rare occasions when John McNeil was in Rockville instead of Thailand, he took refuge in his office at 1 Taft Court, a demilitarized zone between Burke and Redfield. Although few of Redfield's people even knew John by sight, they demonized him as the preventive vaccines guy who was siphoning off funding that was rightfully theirs. When morale ebbed, they probably even blamed John for the crappy phones and the computers that didn't work.

●

No matter how dark his situation in Rockville, Redfield was a star when the Eighth International AIDS Conference kicked off in Amsterdam on July 20, 1992. The *Washington Post* called Redfield's report on the Phase I gp160 trial, along with therapeutic vaccine presentations by Jonas Salk and Daniel Zagury, "the most controversial and eagerly anticipated sessions of the meeting." The *Post* played up the National Institutes of Health's recent decision to fund the enrollment of another 300 participants in the Phase II study of gp160, which would double its size. Flushed with enthusiasm the day before his talk, Redfield told the *Post's* reporter, "I believe that we are on the verge of a radical revolution in terms of our armamentarium to treat viral diseases."

When Redfield took the stage on July 21, he had only fifteen minutes to say his piece—typical for a big scientific meeting with a packed schedule. He explained that the study was meant to find out whether immunizing thirty HIV patients with gp160 was safe and whether a series of shots would prevent or stabilize the immune deterioration that occurs as AIDS worsens. Summarizing columns of laboratory data projected from slides, Redfield said that most of the immunized men produced new T cells and new antibodies that were not found in the unvaccinated comparison group. In half the vaccinated patients, Redfield's lab had used a new, exquisitely sensitive technique, called PCR, to measure the amount of virus circulating in the bloodstream. A series of measurements showed that this circulating amount, also called the viral load, either decreased or was unchanged in 93 percent of immunized patients. In a comparison group of untreated people, PCR testing showed that viral load increased in 47 percent of untreated patients. Redfield called the difference between the two groups "statistically significant," meaning that it was not due to chance alone.

"What we've shown, in fact, is that the amount of virus goes down," Redfield told the *Boston Globe*, which ran a story the following day. "Unless we're in a Kurt Vonnegut novel where there's no sense in anything, we think that's very important." Redfield's interpretation of the data buoyed the hopes of many AIDS patients and their families, who were tired of discouraging reports about AIDS treatments that didn't help or brought terrible side effects. NBC was sufficiently impressed to book him on the *Today Show* for a chat about AIDS vaccine research.

John McNeil was in the auditorium for Redfield's talk, and he thought Redfield was talking big for someone with data from only thirty patients. Still, "it's not unusual for investigators to overinterpret or be overenthusiastic about their data," John said. "I didn't think he was trying to gain himself any personal acclaim. I just thought he was very excited and hopeful that this would work."

Redfield's Amsterdam glory was fleeting. He had scarcely unpacked his bags when a bombshell landed at WRAIR. Craig Hendrix and Neil Boswell, air force physicians who were coinvestigators on the gp160 trial, now charged Redfield with falsifying data and misrepresenting study results in his public presentation. In addition, they claimed that someone other than Redfield had altered patient records to make immunized patients in the trial look healthier than they actually were, supporting the idea that vaccination was an effective treatment. Hendrix and Boswell demanded that the army launch an official inquiry into these misdeeds.

As Redfield's immediate superior, Burke could have herded the accusers and the accused into a room and insisted that they review the study data and settle their differences. Instead, he passed the request for an inquiry up the chain of command. And while it was being processed, he brought in a Jackson Foundation statistician to reanalyze Redfield's data. Using different methods, this statistician found no significant difference between viral loads in treated and untreated patients. "Bob's long suit has never been statistics," Burke said in a 1999 interview. "There were all sorts of charges and accusations about intentional or unintentional errors in how the data was represented. I went over the data myself with Bob, and I have no doubt whatsoever that he made mistakes that were unintentional, where he just used statistical techniques that were not correct for the data."

In 1992, however, the threat of an inquiry uncoiled at a slow and torturous pace, as higher authorities weighed its merits and decided how formal the process would be. While this was going on, none of the accusers talked with Redfield, Debbi Birx, or anyone else who worked on the gp160 study at WRAIR. Hendrix and Boswell never asked to examine patient records, lab notebooks, or the reams of data that the lab had printed out. Finally, the complaint resulted in a "commander's inquiry," which is closer to a deposition in a lawyer's office than to a courtroom trial. As anyone who's been deposed is aware, however, this can be burdensome and intimidating enough.

Debbi Birx was sucked into the vortex of the investigation. One of the most damaging accusations made by Hendrix and Boswell was that a physician at Walter Reed had deliberately made an immunized patient look healthier than he was, by arbitrarily changing his designation from Walter Reed stage 5 to stage 3. Although Debbi was not named in the complaint, her initials were beside the alteration in the patient's chart.

Soon Debbi and Redfield faced the first of six Defense Department investigators who would come to 13 Taft Court, one by one, over the next nine months. Redfield was so stunned by what was happening that it fell to Debbi to compile the stacks of written documents that the inquisitors wanted to review. She lost track of the number of daylong, taped interviews they sat for. Over and over, Redfield and Debbi went over the data presented in Amsterdam, reiterating that Redfield had reported what the study showed. People could disagree with the spin on it, that was fair enough, but he had not tinkered with the facts.

When Debbi was asked whether she agreed with Redfield's interpretation, she said her view of the increased helper T cell activity in immunized patients was more equivocal than his. He credited the vaccine for the positive changes seen in some patients; she believed people who responded well to vaccination might simply have had more intact immune systems to start with. Both Debbi and Redfield hoped results of the large Phase II study would eventually show whether the vaccine was really helping.

As for fudging patient records, Debbi said a patient had been labeled a stage 5 after he was diagnosed with an oral yeast infection commonly called thrush. When she interviewed him at the next clinic visit, however, it was clear that he had developed thrush while taking powerful antibiotics. These drugs often trigger yeast infections, and when this happens the patient is rated as stage 3. So Debbi made the change.

Meanwhile, the Phase II gp160 study was enrolling 300 more patients, paid for by the NIH and by Wyeth-Ayerst, which was subsidizing Micro-GeneSys; and the original 300 were coming in every other month for blood draws at seventeen different test sites. Some of the cellular immunology studies had to be done on fresh blood, so Debbi and the lab people hung around late, waiting for the blood to be delivered. With the results of the Phase I trial now under official investigation, the laboratory team had assumed a tense defensive stance. "The one thing we could do was to make sure the trial was above reproach. I didn't want the FDA or anybody to be able to come in and say that it was not done perfectly," Debbi recalled. Little did they know that their troubles were going to get a lot worse, and soon.

●

On September 16, 1992, the Senate Appropriations Subcommittee on Defense held a closed-door session to mark up the annual spending bill. Immediately after the meeting, a Senate staff member who was friendly with Don Burke called to tell him some astonishing news: The bill now included a recommendation that $20 million be set aside to launch a "large-scale Phase III clinical investigation of the drug gp160."

"No, no, no! No fuckin' way! Line in the sand, NO!" Burke shouted into the phone. Once he calmed down, Burke told the Senate aide that a Phase III trial would be premature and "a terrible idea"; gp160 was in a Phase II study, and in his view the vaccine didn't appear to be having much of an effect on the clinical well-being of patients. Burke advocated going ahead with the Phase II study, then analyzing the results and deciding whether gp160 should advance to a larger, more costly study.

"She told me that she couldn't deter Congress, but she could change the wording of the bill," Burke said. Various drafts circulated over the next three weeks, with input from Burke and countless others, and the final version was released on October 5. It provided that the trial would proceed unless the secretary of defense, the director of the NIH, and the FDA commissioner agreed that it should be halted and justified their decision in writing. The bill gave them six months to decide and write it down. If the trial did not go forward, then the $20 million would revert to the army for use in any type of AIDS research program. This raised the possibility that Don Burke would end up with control over $20 million originally earmarked for Bob Redfield's pet project.

Hostile stories about "pork-barrel research" and "Congress playing doctor" hit television and newspapers almost immediately. It was a Capitol Hill story with something for everyone. Connoisseurs of Louisiana politics, where former elected officials immediately turn into inmates or lobbyists, were amused to learn that former Senator Russell Long had been retained to promote the interests of MicroGeneSys. Apparently he did a bang-up job, persuading his powerful Senate friends Sam Nunn and John Warner (D-Georgia and R-Virginia, as though it mattered) to sponsor a $20-million boost for his client's sole product. It was not insignificant that by now the giant drugmaker Wyeth-Ayerst had also jumped on the MicroGeneSys bandwagon.

The major newspapers and scientific periodicals were a bully pulpit for NIH officials, AIDS researchers, and other scientists who inveighed against the danger of having Congress—a group not noted for scientific acumen—pick commercial products for tax-supported efficacy testing. "If we're going to have legislators determining what drugs we test in people, I think that, as physicians and scientists, we're potentially facing as large a moral dilemma as we have ever faced in medical science," NIH director Bernadine Healy thundered after the appropriations bill passed on October 6. Healy promptly announced formation of a blue-ribbon panel to evaluate the merits of a gp160 efficacy trial.

Redfield tried to steer clear of the $20-million mess by refusing all interview requests. Although the public knew nothing of this, he was still being harried by army investigators unleashed on him back in July. His intramural troubles went public in early November, when Jon Cohen, a writer for *Science*, broke the story of the army investigation into Redfield's Amsterdam presentation. The story aired the complaints filed by air force doctors Craig Hendrix and Neil Boswell, but did not mention their names. Don Burke, however, was quoted as saying that he had Redfield's statistics recalculated and now thought there was no statistically significant difference between gp160-treated patients and untreated controls.

The *Science* story was picked up by CNN, CBS *Evening News*, the *Washington Post*, the *New York Times*, and others. For Redfield and the people who worked for him, it was like being clamped into stocks on the village green. They might pop open a beer and slump in front of the TV, only to hear some broadcaster intoning, "He was the man of the hour at this summer's international AIDS conference . . . That was July. Now the army's worried its vaccine, once the leading contender, isn't so promising after all. Colleagues accused Redfield of hyping his results." They opened the morning newspaper with a sense of dread.

"It was a very sad time for my family," said Redfield, who lived with his wife and children in Baltimore. "It obviously saddened me." In the laboratory, Debbi Birx and her colleagues focused on the daily grind of doing the lab work for the Phase II study. They had a bunker mentality: Keep your head down, do your work, don't talk to strangers. Everyone associated with Redfield became so paranoid that if the Coke machine broke, it seemed like part of a vast conspiracy.

On the other side of the moat, in Burke's camp, gloating was not unknown. Many people saw Redfield as pompous and condescending, the kind of guy who deserved to get his comeuppance. Regardless of whose side they were on, most people recognized they were not part of a normal, healthy workplace. They began to call WRAIR's Rockville campus "the Land of Oz," because weird things happened all the time, there were good and bad witches, and houses fell and crushed people with no warning. For some of them, it would soon get even worse. As their misery deepened, it seemed to the denizens of 13 Taft Court that the whole world was watching this humiliating spectacle.

●

Chris Beyrer, however, knew nothing about what was happening at WRAIR. In August 1992, as soon as he finished his residency in preventive medicine at Johns Hopkins University in Baltimore, he left the rat race of academic medicine behind. He moved to a friend's house on Fire Island, and by October he was far too relaxed to trouble himself over the gp160 brouhaha that was churning up the AIDS establishment. AIDS vaccines were nowhere on Chris's radar screen when he got a call from an old friend in Baltimore, saying that Johns Hopkins had new NIH money for a program called PAVE, which stood for Preparation for AIDS Vaccine Evaluation. It offered a great job opportunity—for a field director with medical and public-health credentials, which Chris definitely possessed, who would pull together and study groups of high risk, HIV-negative people who might later enroll in vaccine trials. There was only one catch: The job required relocating to Chiang Mai, Thailand, immediately. Chris's friend hoped that the location and the urgency wouldn't cause Chris to say no.

On the contrary: "As soon as I heard, I thought yes, that is the next round." It was as though Chris had been poised for a sign, waiting for the right mission to present itself, and here it was. The NIH, like the army, wanted to find places where AIDS was spreading fast, where there were reputable hospitals and laboratories, and where vaccine trials might yield speedier answers than in the United States. So the NIAID was funding eight PAVE sites in different parts of the globe, and Chris was exactly the kind of scientist they hoped would run these operations.

Within one week of the call, Chris was in Chiang Mai, meeting with the Thai researchers for the project, everyone interviewing and sizing up everyone else. All agreed he was the right man for the job, and by November 1992, Chris Beyrer had embarked on a new life in Thailand's second-largest city, where he saw the epidemic exploding in an all-too-familiar way.

Chris had been part of New York's gay community when AIDS struck in the early 1980s. As a medical student at State University of New York Health Sciences Center in Brooklyn, his first AIDS patients were not gay men, however, but poor people of color. They lived in East Flatbush, and many were IV drug users or Haitian immigrants, a group that had been colonized early by the virus. "I had the unique and tragic experience of dealing with the HIV epidemic in the developing world, but it was happening in Brooklyn," Chris said.

Across the river in Manhattan, where Chris lived with his actor boyfriend, a 1985 sampling of gay men in New York indicated that half were already infected with HIV. Chris and David talked it over and decided not to get tested, because there were no treatments at that point and they were already monogamous. Three years later, after they had moved to Madison, Wisconsin, where Chris was doing an internship in family medicine, David developed AIDS. He had no insurance, and his first stay in the hospital cost $36,000, wiping out the couple's savings. They moved back to the East Coast, where they had more social support, and for the next three years Chris took care of his lover while going to grad school in public health, doing a residency, and moonlighting in emergency rooms to make money. "I never slept," Chris recalls. "And then it was over."

One year after losing his partner, Chris was learning his way around the most disreputable back alleys in Chiang Mai, where female sex workers plied their trades in bars festooned with strings of Christmas lights, or bumping over rough mountain roads to locate men who had been treated for sexually transmitted diseases. His mission was to figure out whether HIV vaccine trials could be done successfully among several different groups: female sex workers, men who visited sexually transmitted disease (STD) clinics, active-duty soldiers, and men recently discharged from the army.

There were many questions to be answered, including the incidence of new HIV infections in each group, behaviors that were spreading infection, what viral subtypes were common, and how likely people were to keep scheduled clinic appointments. Chris was the sole Western scientist on the PAVE project, and he sat in on interviews conducted by his Thai colleagues and worked diligently to learn this polytonal, difficult tongue. Chris took to Thailand and its people immediately: He was already a Buddhist, he had studied Asian history in college, and he had lived for short periods in Sri Lanka and India. It was an excellent fit.

The PAVE project had an office at a public-health research facility attached to Chiang Mai University, called the Research Institute for Health Sciences, or RIHES. Although it had some good labs, RIHES wasn't equipped for the kind of sophisticated viral characterization that the army labs at AFRIMS, down in Bangkok, could do. Chris heard about John McNeil, who had helped the Royal Thai Army set up its HIV surveillance system. The PAVE project used some of the data collected by the RTA system, and Chris got a graduate student from WRAIR, who was on temporary assignment at AFRIMS, to do virology work on the recently discharged soldiers PAVE was studying.

When Chris and John McNeil eventually met, John quickly saw that the PAVE study lacked the money and staff to carry out the virology studies Chris needed. At first the army helped in an informal way, but gradually the collaboration became more formal.

Thailand was a hotbed of AIDS vaccine activity when Chris arrived. In addition to John's work on behalf of the army and Chris's new job with Johns Hopkins and its partner, Chiang Mai University, the World Health Organization and the U.S. Centers for Disease Control were also weighing Thailand as a place to study vaccines.

At first, many of the Thai scientists seemed perplexed by all this international attention. The Thai medical community is a socially elite group, as in America, and the first waves of AIDS patients were from marginalized populations—sex workers in low-class brothels, gay men, IV drug users. These people had little to do with the doctors themselves. But as an ominous picture emerged from their own surveillance data, Thailand's medical establishment realized that in fact their country might be headed for a worse epidemic than the United States. In 1991, the Thai Ministry of Public Health mounted a massive health education effort called the "100-percent Condom Campaign" as a first line of defense against AIDS. The ministry also met with everyone interested in HIV vaccine research, as top officials began to consider not only the public-health benefits that HIV vaccines might have but also how partnering with foreign companies might advance Thailand's own technological and business development.

Back in Rockville, another of Don Burke's periodic reorganizations had promoted John McNeil to chief of vaccine development for WRAIR in February 1993. That year he made nine trips to Thailand, spending almost as much time in Asia as at home. Living this way had its good and bad points. The bad side was stepping off a plane in Washington and having the younger of his two daughters, not yet three at the time, look at him as if to say "Who in the hell are you?" The good side was that he missed the final act of the tragicomedy in Rockville.

●

The meeting room was filled with physicians, nurses, and technicians from the seventeen sites participating in the Phase II trial of gp160. They had traveled to this nondescript hotel on the Washington Beltway to hear an update on the trial from Bob Redfield, the principal investigator, and Debbi Birx, who was running the central immunology lab. In the corridor outside, Redfield and Debbi had been waylaid by the Wyeth-Ayerst physician who was in charge of the manufacturer's part of the enterprise.

His message was simple: "Wyeth-Ayerst is pulling the plug. As of thirty days from now, we're stopping all fiscal support for the trial." Wyeth-Ayerst's investment in MicroGeneSys and its gp160 vaccine had reached the level of nearly $6 million per year, and what were they getting in return? Nothing but a bombardment of disastrous publicity about backroom deals on Capitol Hill, NIH meetings where their product was dismissed as useless, and a principal investigator who was accused of scientific fraud. The big company wanted out, and there was no way to bar the door.

In the wake of this short but deadly exchange, Redfield and Debbi had to go into the investigators' meeting and act as if nothing was wrong. Even as they fielded nuts-and-bolts questions about the minutia of the trial's procedures, Debbi's brain was in overdrive. Her first thought was, "We have 608 volunteers on study. We are halfway there and it has to be completed. We see these patients all the time. The one thing I could promise every patient was that we were going to get interpretable data, positive or negative. After all, half these HIV infected patients were on placebo, and they agreed to this because they wanted to see what the answer was."

By the time they got back to WRAIR, Debbi had a plan. She figured the trial could go forward if they cut out all the interesting but extra immunology experiments her group had been doing and stuck to the bare-bones assays the FDA expected to see. The money saved on lab work could be used to reimburse the clinics for patient visits and to pay for the data monitoring and quality assurance required by the FDA. Debbi gathered the lab staff and told them what had happened and how the trial could be salvaged. Fifteen of them volunteered to drop what they'd been doing and take on new jobs, ranging from keyboarding data into computers to retraining as monitors, who visit sites and scrutinize every detail in patient charts.

Her plan succeeded, and Debbi herself got a crash course in vaccine development; with Wyeth out of the picture, she now worked directly with the FDA on data reporting and the intricacies of quality assurance and control. There was another lesson from all this, too. "I learned that people really are our most valuable resource. Everybody worked fifteen- or twenty-hour days for almost a year and a half. They'd never been to the clinic before this happened, but they understood that it was important to finish the trial," Debbi said.

None of this unglamorous labor drew the media's attention, which was understandably diverted by the misadventures of the $20 million that Congress had set aside for the controversial efficacy trial. NIH's blue-ribbon panel said NIH would take some of the money and team up with the Department of Defense to compare gp160 with other unspecified vaccines. If you're so interested, the DOD answered, take the whole $20-million hot potato. Wait a minute, chimed in Wyeth-Ayerst, we're not giving NIH our vaccine so they can compare it with stuff made by our competitors. And NIH told the DOD, if the company won't cooperate, then you might as well take the money. We'll take it, responded the DOD, but there's not enough to pay for a multivaccine trial, so we're only going to test gp160. You can't do that, shrilled the NIH. That's what got you in trouble in the first place!

When the tumult and shouting was over, the $20 million quietly rolled over into WRAIR's AIDS budget for the next year. Don Burke's division solicited proposals to promote "start-up science" for making HIV vaccines, using some of the money to back novel, early vaccine research, including Bob Johnston's transformation of Venezuelan equine encephalitis into a live vector. In Burke's view, these were far better investments than a gp160 trial would have been. "I'm very proud that I stepped in front of the goddamned freight train. I lost a friend, and I had a rocky career, but I made what I believe to be some excellent decisions at the time."

Meanwhile, the commander's inquiry cleared Bob Redfield and the unnamed physician, who was actually Debbi Birx, of misrepresentation, fraud, or malfeasance of any kind. The news of their innocence barely had time to sink in, however, before there was another startling development. Neil Boswell, one of the air force doctors who had brought charges against Redfield, was recruited by Burke to be deputy director of the Division of Retrovirology.

"I needed the program to be truly tri-service, and I needed somebody who was a butt kicker. And Neil was a butt kicker, and he was available, and he was air force. In retrospect, I don't know whether it was a smart idea or not. Hard to say," Burke mused a few years later.

Redfield was outraged. "Here's somebody who falsely accused me, and the army concludes that he falsely accused me. And then Don Burke hires the guy to be my boss. You had to ask, what's going on here?" What was happening, of course, was that therapeutic vaccine research was history. WRAIR was no longer a place for Bob Redfield. In mid-1994, he left Debbi Birx in charge of his research department and returned to the clinic at Walter Reed, where he cared for AIDS patients full-time.

It took until 1996 for Redfield to retire, and after returning to civilian life, he claimed not to be bitter against those who, in his view, drove him from the army. Still, he said, "I am disappointed in the institution, the army, for not going back and holding these individuals accountable for what I consider conduct unbecoming an officer."

●

Having vanquished the leading proponent of vaccines as treatments for AIDS, Don Burke refocused WRAIR's efforts on the more traditional mission of developing a vaccine that would protect healthy troops against HIV. Because the armed forces viewed both homosexuality and IV drug use as incompatible with service, what they wanted to guard against was heterosexual transmission. Therefore, they needed to test potential vaccines in a place where HIV was spreading mainly through heterosexual contact. Thailand, according to studies carried out by the Royal Thai Army, Chris Beyrer, and others, was just such a place.

In fact, John McNeil wrote in a bold pitch that he sent to Chiron and Genentech, "There is a globally unparalleled confluence of epidemiological, virological and sociological circumstances in Thailand favorable for vaccine trials." When the companies received this letter in May 1993, they were leading the domestic vaccine race. Although it was a great coup to have their products in Phase II studies sponsored by NIH, they knew NIH was seething with internal debates about the scientific merits, costs, and political complications of doing an expensive efficacy trial in the United States. Whether NIH went ahead with a Phase III trial or not, it was always smart to have a Plan B—and that's what John proposed.

According to John, Thailand met all the basic requirements for a good trial site, and then some. First, it had a serious AIDS epidemic that was affecting many groups of people living in many locations. Its relatively high, relatively stable incidence was an ideal setting for determining whether immunization would make a difference. Second, Thailand had laboratories and research institutions that could carry out some of the immunology testing needed to measure vaccine activity. Finally, the political and social conditions were right: The government had already vowed to participate in international AIDS vaccine research, there was a procedure for making sure that trials were conducted in an ethical manner, and there was a history of successful vaccine collaborations between Thailand and the U.S. Army. Beyond that, the obvious advantage of John's proposal was that the U.S. military would sponsor efficacy trials in Thailand and pay most of the costs.

One part of the proposal, if they signed on, would cost the companies money: John strongly suggested that they come up with a version of gp120 that mimicked the envelope protein of the Thai subtypes that Francine McCutchan had identified in her lab at WRAIR. At this point there were two distinct epidemics in Thailand, subtype B and Thai E, and no one knew whether a vaccine designed to prevent infection with one would also guard against the other.

Another unanswered question was whether antigens from one subtype might stimulate more broadly protective antibodies than antigens from the other. Kathy Steimer had recently found that antibodies elicited by Chiron's original gp120, based on a subtype B virus, failed to kill newly isolated B type viruses in test tubes. Would antibodies stimulated by an E-based vaccine be more powerful? If the companies were willing to make subtype E vaccines, they could be pitted against B and E viruses in real-world encounters, and so could the original subtype B vaccines. Thailand's double-barreled epidemic gave companies an opportunity to answer more research questions, more quickly, and at lower cost than in the United States.

John closed his letter with an appeal for the companies to reach out to the "less affluent regions of the world where the HIV pandemic is most burdensome." He enclosed maps and statistics showing the swath that HIV had cut through Thailand, inviting the companies to visit and see for themselves. Raised in the South, where the exact wording of an invitation matters, John knew that there was a big difference between "please come see us sometime" and "please come for dinner on Friday of next week." So he invited Chiron and Genentech scientists to come to Chiang Mai for a workshop on September 19 through 22, followed by a visit to AFRIMS in Bangkok. They were asked to make scientific presentations about their vaccines to an audience of Thai researchers and public-health officials, who in turn would discuss their latest findings about HIV in Thailand. There would also be field trips, John promised.

And so it happened that Kathy Steimer, along with Anne-Marie Duliege from Chiron's clinical trials department and other American participants, found herself stepping out of an air-conditioned van and into the fetid, sweltering environs of Chiang Mai Hospital, the teaching institution for Chiang Mai University Medical School. After much ceremonial bowing, staff physicians in immaculate white jackets divided the visitors into groups and herded them through crowds of patients in the first-floor lobby, which is also the outpatient reception area.

Kathy's group packed into a narrow elevator with scarred metal walls, along with patients in various states of misery and undress. Kathy felt massive and ungainly next to the diminutive Thais. Her hands were pinned against her sides and seemed like huge, dangling appendages. Her flaxen hair, so odd and conspicuous in this setting, was being riffled by a breeze. She looked up and saw that a ceiling fan was furiously sucking air directly from the elevator shaft and blowing it straight into her face. At home, Kathy had banned the use of kitchen sponges because they harbor dangerous microbes. Now she was trapped where contagion was probably everywhere.

Finally, the group stepped out on the top floor, which houses the infectious disease wards. Sad-looking people lined up on a wooden bench eyed the *farang*, who were trying to take in the scene. Not twenty paces from the elevators were a half-dozen metal hospital beds in a row, occupied by skinny men in johnnies who were sleeping, staring into space, or eating rice out of plastic bags brought by their families. The *farang* shuffled first into the women's ward. All beds in the large open wards were filled, and more had been set up in the hallways. Most patients lay motionless, even in the bustle of the halls. There were few IV drips, and no beeping bedside monitors.

Do all of these people have HIV? the visitors wanted to know. Not all, the doctors said: About 80 percent of the hospital's admissions are related to HIV, but many of the people you see have tuberculosis—some also have HIV, some do not.

Unlike HIV, TB is an airborne bug. Although the windows were open and huge roaring fans mounted near the ceiling circulated the hot air, quarters were close. There were a lot of sick people here, and if the visiting Americans could have held their breath indefinitely, they would have.

The men's ward down the hall was not quite so crowded, but almost everyone had AIDS and some of the patients were comatose, looking not long for the world. Everyone in the tour group sweated freely, even the hospitable young doctors in their starched white coats. When the tour was over and the visitors poured into the crowded street beside the hospital, they gulped the diesel-heavy air as though it was a zephyr.

The next day, most of Kathy's presentation to the workshop focused on Chiron's clade B vaccine. She also mentioned that the army had given her samples of Thai E viruses, and that she had begun fiddling with them in the lab, thinking about which parts of the envelope gene might code for the most potent antigens. When she was finished, John McNeil rose beside his chair. "I'm sorry to put you on the spot in public, but I am going to put you on the spot: Does this mean that Chiron is committing to developing a Thai gp120?"

Kathy hesitated for a moment, and then she said, "Yes."

John was elated. "That was the first time that we knew we were going to have a Thai-specific candidate vaccine."

Jack Obijeski of Genentech, on the other hand, was in no hurry to make a clade E vaccine for Thailand. Jack, the self-described gumshoe virologist who was once with the CDC, wasn't sure that assigning viruses to arbitrary genetic subtypes really mattered. It might be that certain parts of the HIV envelope would be the same for every genetic subtype. If a clade B vaccine contained some of these common epitopes, in theory it could elicit antibodies against other strains of virus as well, a phenomenon called cross neutralization.

"That's what I proposed at the Chiang Mai meeting," Jack said in a later interview. "I said 'Lookit here. In order to make the E, we then have to scale up production, we've got to do this, we've got to do that, and it's going to be at least a couple of years before we have it in hand. I don't know if I can convince the management at Genentech to do it, okay? But we've got the MN (subtype B) vaccine, and who knows? You might get cross neutralization—and the trial will prove it or not prove it, you see?'"

The trial that Jack was thinking about would not be an army-sponsored study, but an alternative plan that he had heard about from William L. Heyward, an old buddy from the CDC who was now working with the World Health Organization in Bangkok. Jack and Bill had gone out for dinner on their own during the Chiang Mai workshop, and over a bowl of very spicy soup, Bill had described an opportunity that he saw developing in Bangkok. Clade B was the predominant virus among injecting drug users there, and WHO was already funding a study to find out whether participants in the city's huge drug-treatment program might be suitable for a vaccine trial. The data weren't in yet, but if it turned out that the participants would be willing to volunteer and were reliable enough to show up for the necessary clinic visits, then they would be perfect for testing a subtype B vaccine—which Genentech had already made. Jack found this proposal much more attractive than what the army had in mind. And Thailand was a big country. He and Bill agreed: There was room for more than one efficacy trial of an HIV vaccine.

Back in the states, after the Chiang Mai meeting, Kathy's bosses at Chiron wanted to know more about Thailand's need for an E-based vaccine. So she invited John McNeil and Don Burke to give a seminar at Chiron and to have dinner with founding scientist Bill Rutter and the other top executives. After meeting with the army representatives, Chiron's leaders gave Kathy the green light.

Years later, former Chiron CEO Ed Penhoet recalled how passionate Kathy had been about making and testing a vaccine for Thailand. It would not cost all that much to make a Thai E vaccine, and the epidemic there was so severe that "even a partly efficacious vaccine could make an important preventive contribution. That was the primary human reason for pursuing this."

It was a hopeful sign that an American company was willing to invest in a vaccine for use not in the lucrative U.S. market but in a country nearly halfway around the globe. And if Thailand could support not one but two vaccine-efficacy trials, one among heterosexuals in the North and another among Bangkok drug users, that would ultimately benefit Thailand and might also speed development of vaccines for other parts of the world. When John McNeil stepped back and looked at where HIV vaccine research stood at the end of 1993, he could not help but be encouraged.

II

THE WATERSHED

April–June 1994

●

7

NOTHING VENTURED,

NOTHING GAINED

A T 7:28 ON THE MORNING OF FEBRUARY 2, 1994, Phil the ground-hog emerged from his burrow on Gobbler's Knob, near the town of Punxsutawney, Pennsylvania. Legend holds that there will be six more weeks of wintry weather if February 2 is a sunny day, causing the bucktoothed, brown-furred creature to see his own shadow when he emerges from hibernation. Hundreds, sometimes thousands, of groundhog aficionados gather to witness this annual event. In 1994, Phil saw his shadow right away. There would be bad weather ahead.

But snow and ice were nothing compared to the deadly shadow cast five weeks later, when the nation's annual surveillance report on AIDS emerged from the Centers for Disease Control. In March 1994, CDC's forecast was far more chilling than Punxsutawney Phil's: Years of death and disease lay ahead. The number of AIDS cases in the United States had rocketed to 106,949 in 1993—double the number for the previous year. CDC said that nearly 133,000 people were living with AIDS in the United States, and 51,439 more were known to be infected with HIV but had not yet developed full-blown AIDS. As to how many were already infected but hadn't yet been tested, scientists could only guess. Their best estimate put that number at around 850,000. Already, the disease had killed 218,000

Americans; now CDC's numbers made it clear that more deaths were to come.

Part of the past year's dramatic increase in AIDS cases came about because CDC was finally counting women more accurately. In previous years, many women with AIDS had been excluded by CDC's reporting system. This happened because the list of medical criteria that health departments used to distinguish AIDS from HIV infection did not include the very illnesses that women with AIDS were most likely to develop, such as pelvic inflammatory disease, vaginal candidiasis, and cervical cancer. Only people who met CDC's criteria were counted as having AIDS, no matter how sick they were. As a result, men were more likely to be diagnosed and to qualify for disability benefits, subsidized care, and experimental treatments than women. The case definition was expanded after years of protests and lawsuits by women activists who were outraged by these inequities.

Once the official AIDS tally more accurately reflected what was happening among women, epidemiologists began to realize that the epidemic was not as gay, male, and white as they had thought. According to the new way of counting, heterosexual transmission now accounted for 9 percent of new infections in 1993, up from 1.9 percent back in 1985. Intravenous drug use also loomed larger, explaining 28 percent of new cases, up 3 percent over the previous year. Now that women were on the radar screen, it was obvious that AIDS was afflicting disproportionate numbers of black and Hispanic people. The global shadow of AIDS was even larger and darker than it was in the United States: 16.6 million people were infected with HIV, and nearly 12 million of them were in sub-Saharan Africa.

While the Atlanta-based CDC was responsible for counting the bodies, the National Institutes of Health held sway over AIDS-related science—and better treatments were the number-one item on the NIH research agenda. As increasingly powerful activist groups constantly reminded Tony Fauci and other top officials, HIV-infected people who didn't need treatment today would need it tomorrow—and they expected the NIH to come up with more and better options. The first HIV antiviral drug, AZT, had been available since 1987, followed by only a handful of others.

It was obvious to patients and their doctors that the current AIDS treatments didn't help everyone, had severe side effects, and often stopped working after only a short time. Virologists attributed this to the high rate of mutations in HIV, which unlike some other viruses does not proofread for accuracy when it copies itself in human cells. As a result, random changes in its genetic makeup take place all the time. Some of these mutations enabled the virus to dance away from drugs that were none too nimble.

By 1994, treatment failure—like HIV infection itself—had many faces. Indiana hemophiliac Ryan White, who was denied public schooling after he was infected by contaminated blood products, was dead at eighteen. So was tennis champion and Davis Cup captain Arthur Ashe, who contracted the virus from a blood transfusion during open-heart surgery. And so were many thousands of relatives, friends, and lovers of ordinary Americans. Throughout the United States, organized groups of HIV-positive activists—most of them gay white men—urged the NIH to back basic research on the HIV virus and the human immune system. Their hope, of course, was that increased knowledge would translate into better treatments—if not in time to help them, then perhaps for their friends.

AIDS activists found the Clinton administration far more sympathetic to their cause than Reagan's people had been, and their lobbying was paying off. NIH's budget for AIDS was only $300 million back in 1984, the year that Tony Fauci became head of the National Institute of Allergy and Infectious Diseases. By fiscal year 1994, it had quadrupled to nearly $1.3 billion. The bulk of the money was going for basic science, always a point of pride for the NIH leadership, with especially lavish grants made to researchers who linked their sometimes arcane laboratory experiments to the hot topic of the moment—"novel AIDS therapies." Prominent among these were the protease inhibitors being developed by several companies, including the Merck effort led by Emilio Emini.

Vaccines, on the other hand, had no outspoken public constituency. No organized groups of healthy people prowled the corridors of power on Capitol Hill or picketed at NIH, demanding a vaccine that would protect them against AIDS. Without public scrutiny, the pace and scope of vaccine research were largely controlled by Tony Fauci and the Division of AIDS staff. If they wanted advice about vaccines, they asked for it; advice was rarely thrust upon them by activists or editorial writers.

The vaccine program was dwarfed by treatment research: The FY 1994 budget for vaccine research was $110.6 million, or 8.5 percent of total AIDS spending at NIH. This was 38 percent higher than the previous year's allocation, and the increase was earmarked for the country's—indeed the world's—first efficacy trial. The Division of AIDS was finalizing HIVNET contracts, worth $42 million, to pay for clinical research at eight U.S. and nine overseas sites, as well as the myriad administrative and laboratory services that a huge trial requires. HIVNET was standing by: It would shift into gear just as soon as NIAID approved a vaccine for large-scale testing.

●

When DAIDS sought advice about vaccine research, one place the agency turned was the Vaccine Working Group. Less rigidly constituted than most NIH advisory committees, the members of the VWG were drawn from universities, companies, AIDS advocacy groups, and even from the DAIDS program itself. This was an unusual opportunity for DAIDS scientists, who implemented policy decisions but rarely got to sit at the tables where they were made. The VWG's twenty-eight members were chosen for their expertise in fields such as basic virology or immunology, animal models, clinical trials, and vaccinology. Maurice Hilleman, the grand old man of Merck vaccines, was part of the group. So was Larry Corey, the University of Washington professor who had delivered gourmet food and videos to participants in the first human trial of a vaccinia-based HIV vaccine.

The VWG was cochaired by Peggy Johnston, who was acting deputy director of DAIDS, and Duke University virologist Dani Bolognesi. Bolognesi, who bore a burly resemblance to Kojak, not only ran the central immunology lab for NIH-sponsored vaccine trials but also was an old friend of NIAID director Tony Fauci. In fact, he was probably one of few people who could coax Fauci, a noted workaholic, to take time out for an occasional fishing trip. Bolognesi's bluff, hale-fellow style was a counterpoint to Peggy's more reserved, by-the-book demeanor.

The VWG usually met to chew things over and make general recommendations about what sorts of vaccine research DAIDS should emphasize. Typically the members worked in small groups, then came together to review what was going on in various scientific areas. Their recommendations were usually no more specific than "you should do more of this and less of that." The meeting that began on the morning of April 21, 1994, however, was going to be different.

According to a process that DAIDS had laid out six months earlier, the VWG's charge was to review scientific data about the gp120 vaccines made by Chiron Biocine and Genentech, both being studied in Phase II trials, and recommend whether either or both should be advanced into an efficacy study. Instead of breaking into small groups, they were going to spend two days around one large table. The VWG assessment would be sent to Fauci and would be summarized at a joint meeting of the AIDS Research Advisory Committee, called ARAC, and a subcommittee of the NIAID Council. This combined group would meet eight weeks later, on June 17. Their job was to consider efficacy testing not in isolation, but in the context of NIAID's total AIDS program. Their recommendation would go to Fauci, who would make the final call.

Never before had the VWG had been handed such a specific, high-stakes issue, and the atmosphere was expectant as committee members, a handful of invited speakers and observers, and a few staff filtered into Ballroom III at the Dulles Renaissance Hotel near Washington. The meeting was not open to the press or other outsiders, and the delegations from Chiron Biocine and Genentech were not due to arrive until later in the morning.

Sharing the gavel with Peggy Johnston was Ashley Haase, pinch-hitting for Bolognesi. Less colorful than Bolognesi, Haase was a tall, square-jawed physician and virologist who headed the microbiology department at the University of Minnesota. He was also chairman of ARAC, the next group the vaccine makers would face on the way to an efficacy trial. Haase had never worked on an AIDS vaccine, which made him an ideal substitute for Bolognesi—who was not allowed to preside because he consulted with Pasteur Mérieux Connaught on its canarypox vaccine against HIV.

The rest of the VWG members, who did not have direct personal investments in what happened to the gp120 vaccines, nevertheless took this meeting very seriously indeed. "There was so much focus on what was the correct next step, that the majority of people saw this as an incredibly important intellectual exercise. All of us understood that this next step was going to have big implications, whichever way it went," said Susan Zolla-Pazner, an immunology researcher at the Veterans Administration Medical Center in New York. Like Haase, she also served on ARAC, which meant that she would vote on this issue again in June.

The first speaker was Jack Killen, a forty-five-year-old physician who had recently been promoted to director of DAIDS, after six years as deputy director. He was a genial, good-looking gay man, about Fauci's height, who had arrived at NIH shortly after completing his training as an oncologist. Killen held what many regarded as a thankless job—one with a great deal of apparent responsibility but little real power. He reported directly to Fauci, whose entire star-studded career as a researcher, public-health expert, and NIH empire builder was founded on AIDS. Although Fauci kept close watch over the other NIAID divisions, their directors had at least a bit of wiggle room. But where AIDS was concerned, it appeared that no decision of any consequence would ever be made by anyone other than Fauci.

If Killen shared this view, and if it nettled him, he would never let on. Although many scientists are aroused by the thought of a good fight and enjoy sparring with one another in a room filled with their peers, this is not Killen's style. When researchers are at swords' points during a meeting, when it is obvious to everyone in the room that they do not agree even on what day it is, Killen will take off his horn-rimmed glasses, lean earnestly onto the table, and say softly, "I don't think the two of you are really so far apart on this." Clearly, he is not a man who likes a fight. Perhaps because he abhors conflict, or perhaps because he honestly feels this way, Killen says his working relationship with Fauci has always been "superb," adding "I certainly don't see him as a micromanager."

When Killen rose to introduce the goals of the VWG meeting, Fauci was sitting in a chair on the perimeter of the room, among the observers and staff. Although he would not stay for the entire two-day event, and never addressed the gathering, his presence signaled that this was a meeting of consequence. Killen told the group their mission was to conduct a comprehensive review of the scientific data about the vaccines and recommend how DAIDS should proceed. This was not the same, he explained, as being called on to make any kind of decision about an efficacy trial—the director of NIAID would take care of that. Although the VWG's task might not have qualified as a "decision" in Killen's bureaucratic lexicon, no doubt many in the group took his remarks with a grain of salt. Whether the future of the two vaccines was ultimately in their hands or not—and they knew it was not—this was still a momentous occasion for them.

Just as Killen was always willing to pour oil on the waters, the next speaker was always willing to stir things up. Born into a Texas ranching family, Mary Lou Clements was endowed with a formidable intelligence, considerable ambition, and no tolerance for anything that struck her as foolish or ignorant. Ever since she and Don Francis had worked on the World Health Organization's smallpox eradication program in India, she had been a powerful advocate for vaccination as a force for public good. If there was anyone who believed that a vaccine was the best hope for diminishing the shadow of AIDS, it was Mary Lou.

At forty-five, she was a short woman with attractive features, disconcertingly frank blue eyes, and a thick head of auburn hair styled in a way that would resist all but a stiff breeze. When she spoke in her throaty alto, with its underpinnings of Texas twang, the passion of her opinions was unmistakable. Mary Lou had been invited to provide the VWG with a historical perspective on vaccine development—right up her alley, since she had led or helped conduct nearly 100 clinical trials of vaccines against dozens of infectious diseases. She was no stranger to AIDS, either. At Johns Hopkins University, where she founded the Center for Immunization Research, she was the principal investigator on the first NIH-sponsored Phase I trials of Genentech's gp120 and PMC's canarypox, and had worked on clinical trials of Chiron's gp120 and a half dozen other experimental HIV vaccines. Mary Lou had also helped scientists and public officials in Thailand and Uganda formulate national plans for HIV vaccine development, so they would be ready when American companies approached them about hosting clinical trials.

An ideal AIDS vaccine, Mary Lou told the VWG, would protect against lots of HIV strains, would elicit high levels of neutralizing antibodies and cellular immune responses, and would block sexual transmission by setting up immune responses in the vagina and other mucosal surfaces. And, in a perfect world, a large and expensive human trial would be launched after scientists had determined—from experiments in test tubes and ani-mals—exactly what the immune system needed to do to fight off disease.

But this was not a perfect world and never had been. Historically, vac-cines against diseases other than AIDS had entered efficacy trials on the basis of scantier information—generally after small studies showed that a vaccine appeared safe and stimulated an immune response that might reasonably be protective. Many widely used vaccines that have saved mil-lions of lives, Mary Lou said, demonstrated protection in large studies with humans before there was any proof they worked in animals and long before scientists knew what immune response they should stimulate.

In her view, the current crop of HIV vaccine candidates was typical—no better and no worse than experimental vaccines against other infec-tions. History showed that the earliest clinical trials of a new type of vaccine often don't demonstrate protection. Pertussis vaccines, which prevent whooping cough, had required a dozen large trials in many coun-tries. But even unsuccessful trials sometimes hold clues to improvements in vaccine design or to better dosing or immunization schedules. When new data are gathered at government expense, this often stimulates pri-vate industry to develop more sophisticated products. The bottom line of Mary Lou's talk was simple: If a candidate vaccine is safe and if it stimu-lates an immune response that might be protective, then it makes sense to try it in a trial large enough to find out whether it works.

During the discussion that followed, not everyone agreed. Maurice Hilleman, whose vaccine experience started in the 1950s and trumped that of Mary Lou or anyone else in the room, sounded a cautionary note. The earlier vaccines that turned out to protect people, despite low scien-tific expectations that they would, were "the easy ones" that guarded against diseases less serious than AIDS, said Hilleman. HIV was unique in its ability to colonize and then demolish T cells, and it was the most genet-ically diverse virus that had been studied so far. "Don't go by precedents," he advised.

But Mary Lou's argument that it made sense to test safe and plausible candidates struck a chord with others at the table. An old joke among basic scientists is that the best conclusion for a journal article or research paper is "more research is needed." Woe unto the academic scientist who declares that he has solved his particular riddle, for that is a scientist whose lab may soon be out of business—unless he has another mystery on deck. As a result, researchers may obsessively pick the bones of a small, desiccated problem, oblivious to a herd of live animals thundering toward them. Mary Lou seemed to be telling the VWG members to lift their eyes from their individual lab benches and to consider moving these vaccines into clinical trials before the AIDS juggernaut crushed millions more people. Humanitarian benefits aside, such an experiment should also yield a wealth of new data for bench scientists. This message hung in the air as committee members stretched, took their first break in what was going to be a long day, and anticipated presentations from Chiron Biocine and Genentech.

•

Chiron had the floor when the VWG meeting reconvened, and Kathy Steimer sat back and listened to presentations by Dino Dina, president of the Biocine operation, and by Anne-Marie Duliege, a French physician who had left Genentech to run vaccine trials for Chiron. The story they told was a positive one, and it began with ample reassurance that the company's gp120 was safe—the first and foremost requirement for any product intended for use in millions of healthy people. In 600 adult volunteers and forty infants who had been immunized in Phase I trials, it appeared completely harmless. Nor had any adverse effects showed up in the Phase II study currently underway, where some volunteers received Chiron's gp120 and others got Genentech's rival product.

Even better, the Chiron gp120 elicited a robust immune response when it was injected in a mixture with MF59, an adjuvant that Chiron scientists had invented as a way of boosting the immune system's response to the vaccine itself. A widely used commercial blood test, called an ELISA, detected HIV antibodies in 100 percent of volunteers who had received three immunizations. This meant only that the immune system had made antibodies; it said nothing about their impact on the virus.

When other tests were used to examine the antibody response more closely, all the volunteers had antibodies that would neutralize and thus disable SF2, the lab-adapted HIV strain Kathy had used as the starting point for the vaccine. Two-thirds of the immunized volunteers also made antibodies against a second lab-adapted virus, the MN strain that Genentech had used as the basis for its gp120. When volunteers were tested several more times, the antibodies persisted for at least six months after the final shot.

The catch, of course, is that in the world of HIV, these lab-adapted strains are considered tabbies, not tigers. And it must have been torture for Kathy to listen to this happy talk about the vaccine she invented, knowing that within minutes she would be unfurling the darker side of the same story. Since the previous October, Kathy had been reporting to different scientific groups that antibodies from immunized volunteers did not neutralize so-called primary isolates—HIV samples that are collected from infected people and then grown in fresh blood cells drawn from healthy people. At least she could detect no neutralization in her experiments, which she viewed as some of the finest technical work she had ever done.

Her desire to do everything well stretched Kathy thin. As head of the viral immunology department, she supervised twenty people working directly on HIV vaccines; as head of analytical viral immunology, she supervised twenty-nine others who developed and performed assays for clinical trials of vaccines against HIV and a half dozen other infectious diseases. Despite the heavy demands of these two managerial positions, she could not seem to give up the bench work that she loved. Kathy personally devised the assay for detecting antibodies that would destroy primary isolates and did many of the experiments herself—a task many scientists at her level would have delegated.

In the lab, Kathy worked shoulder-to-shoulder with Faruk Sinangil, a Turkish-born virologist whom she had recruited in 1990, shortly after he obtained his Ph.D. at Columbia University in New York City. Temperamentally, they were an excellent match. Both were impatient with endless meetings and disliked pushing papers, and when they decided to try something in the lab, they threw themselves into it—working nights and weekends, changing direction when their results demanded, improvising as needed. "There was all this incredible movement, which was for some people very annoying. But for me it wasn't," Faruk said.

Unbeknownst to Faruk, Kathy's workaholic behavior during this period probably crossed the line into illness. Her husband and at least one of her physicians believed that she was exhibiting clear signs of bipolar disorder, otherwise known as manic depression. She had always been a creature of extremes—sometimes working tirelessly for days, then sinking into such a blue funk that dragging herself out of bed was a major victory. This pattern intensified when she got disappointing results in the lab, and it was compounded by a welter of physical complaints: She couldn't sleep, her heart raced, and she must have felt that she was falling apart.

Her personal calendar for 1993 was crammed with doctors' appointments—sometimes as many as three different specialists on a single day. Kathy feared that she might have heart disease, but in October she abruptly canceled a special high-tech treadmill test when she was summoned to Washington. She had been asked to fly across the country and preview her primary isolate findings for an earlier meeting of the VWG. After the group heard Kathy's report, Peggy Johnston wrote in a memo to Tony Fauci: "The group's enthusiasm for moving the current phase II gp120 products into a phase III efficacy trial has been significantly dampened by the neutralization results."

In November, one of Kathy's physicians persuaded her to try Depakote, a drug used to treat the manic episodes associated with bipolar disorder. If it didn't appear to help, she could stop. But if the drug was effective for her, it would lessen the hyperactivity and insomnia, restrain runaway flights of thought, improve judgment, and calm feelings of hostility. Whether it accomplished all these miracles for Kathy is impossible to say.

Although it is always painful to expose your failures in public, it was a pain that Kathy knew well by the time she addressed the VWG in April 1994. She described the experiments she and Faruk had performed, what they had found, and what the limitations of their methods might be. It was possible, for example, that the blood samples from volunteers really did contain neutralizing antibodies but that Kathy and Faruk's test was not sensitive enough to detect them. Or something in the setup of the assay might be interfering with the interaction of antibody and virus, which could mean the primary isolates resisted neutralization in the test tube, even though they might be easily neutralized in the body of an immunized person. Kathy and her colleagues had thought of a dozen possible reasons their results might be wrong; unfortunately, they had no way of knowing whether any of their theories were true.

The remainder of Chiron Biocine's presentation, which fell to Kathy's colleagues, was a mixed bag. In Phase I trials, three volunteers who had been injected with gp120—as opposed to inactive shots used for comparison—had become infected with HIV. Two of these people were infected after receiving two of the four shots called for in the study; one had completed the series. All were gay men who engaged in risky sexual behavior, and no one had expected the gp120 vaccine to be 100-percent effective; after all, no vaccine was perfect. Still, this was sobering news. On a more positive note, in small experiments using chimpanzees and baboons, gp120 immunization appeared completely protective in a few cases and partly so in others.

Two and a half hours after they started, the Chiron speakers wrapped up their presentation before the VWG. They had discussed not only their successes, but also their distressing and painful failures. In *The Iliad*, Homer tells how Chiron taught the hero Achilles how to use herbs to stanch bleeding and heal the wounds of his soldiers. For this, Homer calls Chiron "the most righteous of all the centaurs." As representatives of the company named for the good centaur, Kathy and her colleagues knew it was right to go public with negative results about their own vaccine. No true scientist could do otherwise. The VWG members, every one of whom knew what it was like to have an experiment fail, respected Kathy for the precision of her experiments and the completeness of her disclosure. As for Chiron's gp120 vaccine, they would not pass judgment on its future until later.

●

After lunch, it was Genentech's turn. If Chiron came across as the righteous centaur, Genentech's delegation was more like the Four Horsemen—not of the Apocalypse, but of the University of Notre Dame. Don Francis was the marquee quarterback, a household name thanks to Randy Shilts's book *And the Band Played On,* which portrayed him as a hero for his leadership in fighting the spread of the AIDS virus; the film added Hollywood glamour. Jack Obijeski provided extra muscle as head of the company's vaccine program and a key player in recruiting Don. Phil Berman and Tim Gregory were the guys who had designed and made a gp120 vaccine against AIDS. This team entered the room with their game faces on, cocky and expecting to prevail.

And why not?

Genentech was one of the world's top biotech companies in early 1994, not just because it had brought products to market and generated revenue—which most of the industry had yet to accomplish—but also in terms of scientific clout. A multiyear ranking of "hot" scientific articles showed that Genentech's publications on AIDS research were being cited more often by other scientists than those from many of the world's most prestigious universities. The company's highest impact publications were mostly on the gp120 gene and its protein, and Phil's name was on almost all of them. Ever since 1990, when the purloined chimpanzees had been protected against HIV in Phil's clandestine experiment, what he called an "era of unbelievable optimism" about gp120 had prevailed at Genentech. The company was so confident that the NIH would authorize a Phase III trial that it had already packaged 15,000 doses of gp120 in vials and had another 300,000 doses in bulk storage.

The only fly in the ointment was that a scientist at Genentech, like Kathy Steimer at Chiron, had also done experiments showing that gp120 didn't neutralize primary isolates. Phil had not done this work himself and his reaction was that the assay must be wrong. As a result, Genentech researchers didn't say much unless they were asked. This apparent reluctance to talk about negative results led some researchers to feel that the Genentech team couldn't be trusted to put science above the company's self-interest.

Like everyone else invited to the VWG meeting, Jack Obijeski knew that the neutralization studies were going to be a big deal. And he anticipated this was the kind of scientific issue that could really bog down a group like the VWG, which was larded with academics and government scientists—people for whom more research is always needed. Jack had ruminated for weeks about how he could encourage the group to keep its eyes on the goal of making a successful AIDS vaccine instead of losing itself in the minutia of laboratory testing. Jack's job was to clear a path for Don Francis, the star player on Genentech's team.

Perhaps a simple graphic, the sort of thing that an ad agency might use to sell a product on television, would do the trick. More than anything else, Jack needed a simple way to show how clinical trials contributed to scientific progress against HIV. He started by sketching a graph with time on the horizontal axis, across the bottom of the picture, and knowledge on the vertical axis. He drew a steep rise in knowledge gained from laboratory science, beginning with the discovery of the virus in 1983 and climbing until the early 1990s, when the line leveled off as the pace of discovery slowed. And then, in a second color, he drew a different slope showing advances in clinical science. Its upward trajectory soared into the future, as a Phase III vaccine trial was launched and began generating new data that laboratory researchers could dissect.

When Jack projected this new slide at the VWG, he argued that an efficacy trial would be the best way to get what he called "the next big increment of knowledge." Scientists would be able to compare their laboratory tests against what happened in the field, and if all went well, they would eventually know exactly what immune responses a successful vaccine needed to elicit. Jack was a big, brawny, confident presence as he stood before the group, a true believer in the vaccine and its future. If there were skeptics in the room who didn't buy Jack's line of argument, he didn't notice them. He came away thinking, "we led them by the nose."

Whether that was true or not, Jack probably did clear a path for Don Francis. If some quarterbacks are said to have a throwing arm like a rifle, Don has a mouth like an Uzi—a rapid-fire burst of passionate verbiage about his role in humanity's victory over smallpox, his role in the successful testing of a vaccine against hepatitis B, and the urgent need for an AIDS vaccine. At fifty-two, Don was the leanest and most tightly wound of the Genentech foursome, with a forelock of dark blond hair that flopped down over his bright blue eyes.

Like Mary Lou, with whom he had worked during the global smallpox eradication campaign, Don emphasized that many successful vaccines had been tested and approved long before anyone knew exactly how they protect against disease. Although there was a lot of talk at this meeting about neutralization assays, he let it be known that in his mind there was no contest—animal studies took precedence over lab tests any day of the week. In 1990, Phil Berman showed that two chimpanzees immunized with his original gp120, which was based on HIV_{LAI}, did not become infected when they were challenged with the same strain of virus. This was the experiment that restored corporate confidence in the vaccine project and allowed the work to continue. Phil's second version of gp120, derived from the MN strain, was first tested in chimpanzees in 1992. When the time came to challenge these animals, they were injected with a variant of HIV_{SF2} that had been grown in fresh blood cells, much like the primary isolates that Kathy and others had found impossible to neutralize in the lab.

This chimp experiment, in Don's view, made anything that happened in test tubes profoundly irrelevant: The immunized animals were protected against what he called a "whopping dose" of SF2 virus. The single control animal, on the other hand, was infected. And here was the kicker: In the lab, sera from the vaccinated animals had not neutralized the SF2— even though these same animals were protected and no sign of HIV could be found in their bodies. At the VWG meeting, "anybody in their right mind would have known that neutralizing antibody was not predictive of protection," he said.

Others in the room thought that no one in their right mind believed that chimps were a good model for studying AIDS vaccines. These great apes are better at fighting off HIV infection than humans; if they do get infected, the virus doesn't grow very well in their bodies, and often they clear the virus from their systems without any intervention at all. One of the most influential critics of the chimp model, Harvard primate expert Norman Letvin, was sitting at the VWG table while Don spoke. Letvin, a small man with a narrow face and a dark beard, makes quick gestures much like the Asian macaques he favors for testing potential vaccines. Anybody who talked with him for longer than five minutes would have known that he was contemptuous of chimp studies and saw macaques as a far superior animal model.

Although Don and his teammates believed that the chimp data constituted a winning hand, they didn't stop there. They hedged their bets by touting the safety of their gp120; like Chiron's vaccine, it had caused no problems in hundreds of healthy volunteers. Genentech sought to set its product apart by emphasizing that it was formulated with alum, the only adjuvant licensed by the FDA for use in the United States. Alum had a long track record and had been used to enhance the immune response to other vaccines. Chiron's gp120, in contrast, was formulated with MF59, an experimental adjuvant the company hoped to have licensed soon. If the NIH chose to advance only one of the two products into Phase III trials, Genentech was determined to be the chosen one. If using an established adjuvant tipped the scales in the company's favor, fair enough.

●

A panel discussion followed Genentech's presentation. At this point, the VWG members had sat through five hours of corporate verbiage with little chance to talk back. Now the meeting schedule gave them one hour to vent, and they unleashed a volley of concerns about the size, expense, and possible social costs of going ahead with a huge efficacy trial. Many were troubled by unanswered questions about possible efficacy of the vaccines and how big a trial might have to be. If the gp120 vaccines protected only one-third or one-half of immunized people, then a very large study would be needed to detect such a low level of efficacy. And what if a giant gp120 trial used up most of the potential volunteers in the United States? Would there be enough volunteers left for future studies of products that might be more effective?

One of Tony Fauci's precedent-shattering innovations as director of NIAID had been to bring AIDS activists into the government tent. Some of the men who had once accused Fauci of trying to kill them—because he wasn't pushing fast enough for new drugs to treat AIDS—now belonged to the advisory groups that were weighing the future of the gp120 vaccines. Many of the activists were cut from the same cloth as the government and academic scientists they served with—they were white men who had attended elite colleges and pursued professional careers. And now that these sophisticated advocates had a seat at the official table, some lobbied Congress very effectively on behalf of NIH in general, and NIAID in particular. Self-interest and the public good were one.

When activist Derek Hodel spoke during the VWG's panel discussion, he focused on how a vaccine efficacy trial might affect various segments of the urban gay community. It was a world he knew well: Hodel had become an AIDS activist in New York during the 1980s, working with Gay Men's Health Crisis during its early years. Now he was policy director for AIDS Action, a major organization based in Washington, and wore a coat and tie as well as an earring.

The new HIVNET system would be doing most of its recruiting among gay men in big cities. As data from Chiron and other labs showed, gp120 immunization caused most people to test positive on the blood test commonly used to diagnose AIDS and screen blood. Some homosexual men might shun the trial for fear that testing positive would cause them to lose health insurance, or perhaps even their jobs. Others might worry that the vaccine would not protect them and might speed the course of disease if they later became infected. There was no evidence that this would happen, but scientists couldn't rule it out. On the other hand, it was possible that men who had no intention of practicing safe sex would rush to volunteer, hoping that the experimental vaccine would keep them safe— even though there was no evidence for this, either.

Most of the world's AIDS sufferers weren't the gay men that Hodel spoke for, of course, but poor people with far fewer options. The developing world's urgent need for a vaccine was articulated by José Esparza, a Venezuelan physician who headed HIV vaccine development for the World Health Organization's Global Programme on AIDS. Although Esparza was officially based in Geneva, he gave the appearance of living on airplanes. He was a tousle-haired, slightly rumpled figure who turned up at vaccine meetings around the globe and seemed to know everyone. His ability to schmooze, synthesize, and help people make deals and connections gave Esparza influence that far exceeded his program's small budget.

On this occasion, he argued that the developing world would be a highly desirable setting for efficacy trials. More than 90 percent of infections are in developing countries, and countries with rapidly growing epidemics could benefit more than industrial nations from a successful vaccine trial—assuming, of course, that it led to an affordably priced product. Trials in developing nations could test the merits of vaccines more cheaply and rapidly than studies conducted in the United States, where the incidence of disease is generally lower.

One principle of Statistics 101 is that the more frequently an event occurs, the smaller the sample needed to study it. A vaccine's protective effect would be easier to see where the incidence of AIDS is high than where the disease is spreading more slowly. In fact, HIVNET was already planning to test vaccines in high-incidence areas like Thailand, Africa, and the Caribbean. But if NIH decided not to go forward with efficacy trials, it would be a long time before most of these places saw an HIV vaccine. The army was working toward a trial in Thailand, which it would fund. Beyond this, there was scant hope that private companies would pay to carry out clinical trials in faraway places.

This discussion eventually led a VWG member to ask the corporate scientists, who were available to field questions, what their companies would do if the NIH decided against sponsoring an efficacy trial. Chiron's response was that it would probably shelve gp120, then change gears and pursue a different approach to HIV vaccines. The DNA concept, which was very popular with NIH leaders at the moment, would be the most likely choice. But Chiron Biocine could not have such a product ready for testing in less than four years, and there was no guarantee that top management would authorize such a long and costly undertaking.

The idea that there might not be an efficacy trial catapulted Don Francis into full Cassandra mode. "If you do this to us, we're telling you that the corporate decision is going to be to shut us down," members of the committee remember him saying. He thundered at the members of the VWG, insisting that voting against an efficacy trial would cause all the biotech companies and pharmaceutical giants working on HIV vaccines to drop out of the field. Whatever the committee thought about the value of the two gp120 vaccines, they had to realize that stopping the momentum of clinical trials at this point would have dire, far-reaching consequences for all the companies—not just the two whose products were in the docket today. It was as though Don was a guest chef who had marched into the kitchen, cranked up all the burners as high as they would go, and filled the room with flames and smoke in his haste to get his message out. The committee was largely made up of scientists who are not at home in such a hot kitchen.

Maurice Hilleman lowered the temperature and, in his own laid-back, Montana via Merck style served up the same message without the pyrotechnics. The most compelling argument for going forward was that this would encourage industry to remain involved in HIV vaccine development. Corporations would be motivated by the NIH's willingness to invest in large field studies of products created with private-sector money. As for gp120 itself, "it's not bad enough not to consider," Hilleman said, having the last word as usual.

●

To be part of an AIDS vaccine meeting in a place like the Dulles Renaissance Hotel is to be suspended in a strange bubble, speaking a private language, surrounded by sales meetings and personal growth seminars whose participants would find the arcana of vaccines as unfathomable as Urdu poetry. The VWG meeting had begun at 8:30 in the morning and didn't break up until after 7:00 P.M. Meetings like this are so intense and exhausting that it would make sense, at the end of the day, for people to retreat upstairs to their private rooms, to order room service or call home or watch TV or do anything to escape the litany of vaccines, vaccines, and more vaccines. But what really happens is that vaccine people can't break out of the bubble. Some of the scientists stream into the bar, which is usually just off the lobby or tucked away on the mezzanine. Most break into pods and eat dinner in the hotel's high-end restaurant, which is never as good as a real restaurant, but good enough under the circumstances.

Depending on how she was feeling, Kathy Steimer sometimes dined alone at the hotels where vaccine meetings took place. She would fend off company with a book, usually a novel of some literary repute, and drink the best by-the-glass wine with her solitary dinner. On this occasion, however, she joined Susan Zolla-Pazner and some of the other VWG members at a big round table. It had been a tense day. Kathy and her company had so much riding on their presentations, and no control over the outcome. The committee members knew their recommendation would have a major impact on the future of vaccine development, whichever way they voted. And Don Francis's lecture essentially stated that a vote against the proposed efficacy trial would pound a stake through the heart of vaccine development.

At dinner, the stress and seriousness of the day gave way to a level of giddy hilarity rarely seen at gatherings of serious-minded midcareer scientists. No matter what anyone said about anything—about work or family or food—it was hysterically funny. They laughed and laughed and laughed until the meal was done.

Eventually they went upstairs, where some no doubt slept easier than others.

●

When the VWG meeting resumed at 8 o'clock on Friday morning, the first speaker was virologist James Bradac, who was in charge of the HIV viral diversity program within the Division of AIDS. In this capacity, Bradac had become a connoisseur of exotic strains from around the world. So far, his lab had received more than 300 samples from HIV-infected people, about half from outside the United States, and had isolated and prepared about 100 of them. These Bradac would send, like books from a library, to scientists who needed them to design new vaccines or test ones already made. It was useful to have all these different HIVs available, because researchers could use them to figure out how broadly protective a given vaccine might be. AIDS was a worldwide pandemic, he emphasized, and it was important to find out how many vaccines might be needed to contain it.

As Bradac spoke, he turned up the volume on the ominous background noise that had been present throughout the meeting—the apparent inability of gp120 vaccines to generate antibodies that would neutralize primary isolates of HIV. More than concerns about cost, more than worries about a possible shortfall of volunteers, this was the torpedo most likely to sink plans for a gp120 efficacy trial.

Kathy Steimer had an excellent reputation as a scientist. Nevertheless, her failure to neutralize primary isolates with antibodies to gp120 would not, by itself, have been damaging enough to scuttle the proposed trial. Nor would Genentech's similar results have done the trick. But other investigators had independently come up with the same results, and although these had not been published in a scientific journal, which is the preferred way of communicating new findings, they were well known to many members of the VWG.

Four months earlier, at Hilton Head Island, South Carolina, DAIDS organized a workshop for scientists who had been doing primary isolate neutralization studies. Several groups, including Kathy's, reported that vaccinee sera strongly neutralized lab-adapted strains but not primary isolates grown in fresh blood cells. One of these teams was the central immunology lab at Duke University, which did laboratory testing for all NIH-sponsored HIV vaccine trials. The Duke lab was regarded as a quality, unbiased operation with no political axes to grind.

Although all the assays followed the same basic principles, there was plenty of room for variation. Different investigators obtained viruses from different sources, sometimes from patients in nearby AIDS clinics, sometimes from libraries of viral strains. There was no way of knowing how these strains compared in terms of virulence, which is their ability to infect human cells. Furthermore, to be considered primary isolates these viruses had to be grown not in an immortal cell line, like the lab-adapted strains, but in fresh blood cells. These peripheral blood mononuclear cells, usually called PBMCs, were sometimes obtained from blood banks, in other labs from graduate students. Obviously the characteristics of these fresh blood cells would vary. Some would be more receptive to HIV infection than others, for example, and this could affect how the experiments turned out.

An even greater source of variation were the techniques used to provoke PBMCs to divide in the lab, which is necessary for HIV's genetic material to replicate. First, the PBMCs had to be activated with a dose of a chemical mitogen, which is like poking them in the butt with a sharp stick. When these cells get moving, they will take up growth factors, which are added to the mix according to the lab's individual recipe. Once the virus is growing, vaccinee serum is added, to see whether it will neutralize the HIV. Sometimes serum is used straight; sometimes it is diluted with a neutral buffer. Finally, labs may differ in their interpretation of what happened between antibodies and virus: Some scientists say that neutralization occurred if 50 percent of the HIV in the tube was disabled; others hold out for 90 percent.

In assays like these, numerous investigators found that it was easy to neutralize lab-adapted strains of HIV, such as MN and SF2, on which Genentech and Chiron had modeled their vaccines. One theory was that the envelope glycoproteins on these strains, the targets of the vaccine-induced antibody, were "relaxed" after years of growing in the laboratory, where they had no enemies. The envelope glycoproteins on virus freshly drawn from a patient may be coiled in a more defensive posture to fend off immune attack. This might explain why vaccinee sera neutralized lab-adapted strains, but not primary isolates.

Such methodology issues had dominated the Hilton Head workshop back in January. After much discussion of altering the neutralization assays to make them more sensitive, no one could agree on how this should be done or whether it was even worthwhile. At the close of the workshop, participants were evenly divided about whether their results meant that a Phase III trial should move forward or be delayed. "The only certainty is that a difficult decision remains," concluded a journal article about the meeting.

Bradac's presentation forced the VWG members to think about the neutralization issue but did not supply a magic decoder ring to explain what it all meant. So committee members who favored going forward with efficacy trials continued to think the assays were the problem, and neutralization would surely be seen if the lab tests worked better Those who were against expanded clinical trials trusted more in the assay results. If there was one thing these two camps shared, it was regret that there was no scientifically unimpeachable way to break the tie, to know for certain whether the assays or the vaccines were flawed.

As the discussion of Bradac's presentation wound down, a few members urged the group to stop worrying about antibodies and the assays used to measure them. Instead, they advised, put more energy into developing vaccines that activate not antibodies but CTLs, the killer T cells the canarypox and naked DNA vaccines are meant to elicit.

●

The last three presentations of the morning went quickly. Alan Schultz, DAIDS's in-house expert on primate research, summarized experiments with gp120 products and with vaccinia and canarypox vectors. Although each of these types of vaccines has protected some animals in some experiments, he said, it isn't clear whether protection is conferred by neutralizing antibody, a CTL response, or some combination of the two. By the time Schultz had finished describing the confusing, sometimes contra-dictory results obtained so far, it was clear that the chimps and monkeys were not going to resolve whatever doubts VWG members had about gp120 vaccines.

Nor was much guidance provided by Pat Fast's overview of govern-ment-sponsored Phase I and II clinical trials, unless it was that the two gp120 vaccines looked very safe and that their development was at least eighteen months ahead of other candidates. By then, another product might be ready to begin efficacy testing, but it was an unexciting refor-mulation of gp120 with a different adjuvant. Beyond that, the next possi-ble candidate was PMC's canarypox with a gp120 boost. This prime-boost strategy might complete Phase II testing by late 1996, predicted Pat, who was in charge of the DAIDS vaccine program. If canarypox looked good in that study, which had not even started at this point, then it might be considered for an efficacy trial. So far, however, this live-vector vaccine had stimulated CTL activity in fewer than half of the volunteers who had received it.

The final item on the agenda was a short statement from Derek Hodel, who voiced concern that a large vaccine trial would divert resources away from treatment research and other AIDS-prevention efforts. This was a legitimate worry and not a new one for members of this group, some of whom would be directly affected if NIH cut back on treatment research.

The schedule gave the members of the VWG two hours to decide what they were going to recommend to Tony Fauci. Ashley Haase and Peggy Johnston, who were presiding, asked the group to consider the hypothe-sis that gp120 can induce a protective immune response. Should this hypothesis be tested in the clinic? If the group said yes, what was the sci-entific rationale for their decision? And how should the efficacy trial be done? If the group said no, why? And what should the next step be?

All along, Peggy had sensed that the group wanted to go forward with an expanded trial of some sort. Once the participants began talking, clearly this was the case—they focused on what sort of trial should be done, not on whether one should be done at all. What the companies wanted, of course, was a large, definitive trial that would accurately meas-ure efficacy and confirm the vaccine's safety. This was the kind of data the FDA needs to consider licensing the vaccine for sale. Although there were no hard numbers on the table, 10,000 to 20,000 volunteers would probably be required for a double-blind trial in which participants received either the Chiron Biocine vaccine, the Genentech vaccine, or an inactive placebo. A study this size would be powerful enough to detect a level of protection as low as 30 percent. It would also cost a great deal of money, although no one had put a price tag on it yet. It would be the Cadillac of clinical trials.

Another choice was an intermediate-sized study, a Chevrolet-type trial that would be larger than a Phase II but smaller and certainly cheaper than a full-scale Phase III. Such an experiment would provide less precise answers than a bona fide efficacy trial, but members thought that with the right design, it could yield some measure of efficacy and, more important, eliminate a totally worthless vaccine. Even information this crude would help NIH decide on its next move. An intermediate trial might also help researchers interpret the results they were getting from neutralization assays and primate studies. Until scientists could check their lab results against observations of people, many members of the group felt that it was "futile" to continue using animals and lab assays to try to predict how well a vaccine was going to work.

A third option was to do nothing for the present, holding off on an efficacy trial until more promising candidates were ready for large-scale testing. Larry Corey, who was leading the Phase I testing of Pasteur Mérieux Connaught's canarypox vaccine with a gp120 boost, was the most outspoken person on this point. He believed canarypox plus gp120 was superior to gp120 alone, because together they might mobilize both arms of the immune system against HIV. Corey optimistically predicted that the prime-boost approach could be ready for a Phase III study in early 1996, a mere two years hence. Pat Fast, whose program managed the vaccine trials, cautioned that a Phase II study had not yet begun and that results could not be available before late 1996. Neither of them could be certain, however, because PMC was making changes to the product that could result in missed deadlines and delays.

Finally, it was time to decide what the group's recommendation should be. The first question was, in Peggy Johnston's words: "If we can do an intermediate trial, who would be in favor of moving forward?" This proposition assumed that NIH statistical experts could design a trial that would fill some of the persistent and troubling scientific gaps in a cost-effective way. When the vote came, Peggy recalled, "Almost all the hands went up." Twenty-seven voted yes. The only two no votes came from Larry Corey, who clearly thought that the prime-boost strategy was a better approach, and primate expert Norm Letvin, whose laboratory was funded by NIH to test up-and-coming vaccines before they were picked for human trials.

The second question put to the VWG was this: If an informative intermediate trial could not be designed, and the only option was for an all-out efficacy trial, how many would still favor going forward? This time only fifteen people raised their hands. The bottom line was, "I want a car, and if there's a Chevy available, I'll buy it. If the only thing available is a Cadillac, I may not go for it."

It was up to Pat Fast and the rest of the vaccine program staff to figure out whether they could design a Chevy that would take vaccine research where it needed to go. They had a great deal of work to do before June 17, when NIAID's AIDS Research Advisory Committee and the AIDS Sub-committee of the NIAID Council would consider their recommendation about the proposed efficacy trial. Most members of the program staff left happy—they had worked hard to prepare for efficacy trials, and they believed passionately that a vaccine was the only way to slow the epidemic.

Kathy Steimer and the Chiron Biocine team were relieved and elated by the VWG's decision as they flew back to California. Kathy's honesty about the primary isolate neutralization studies had not been the death knell for gp120. Obviously, the VWG was willing to go further to resolve the uncertainty about what these lab findings meant in the real world, where thousands of people were getting infected every day. "We were terribly excited about the decision, that we were moving ahead," recalled Faruk Sinangil, who had worked so closely with Kathy on the neutralization assays.

The guys from Genentech were more blasé about the whole thing. Don Francis saw the members of the VWG as "vaccine experts," which of course meant that they would see things his way. He felt that the chimp experiments had carried the day for gp120, and maybe these findings did sway some of the committee members. But what stands out far more vividly for some participants was Don's prophecy that if the NIH did not pay for expanded clinical trials, then private industry would walk away from AIDS vaccine research.

8

MAY IS THE CRUELEST MONTH

A T their meeting on April 21, 1994, the Vaccine Working Group had taken the first big step toward an efficacy trial for the gp120 vaccines. If the proposed study went forward, it would be the first experiment powerful enough to discover whether one or both of these vaccines could actually protect people against AIDS, as they went about their ordinary lives.

What the VWG members could not have predicted was that two bombs were about to go off in their path, blocking the road to efficacy testing for at least a time. The first detonation was a powerful manifesto about the direction of AIDS research published in the May 12 issue of *Nature*. The second, a news story that broke in the *Chicago Tribune*, would appear at the end of the month.

Although *Nature*'s home office is in England, this journal wields considerable clout in the United States. The *Nature* piece was entitled "AIDS: Time to Turn to Basic Science," its focus was AIDS research sponsored by the U.S. government, and the author was Bernard N. Fields, a renowned virus expert at Harvard Medical School.

In the decade since HIV had been identified, Fields wrote, scientists had come up with drugs that sometimes relieved AIDS complications and enabled patients to live longer. Despite the investment of huge sums, however, science had generated neither a cure for AIDS nor a truly effective means for preventing it. "We need to alter substantially the way we set priorities and fund AIDS research," Fields declared "The focus on drugs and vaccines made sense a decade ago, but it is time to acknowledge that our best hunches have not paid off and are not likely to do so." Instead of being eager to test experimental drugs and vaccines in human volunteers, "we need to put increased emphasis on basic science and broaden our definition of AIDS-related research," he wrote.

Fields made four main points in the article. He argued passionately that NIH should broaden its definition of "AIDS-related" research because insights were as likely to come from unrelated infectious disease studies as from investigations of AIDS per se. His second point was that NIH should invest more heavily in basic pathogenesis studies—investigations of HIV and its earliest, most minute, interactions with human cells. (This was his own specialty as a virologist.) Third, more researchers should be encouraged to study the opportunistic infections that cause most of the suffering and death associated with AIDS. Finally, work should continue on drugs and vaccines. But here the emphasis should be on the scientific merit of experimental products, not on what Fields decried as "politics and the illusion of easy answers." If NIH adopted his recommendations, he foresaw that grant-making committees would soon be picking and choosing from a large and varied crop of "investigator initiated" projects.

Fields emphasized that the "large bureaucracy and infrastructure" that had taken hold during the first decade of AIDS research would be difficult to change. Although he didn't put a price on this elaborate construction, in fact the U.S. government had so far spent more than $20 billion of taxpayer money on AIDS. Few people, aside from religious and political extremists who thought that people with AIDS deserved their fate, had challenged how this money was spent. Neither scientists who already had AIDS research grants nor those who hoped to have them were likely to question the NIH's wisdom. Although researchers might complain among themselves about the types of studies that NIH backed, no one had been willing to publicly tell the leaders of the NIH that they needed to change their ways.

Except Bernie Fields. He was an unusual man in an unusual position.

●

Fields had spent considerable time thinking about AIDS research, even though his lab studied a family of viruses that did not include HIV. He was one of the most eminent academic virologists in the world, the main author of the definitive textbook in his discipline, and for many years chairman of the microbiology department at Harvard Medical School.

In addition to his scientific standing, there was another, more personal reason he didn't hesitate to speak his mind. Fields had been diagnosed with pancreatic cancer two years earlier, and he knew that the disease would eventually claim his life. Before it did, however, he was determined to help shape the scientific battle plan against AIDS. Of all the viral diseases, this was clearly his last great adversary.

During a period when his cancer was in remission, Fields came to Bethesda to interview for the top job at NIH's new Office of AIDS Research. Congress had created this unique office in late 1993, when Tony Fauci had been stripped of his influence over across-the-board AIDS spending. Whoever became the OAR's first director would have a historic opportunity to mold the future of biomedicine's most urgent, high-profile research program. The new office's mission was to analyze the government's annual AIDS budget, some $1.3 billion for fiscal year 1994, and come up with a comprehensive plan for spending it. More important, Congress gave the OAR unprecedented power to enforce its decisions: If an institute insisted on pursuing research outside the plan, OAR could withhold its AIDS money. Although the OAR director would be advised by panels of outside experts, he would be accountable only to NIH director Harold Varmus.

The OAR search committee, chaired by Varmus himself, enthusiastically endorsed Fields as the best candidate for the position. His scientific credentials were impeccable, he was known as a visionary and a compelling leader, and he was a mensch. His warmth, humor, and generous mentoring of students were legendary at Harvard Medical School, where such values sometimes are lost in the pursuit of academic excellence.

The prospect of heading the OAR captured Fields's imagination, and he wanted to give it a shot. He told the search committee there was just one catch: He couldn't say yes unless the odds were good that his health would permit him to do the job. He had been having CAT scans at regular intervals, and so far they had been reassuring. The next scan was scheduled for the following day, back in Boston, and he would let the committee know the outcome.

This time, however, the CAT scan was anything but reassuring: The cancer had returned. Fields called Varmus with the bad news.

Bernie Fields's withdrawal threw the search process into turmoil. There were other good candidates, but for one reason or another, none fit the bill. Finally, Varmus asked William Paul, a member of the committee that had selected Fields, to step into the breach and lead the OAR. It was an interesting choice for many reasons, and one that would have far-reaching effects on the future of HIV vaccines.

Like Fields, Bill Paul was not an AIDS researcher. This was an advantage as far as Varmus was concerned, because he and other elite scientists suspected that most people in the young, highly competitive AIDS arena were too caught up with their own career advancement to step back and make impartial judgments about the big picture. Unlike Fields, a virologist who was well established at a major university, Paul was a fifty-seven-year-old immunologist who had worked for NIH for twenty-six years. In 1970, two years after he came to the Bethesda campus, Paul became chief of the Laboratory of Immunology, a highly respected basic-science lab within the National Institute of Allergy and Infectious Diseases. He had long since been elected to the National Academy of Sciences and was widely known and respected for his research on chemicals that allow cells of the immune system to communicate and to grow. He had a good reputation and an insider's knowledge of NIH bureaucracy.

Like Tony Fauci, Paul had grown up in a New York City borough, but his restrained, cosmopolitan facade and speech belie his background. Paul gives the British pronunciation to words such as "neither" (nyethur) and "figure" (figger). A tall man with a high-domed forehead and an upright bearing, he wears well-tailored clothing, setting him apart from the schlumpy appearance of many researchers. Although he can seem remote on first meeting, he inspires considerable loyalty and affection in people who've worked for him.

Bill Paul agreed with Fields that NIH should change how it handled AIDS research. When the disease first hit, NIH leaders had been right to specify which research areas they wanted extramural scientists to pursue. Certain basic questions about the virus, the immune system, and the deadly tango danced by the two demanded immediate exploration. Lucrative contracts and directed research projects were as magnetic to academics as fresh shrimp at a cocktail party. Not only was the money good, but this was an opportunity for aggressive young investigators, or older ones with time on their hands, to stake claims in an entirely new discipline. Although many excellent researchers were part of the AIDS land rush, others were merely competent. But even the less gifted among them made contributions to AIDS research by pursuing questions dreamed up at NIH.

Now it was time to shift gears. Instead of telling extramural scientists what to study, elite scientists like Fields and Paul believed that NIH should open AIDS research to a larger, and ideally more creative, class of investigators. If NIH did not do this, Bill Paul worried that AIDS research might go the way of the former Soviet Union. "Centrally planned economies have pretty much failed," he said, "and central research planning is not a lot better." It would be profoundly impolitic, of course, for him to tell NIH administrators and program officers that they weren't smart enough to chart the next steps in AIDS research. No one—from Tony Fauci down to the least-known program officer in the Division of AIDS—wanted to be treated like a fading commissar whose next five-year plan was expected to fail.

What the newly hired OAR director would have difficulty saying, however, was no problem for Bernie Fields at Harvard Medical School. Fields's opportunity to take a public stand arose during a conversation with his old friend Barbara Culliton, the Washington-based deputy editor of *Nature*. Soon after Fields turned down the OAR job, the two had a conversation about government AIDS research, the prospects for redirecting it, and the diplomatic challenges that Bill Paul now faced. Culliton invited Fields to lay out his vision in an opinion piece for *Nature,* promising to publish it as soon as possible. It was an offer he could not refuse.

●

On May 12, when Bernie Fields's credo appeared in *Nature,* it was summarized in a long article in the front section of the *New York Times*. His proposals were seconded by some of the biggest names in reporter Gina Kolata's Rolodex, most of whom had read prepublication copies of Fields's article and fell neatly in line behind him.

"We take that as our marching orders," Bill Paul said of Fields's recommended course of action. Echoed Hal Varmus: "Everyone agrees with Bernie's basic precept." Nodding in agreement were sages including David Baltimore and the famous Princeton University biologist Arnold Levine. A slightly more subdued endorsement came from David Ho, the up-and-coming head of the Aaron Diamond AIDS Research Center in New York.

But not everybody agreed with Fields. Noticeably absent from the *Times* article was a response from Tony Fauci, who as head of NIAID was the chief architect of the research establishment that Fields wanted to remodel. Fauci had taken some hits lately: The first blow was when the new OAR was created; then Bill Paul was appointed to lead it, and now an encyclical had been issued by Bernie Fields. As a result, Fauci was not in a good position to comment. Therefore, the job of defending the status quo fell to Ashley Haase, who had chaired the Vaccine Working Group's April meeting and would preside over the AIDS Research Advisory Committee on June 17. Haase had once been a research fellow in Fauci's lab at NIAID, and the two had remained close.

"It's premature to conclude that we are making the wrong bets," Haase told the *Times*. NIH was already sponsoring a great deal of basic science, and he didn't think that the existing research agenda should be tossed out. Still, he wouldn't object if the basic-science budget was fattened with money shifted out of drug and vaccine trials. Asked to comment on the VWG's decision to expand clinical testing of the gp120 vaccines, Haase was of two minds. Even though the gp120 vaccines did not neutralize primary isolates in the lab, a large trial still might show that the vaccines protect people. On the other hand, he told Kolata the VWG vote was "the worst decision I've ever been involved with." Nobel laureate David Baltimore took a more straightforward view of the proposed vaccine tests: He denounced the VWG decision as "anti-science."

●

For every scientist who is invited to write for *Nature* or who is sought out by reporters for the *New York Times*, there are thousands more on the unglamorous front lines. These are not the sleek guys in the stadium sky-boxes, but the players who are trying to grind out a few yards on the muddy field of research. They go to work every day in government office buildings, at corporate labs, and on university campuses. That is as true today as it was in 1994.

At the Division of AIDS, located in a boxy, black-sheathed office building about fifteen minutes north of the NIH campus in Bethesda, vaccine staff members were too busy to spend much time worrying about what had appeared in the pages of the *New York Times* or *Nature* on May 12, 1994. Their marching orders had come from the members of the Vaccine Working Group, not from a professor in Boston. Pat Fast and her staff were on a tight deadline: They had until the June 17 meeting of the AIDS Research Advisory Committee and NIAID Council to write two detailed scenarios for testing the Genentech and Chiron vaccines. The VWG had asked that DAIDS staff come up with detailed plans for both a full-sized Cadillac of a Phase III trial and a more modest, Chevrolet-type version. What could each hope to discover about the vaccines? Exactly how would each protocol be carried out?

By May 3, the in-house team at DAIDS had outlined two possible vaccine trials—a Phase III that would require 3,500 volunteers at the very least, and probably as many as 10,000, and a scaled-down version, what they were calling a "Phase II/III," with somewhere between 1,000 and 3,000 people. Statisticians were plugging numbers into various formulas, calculating how large each type of trial would have to be and how long it would have to last to yield meaningful answers about the gp120 products. In these projections, the size and duration of each proposed trial would depend on factors such as the speed of HIV's spread in the community, the number of people expected to drop out before the study was finished, and the anticipated efficacy of the vaccines. The DAIDS writing team was incorporating all this into draft protocols, which would be analyzed and reviewed by officials at the Food and Drug Administration, scientists at Genentech and Chiron, and selected members of the VWG and ARAC.

On May 13, DAIDS sent drafts to dozens of people who were consulting on the design. Everyone knew the stakes were high. It was crucial that the trial generate data that would help scientists answer vexing questions about how vaccines might succeed, or fail, in protecting against HIV. Even if neither vaccine proved very effective, for example, scientists hoped that results from a large trial would help them figure out what types of immune responses a successful vaccine needed to induce. If they understood what these correlates of protection were, researchers would know what to aim for in designing future products. "A Phase III trial is a big experiment, and we may have to do several of those big experiments before we get a perfect vaccine," Pat Fast said. But that was okay, so long as something new was learned.

The DAIDS staff were like civil engineers on a job site, sweating to bolt together a major highway bridge. From where they stood, the Nobelists and National Academy members quoted in the *Times* were as remote from their work as theoretical physicists. "Basic scientists sometimes think that they are so smart that they can predict what's going to happen. And sometimes they can. But there's a level at which parts of the biology truly aren't understood," Pat said.

In theory, results from an ideal set of laboratory experiments should enable scientists to predict how well a vaccine would protect humans. This was what the big thinkers in the field hoped to see. But what were these ideal experiments? Were they neutralizing antibody assays? Were they the finicky, difficult-to-replicate tests of killer T cell activity? Many of the scientists in the trenches believed that none of these could be trusted to accurately predict a vaccine's performance in people.

Each type of assay represented a narrow slice of reality, but none captured the noisy, complex drama of the whole human immune system. If scientists homed in on the wrong test result, the danger was that they might discard a truly useful product before it got a chance to prove itself. So Pat and other program scientists thought that plausible vaccine candidates should be tested in people while basic research continued. Like any other experiment, an efficacy trial would be an exercise with an uncertain outcome. It was not guaranteed to be a victory lap.

Pat's modus operandi was to figure out what needed to be done and to do it. Her willingness to make decisions and to take risks often put her at loggerheads with Jack Killen, her boss, who was more likely to play it safe.

Whereas Killen was always willing to listen to the "more research is needed" crowd, Pat sometimes lost patience with this. "The day before the efficacy trial of the final vaccine that works really well, there are going to be people arguing for and against. And some of those people are going to be wrong," she said. So Pat's team continued to draw up plans for efficacy trials, as the VWG had asked, regardless of Bernie Fields's manifesto in *Nature.*

It was possible, of course, that Fields's article and the attendant news coverage would turn members of ARAC and the NIAID Council against a large vaccine trial. If this happened, it might not matter how solid DAIDS's presentation was at the June 17 meeting. Peggy Johnston, who had cochaired the VWG session in April, didn't think that Fields's "back to basics" message would close the door on expanded testing for the gp120s. "Bernie wasn't in the AIDS field and he wasn't in the vaccine field. He was a well-known and extremely well-respected pathogenesis expert," Peggy said. Nearly all scientists believe that their own specialty deserves additional funding, so it was not surprising that Fields wanted to expand research on viral pathogenesis. There was nothing wrong or unexpected about that. But AIDS was an urgent, worldwide public-health problem, and Peggy didn't expect the ARAC and Council members to freeze vaccine trials at this stage of the game.

●

Genentech's corporate headquarters commands an entire hilltop in South San Francisco. Its offices and laboratories overlook the seemingly endless suburbs that reach southward to San Jose and beyond, the ever-changing surface of the Bay itself, and—if air quality permits—the undulating hills across the water. From this vantage point, Bernie Fields's manifesto about the future of AIDS research, in addition to whatever the *New York Times* had to say about it, was small and far away. It would be easy to see it as some sort of East Coast egghead phenomenon.

Jack Obijeski, the big-shouldered, slim-hipped man who felt so confident about his presentation to the Vaccine Working Group, shrugged it off. NIH traditionally saw itself as an institution "driven by good science," Jack said, and it seemed to him that Fields's message was totally in line with that high-minded view. AIDS vaccine research was full of "too many people with too many opinions and no vaccinology experience," in his estimation, and there was no point in panicking every time one of them jumped up and barked. Jack had been working on vaccines since 1980, first at CDC and then at Genentech, and he was pretty sure he knew what was what.

Although vaccine inventor Phil Berman respected Bernie Fields as an eminent virologist, he didn't see him as an HIV expert. "I'd been going to AIDS meetings for ten years, and Fields was never at one of them," Phil said. The subtext of Fields's argument appeared to be that the government also needed to fund research on medically important viruses that had been eclipsed by HIV. This was hardly a new concern. In the field of virology, "everybody was afraid that all the money was going for AIDS and being diverted away from more basic research. I think he [Fields] was trying to defend supporting programs on other viruses, which I fully support."

Don Francis and his colleagues in Genentech's clinical trials department didn't have time to worry about Fields because they were working overtime on their own version of a Phase III trial. The DAIDS draft scenarios were wending their way through the review process, and it appeared that the smaller, Phase II/III trial would be presented to ARAC as the first part of a "stepped" design. The idea was that two years would be spent on a small, 4,500-person trial, which would screen candidates before a definitive, 9,000-participant trial would be launched. The stepped approach was like leasing a Chevy for two years, and if that turned out okay, then deciding to buy a Cadillac after all.

Although the stepped design had the advantage of costing less up front, it was not perfect. The small initial trial could identify a highly effective vaccine or a worthless one, but it would not have the statistical power to detect a product that kept 30 percent or 40 percent of people safe. That meant that a moderately effective vaccine, which could save millions of lives in the hardest-hit parts of the world, might go undetected. Another drawback was time: The small trial would take two years, and only then could the definitive, three and a half year efficacy trial get started. There would be no real answer about the vaccines for approximately five and a half years—which Don thought was too long to wait.

As an alternative, Genentech was designing a "large simple trial" that could provide a definite answer in three years. It would also generate data the FDA would require before approving a vaccine for sale. This protocol would recruit 8,100 high-risk volunteers, each of whom would receive four injections. They would be getting one of the gp120 vaccines or a placebo, and no one would know which until the study ended. Don and his statisticians calculated that this trial would have a 90-percent chance of detecting a vaccine that protected 40 percent of immunized people. It would cost more at the beginning than the stepped trial, but it would yield an answer two years earlier. And if either or both of the vaccines worked even moderately well, lives could be saved.

●

Don Francis sent Genentech's Phase III proposal to DAIDS on May 20, where it landed on a heap of other suggestions sent by reviewers throughout the country. Pat Fast and the protocol writing team went through them all. One of the DAIDS scenarios was for the two-step design that would take five and a half years to complete. Their other protocol kept growing and was now slightly bigger than Genentech's proposal—a large-scale definitive efficacy trial that would recruit 9,000 volunteers and yield an answer in three and a half years

As important as these protocols were, they took a back seat to an even more inflammatory issue. So far, nearly 1,000 participants had enrolled in the Phase I and II trials of the gp120 vaccines. Of those, seven previously healthy volunteers had seroconverted, meaning that they now tested positive for HIV. A laboratory test that can distinguish vaccine-induced antibodies and those due to infection left no doubt that these people were now infected with HIV.

Some of these HIV-positive people had received vaccine; others had been injected with adjuvant alone, which could not be expected to protect against infection on its own. When interviewed, all reported having sexual contact with people who were, or might have been, infected. Further testing showed that one of the volunteers who received vaccine had undergone a dramatic loss of CD4 cells, the helper T cells that are especially vulnerable to HIV attack. In general, the fewer CD4 cells a patient

has, the sicker he or she is. There was no way to tell what role the vaccine
had played in this volunteer's CD4 cell loss. But if immunization somehow made people more vulnerable to HIV infection, or accelerated progression to full-blown AIDS, then it was imperative that volunteers be
warned about these possible risks.

DAIDS asked the trial sites to stop enrolling new participants until
they consulted with the study's Data and Safety Monitoring Board, or
DSMB, an independent panel of experts responsible for making sure that
volunteers aren't harmed in the course of human experimentation. The
ethical covenants that govern clinical trials require that participants be
warned, in writing, about anything that could possibly go wrong. No
matter how unlikely an adverse event is, it must be included in the consent form that volunteers sign before the experiment starts. Now these
"breakthrough" infections caused the DAIDS vaccine team to wonder
whether the consent form was adequate.

On Tuesday, May 24, Pat Fast had a conference call with the eight-
member DSMB for HIV vaccine trials. The previous day, they had been
sent two proposed wording changes for the consent form. The first
strengthened the warning against unsafe sexual activity or drug use: "It is
very wrong to think that this vaccine will protect you from infection. It is
very, very important that you be careful and not do anything that might
cause you to become infected with HIV."

The second addition reflected the uncertainty that scientists now felt
about the possible risks of immunization. Although there was no evidence from earlier studies that the gp120 vaccines did any harm, the
plummeting CD4 cells in one newly infected volunteer could not simply
be dismissed. Newly added text read: "If you do become infected with the
HIV virus, we do not know what effect receiving the vaccine might have.
It could make the course of your illness worse." This was followed by
another warning about the importance of avoiding exposure to HIV.

Before they could decide whether these proposed revisions made
sense, DSMB members needed to know exactly what was going on with
the volunteers who had seroconverted. DAIDS had collected individual
data about them from the trial sites and had also gathered summary statistics about CD4 cell decline from large studies of HIV-infected patients.
All this information was discussed in the strictest of confidence. DSMB

members are charged with safeguarding thousands of private citizens who step forward as research subjects, and they take their job seriously. In addition to this humanitarian responsibility, their decisions can have far-reaching economic consequences as well. If the DSMB believes a drug or vaccine is dangerous, it can shut down development of products that have already cost hundreds of millions of dollars to bring this far.

Fortunately for Chiron Biocine and Genentech, the DSMB decided that the gp120 vaccines were not unsafe and that enrollment in the Phase II trial could resume. They agreed that the consent form should be beefed up and recommended that the revised form should be signed by people who were already being immunized as well as by new recruits. The board asked for more detailed studies of risky behavior among volunteers, to try to discover whether people were taking more risks because they believed the vaccines would protect them. Finally, they suggested that participants' CD4 levels should be checked every several months.

Within days of the DSMB conference call, Pat Fast phoned the AVEG investigators in Seattle, Baltimore, St. Louis, Nashville, and Rochester. They could resume recruitment immediately, and her office would send them the new consent wording and the other DSMB recommendations early the following week. In the meantime, happy Memorial Day.

Alas, the second bomb was about to drop.

●

Not much generally happens on the Sunday of Memorial Day weekend. The newspapers typically focus on stories about cars moving extremely fast on the speedway at Indianapolis, or cars moving hardly at all on highways clogged with vacationers. But the *Chicago Tribune* of May 29, 1994, was different: "New Doubts on AIDS Vaccine; 5 Study Volunteers Infected; U.S. Debates Future of Trials," read the headline on page one. The writer was John Crewdson, a well-known investigative reporter based in the newspaper's Washington bureau.

"At least five volunteers in the government's principal AIDS vaccine study have become infected with the AIDS virus despite receiving the vaccine, raising concerns not only about how well the vaccine works but whether it may have increased the likelihood of their infection and—in one case—even accelerated the progression of disease," the article began. The rest of the story contained surprisingly detailed information about how these individuals had become infected, what gender they were, and even the city where one lived. Regardless of how accurate any of this was, it was exactly the type of confidential data that clinical researchers swear not to divulge to anyone not intimately involved with the study. It was the stuff that members of the DSMB had pledged to keep secret.

Crewdson wrote that although none of these findings had been reported in the scientific literature, they had been discussed at scientific meetings, including the Vaccine Working Group, which he did not name but referred to as a "closed-door session in Washington last month." Although these breakthrough infections had been discussed in general terms during the VWG session, many of the clinical details in the *Tribune* story had not come up at that time.

The story was built around interviews with DAIDS Director Jack Killen, Don Francis of Genentech, and Barney Graham, the clinical investigator in charge of the Vanderbilt University test site for the gp120 study. Killen said the seroconversions were causing researchers to doubt the value of the gp120 vaccines and that he didn't know whether testing would be expanded. Don Francis urged that the trials go forward, at the same time acknowledging that immunization might theoretically leave people more vulnerable. Although there was no way to rule out this disturbing possibility, Killen was paraphrased as saying, "There is no statistical basis for concluding that the vaccine has contributed an increased vulnerability to infection." This came near the end of the article, and over the next twenty-four hours, it would become clear that many people, including news directors at television and radio outlets around the country, didn't read that far.

●

Rather than fight highway traffic, Susan Zolla-Pazner and her family typically stay home on holiday weekends. And Memorial Day is a prime gardening opportunity for a Californian like Susan, who never lost the urge to grow things. So she was on one of the decks of her New York City brownstone in the East Thirties, with her hands in dirt, when she was summoned inside to take a phone call from a good friend.

"What's this about the AIDS vaccine causing AIDS?" the friend asked breathlessly.

"Come on, Carol, you must have heard that wrong," Susan quickly replied, sure that her ordinarily sensible friend had made a mistake. The friend insisted that she had just heard this on a television news show, however, and before long Susan was channel surfing, and her husband was trying to track down the story on the Internet.

"I knew that it couldn't be true. These were noninfectious materials," said Susan. An immunology researcher at New York University, she had been studying AIDS since the first cases of Kaposi's sarcoma surfaced among gay men in 1981. She had kept up with the gp120 vaccines since their invention, her own lab measured vaccine-induced antibody responses, and only five weeks earlier she had heard Chiron Biocine and Genentech present their latest findings at the VWG meeting. But none of this had anything to do with the news reports that now flashed across the screen. John Crewdson's story had been picked up and transformed into a classic Frankenstein tale of good medicine turned monstrous. Susan sat stunned with disbelief, realizing that her friend Carol had not misinterpreted anything. "What was coming out to the public was the worst possible story, that the vaccine causes AIDS."

If anyone wanted to arouse public opposition to the proposed efficacy trial, this would be one way to do it. The debate over neutralizing antibody assays was hot stuff in the world of immunology, but it was never going to incite public outrage. Major policy decisions would not be influenced by tiny tempests over lymphocyte stimulation or which primary isolates could or couldn't be killed in a test tube. Nor would the public be galvanized by a Harvard researcher's vision for AIDS research, no matter how eloquently expressed in the pages of *Nature*. But innocent volunteers made sick by a product that was supposed to keep them safe? As told on TV and radio, this was a horror story anyone could understand.

The wave of inflammatory news reports hit the West Coast just as suddenly. On the front lines in Seattle was forty-four-year-old Juliana McElrath, director of the AIDS Vaccine Evaluation Unit, or AVEU, at the

University of Washington. Like Susan and her family, Julie and her scientist husband had elected to spend Memorial Day weekend at home with their son, Ben, who was three years old. It had been an uneventful weekend, and she was caught off guard when her pager and telephone started to go crazy on Sunday. Local reporters, excited by hints in Crewdson's article, were bent on discovering whether any of the infected vaccinees were in Seattle, and they were calling her to find out. Equally determined to protect the confidentiality of her volunteers, she stonewalled.

Julie had all the right stuff for her job. She was an infectious-disease doctor who had been treating AIDS patients since the earliest days of the epidemic, she was a strong clinical administrator, and she was an expert on the arcane and difficult measurement of killer T cells, or CTLs, in the laboratory. For the Phase II study of the gp120 vaccines, Julie was the principal investigator for the five-city trial sponsored by NIH.

She also had the right stuff for this sudden media frenzy and its fallout. Julie is a poised woman from South Carolina who is not easily rattled. She's a handsome, square-jawed blond with a husky voice that is Southern in timbre but no longer in accent. The media onslaught was "a really hard time," she says, but she's not vengeful toward reporters. "If you looked at the details in the articles, they were often very accurate. But if you looked at the headlines, they were misleading. And some people never got beyond the headlines."

The toughest calls were from volunteers in the clinical trial. Some needed a great deal of reassurance that the vaccines were not dangerous, which Julie and the clinic staff rushed to provide. One of the most common misconceptions was that the vaccine contained bits of live HIV and that this could cause infection, a notion that Julie didn't find far-fetched even though she knew it was untrue. "People are not stupid here—they know that flu and polio vaccines contain some virus and on rare occasions make people sick," she said. The Memorial Day stories tapped into this reservoir of fear and suspicion.

Fortunately, the AVEU had plenty of goodwill to draw on. "I'm obviously very partial to Seattle," Julie said. "We have a good relationship with people here. And I think that for the most part they felt like they understood what was happening and they were still with us." It was a rough few days, but the damage to the Seattle AVEU was short-lived.

•

Eight hundred miles down the coast in San Francisco, Sunday's *Chicago Tribune* story, greatly amplified by radio, television, and smaller newspapers, rattled Genentech and Chiron like an earthquake. An aftershock came on Memorial Day itself, when an independently reported article appeared in the *Washington Post*. The *Post* and *Tribune* stories disagreed about the numbers of infected people and how they'd been exposed to the virus, disparities that fueled confusion. And even though the *Post* cited studies showing that volunteers reduced risky sexual behavior after joining the vaccine trial, the article played up the idea that they might take more risks because being vaccinated gave them a false sense of security.

From a purely business standpoint, it almost didn't matter what was true, whether being immunized with gp120 actually made people more vulnerable to HIV or more likely to take risks. Just the hint that such things might possibly happen was enough to panic some biotech investors. Even though recombinant DNA technology had been widely used for more than fifteen years, there was a lingering unease in some quarters that recombinant DNA products would run amok and kill people.

Genentech, in particular, did not need this kind of *tsuris*. In recent years, the company's business practices had been investigated by Congress, the FDA, and the Federal Trade Commission. Although these investigations concerned several different products, the common theme was that the company was extremely aggressive at selling its wares, even when wider use might not benefit patients. So far, the company and its stock price had survived these attacks, but its luck could run out at any time. And Genentech was less willing to take risks on a vaccine, which was not part of its core business, than on the lucrative therapeutic drugs that had made it the darling of Wall Street.

Don Francis was not surprised by the two major news stories, because he had been interviewed for both. The Crewdson article, in his view, "said almost everything correctly." He winced at headline that said "U.S. Debates Future of Trials," because it implied that the efficacy trial he was counting on NIH to sponsor was not a done deal, but he was savvy enough to know that reporters don't get to write their own heads. Don's confidence in the vaccine was unshaken by all the coverage, regardless of the anxiety level in Genentech's executive offices. The product had protected chimps against HIV, which to Don was a key piece of evidence. And he believed, as fervently as anyone could, that the way to find out whether it could also protect people was to push ahead with an efficacy trial.

Unlike Don Francis, Anne-Marie Duliege at Chiron had no advance warning about the Memorial Day media massacre. "The Crewdson article was a disaster," said Anne-Marie, the medical director for vaccine clinical trials at Chiron. "The breakthrough infections were sad, but they were not a disaster. But the way it was presented to the general audience was a disaster." There were always a small number of new infections in the course of a vaccine trial, no matter what vaccine was being tested. Some would occur in people given a placebo, some in those who had not yet received all the prescribed injections, and others in individuals who were fully immunized but not protected. No vaccine is 100-percent effective—especially not in its first iteration. In a large efficacy trial, it is by comparing the number of infections in the vaccine and control groups that scientists can tell whether a vaccine works.

By noon on Tuesday, when executives and scientists had returned from the long weekend, Chiron had taken the lead in drafting a letter to Tony Fauci expressing dismay at the "inaccurate and misleading reporting about the HIV vaccine trials." The letter asserted that the articles "appear to be motivated by political interests against proceeding with further gp120 vaccine trials." It went on to say: "Uncorrected, these recent and subsequent articles could engender a negative environment leading up to the June 17 advisory committee meeting." It was circulated for signing at both Chiron and Genentech.

Most shocking was that confidential information about individual volunteers had made its way into the mass media. The trials were blind, meaning that neither the clinic staff who gave the injections nor the volunteers who rolled up their sleeves knew who was receiving Chiron's vaccine, Genentech's vaccine, or a substance that contained adjuvant alone. This was a safeguard intended to keep expectations from biasing the results of the study. Once a person became infected, however, the code could be broken so that researchers could judge whether it was ethical to continue the study. These particular infections had been discussed at meetings attended by the principal investigators from the five AVEG test sites, top company scientists, and scientists and administrators from NIH. All were bound by ethical guidelines that required them to keep this information confidential, so that the trust of individual volunteers would not be breached.

Obviously, someone was not playing by the rules. Don Francis suspected that the story had been leaked to Crewdson by someone at NIH who wanted to undermine the proposed efficacy trial. Don was so committed to going ahead that it was inconceivable to him that the trial would be derailed. He expected ARAC to respect the VWG's recommendation that the trial go forward, and to act on it. Between now and the June 17 ARAC meeting, Don planned to pull together the most effective presentation he could.

Anne-Marie Duliege was less confident about the upcoming meeting. "We knew enough of AIDS to know how complex it is, how difficult the science, and how political this field is at many levels—whether it's Washington-based politics, or politics among the scientists, or politics at the general audience level, like the Crewdson article."

●

Vaccine program staffers at DAIDS were as surprised as Anne-Marie Duliege when they were hit by the one-two punch of the *Tribune* and *Post* articles. The previous Friday afternoon, only hours before she left the office for Memorial Day, Pat Fast had seen John Crewdson go into Jack Killen's office and close the door. Her office and Killen's were at opposite ends of a corridor lined with low-walled cubicles, and by chance she had been looking down the hall as he went in.

Crewdson was a big burly man with a beard and a formidable reputation as an investigative reporter. Although he had won a Pulitzer Prize for national reporting in 1981, his fame soared in November 1989 when the newspaper ran his mammoth article on the race to identify the AIDS virus. Crewdson made a strong case that Robert Gallo, despite being hailed in 1984 as the American discoverer of the virus, had very likely isolated it from a sample that French researcher Luc Montagnier had sent to Gallo's lab as a courtesy.

Although rumors that Gallo had stolen the virus from the French had circulated since the beginning, Crewdson came up with a great deal of circumstantial evidence to substantiate the claim. His article was a harsh indictment of Gallo and the NIH establishment that protected him, and it helped trigger an onslaught of investigations by NIH, Congress, and the National Academy of Sciences. All this dragged on for nearly five years, paralyzing Gallo's research activities, embarrassing the NIH, and touching off an international patent dispute.

In the wake of all this, John Crewdson could not go unrecognized at the Division of AIDS. When Pat Fast saw him, she had no idea why he was there. After the reporter had left the building, Jack Killen said nothing. Although he could have called together the DAIDS vaccine staff and warned them about what was coming, he did not. As a result, Pat Fast, who was head of the vaccine program, and Peggy Johnston, who was second in command to Killen, were caught by surprise when their phones began to ring on Sunday.

As Crewdson's story was picked up everywhere, suspicion spread among AIDS researchers that he had been tipped off by someone who wanted to frighten the public into thinking that it would be a ghastly mistake to inject thousands of volunteers with gp120. If ordinary citizens, especially gay men who would be recruited to participate, believed that the risks of doing the efficacy trial outweighed its possible benefits, then there would be no political costs associated with canceling it.

If Tony Fauci's inclination was to abort the proposed efficacy trial (and he acknowledged wanting to a few years later), then the bad publicity about gp120 would make this decision easier and less controversial than it might have been. No one who knows the meticulous Fauci believed that he would have done anything so crude as leak the story himself. It is far easier to imagine that he nudged a rock that rolled down the hill and stirred the fault that shook things up from coast to coast. And the rock that he nudged, many think, was the loyal Jack Killen.

Only two people know if that's true, of course, Killen and a Pulitzer Prize–winning reporter who is honor bound not to reveal his sources. For his part, Killen says that he doesn't remember how Crewdson's visit to his office was arranged. He reflected some years later: "He came into my office, asked a number of questions, of which I really don't recall the specifics now, but I certainly had the impression that he had his story basically written. I recall specifically at the end of the interview, him saying something to the effect of 'I'm sorry to have to do this to you, but we'll be publishing the story this weekend.' It seemed clear to me in the interview, and thinking back on the story, that his focus was that there was some kind of cover-up and he wasn't interested in information to the contrary."

Crewdson will not say who put him onto the story or who revealed highly confidential information about individual volunteers. All he would say, questioned years after the fact, was that his Friday-afternoon talk with Killen was pivotal. "My interview with Jack Killen gave me what I thought I needed to write the story. And I wrote it."

●

The shock waves of May 1994 were felt as far away as Thailand.

The Research Institute for Health Sciences at Chiang Mai University, usually called RIHES, is a narrow four-story box hunkered across an alley from Chiang Mai Hospital. Both the towering hospital and the squat research building were originally gleaming white stucco; now they are permanently stained like the collar of a dress shirt worn too long in the steaming tropical heat. Dirt-laden thermals rise from the alley, where diesel delivery trucks and noisy swarms of motorcycles belch noise and exhaust.

Nearly two years had passed since Chris Beyrer arrived at RIHES to help set the stage for AIDS vaccine trials in northern Thailand. He had come to love Chiang Mai, an ancient walled capital that had mushroomed into a tumultuous commercial hub for several hundred thousand people. By the spring of 1994, Chris was entirely caught up in Chiang Mai and in the battle against AIDS, which was spreading faster in the North than anywhere else in Thailand.

The halls of RIHES were painted a shade of green that has a Proustian effect on middle-aged American scientists, transporting them to elementary schools of the 1950s. The sense of having traveled back in time is enhanced by the electric fans that are the only relief from the heat in much of the building. Behind certain tightly closed doors, however, are laboratories crammed with up-to-date equipment and cooled to the point of frigidity. Gary Larson cartoons of geeky scientists and blobs exploding from test tubes are taped to the polished metal fronts of refrigerators—proof that at least some Chiang Mai researchers are fully integrated into modern science.

Chris met John McNeil soon after he arrived, and now he had an ongoing collaboration with the military virus lab operated by the U.S. and Thai Armies in Bangkok, 400 miles to the south. RIHES scientists also had regular telephone and e-mail contact with their stateside colleagues at WRAIR, Johns Hopkins, and NIH. As a result, they knew as much as most U.S.-based researchers about what was going on with HIV vaccine trials. Besides Chris, the others who kept close tabs on what was happening in the States were Dr. Chirasak Khamboonruang, director of RIHES, and Joseph Chiu, an American physician who had been working in Thailand off and on since 1981. All three were disturbed by what unfolded in May 1994, as Bernie Fields's article in *Nature* was followed by John Crewdson's story in the *Chicago Tribune*.

Whatever happened in the United States would have serious repercussions for Thailand. In developing countries or newly industrialized ones like Thailand, governments often take their scientific lead from U.S. agencies like the NIH and the FDA. Because these agencies are respected for their high standards, a new drug or vaccine that is licensed for use in the States will usually sail through approval in Thailand. Conversely, a product that fares poorly in the U.S. system might well be dismissed out of hand.

In the case of the gp120 vaccines, Chris and his Chiang Mai colleagues worried that the proposed U.S. efficacy trial might be turned down, not on the basis of any firm scientific evidence but because NIH officials thought it would be politically risky to go forward. Such a decision could easily cripple the prospects for doing vaccine trials in Thailand, even though the potential benefits were greater in Thailand because AIDS was spreading so fast. "The public perception would be 'Oh, this product wasn't good enough to test in the U.S. Now you want to test it in us,'" said

Joe Chiu. The Thais are a proud people, whose country has never in its long history been overrun by a foreign power, and they were understandably sensitive to any hint of exploitation.

Thailand had already created a system for approving HIV vaccine trials, wisely believing that they should have guidelines in place before they were asked to authorize a specific product for testing in Thai volunteers. In 1992, shortly before Chris Beyrer arrived in Chiang Mai, the country had drafted its first National AIDS Vaccine Plan. A leading architect of this plan was Dr. Natth Bhamarapravati, one of the nation's most influential—and entrepreneurial—academic scientists.

Dr. Natth's career path, even more than the lingua franca of Gary Larson cartoons, illustrates the extent to which elite science has truly become transcultural. He got his medical training at the University of Pennsylvania and is board-certified in pathology in the United States. Prominent on his office wall is the framed title page of an article on dengue fever, his research specialty, signed with a personal greeting from its author, vaccine pioneer Albert Sabin. Dr. Natth sits on international scientific boards including UNAIDS and the World Health Organization's polio eradication program and is on a first-name basis with a pride of Nobel laureates.

For twelve years, Dr. Natth was president of Mahidol University in Bangkok, generally regarded as the nation's top school. One of Natth's proudest achievements was the creation of a new campus dedicated to the study of the sciences and technology. Located in a flat and dusty Bangkok suburb just off an expressway, the Salaya campus resembles the University of California-Davis. When Thailand's strict civil-service law required Dr. Natth to retire at age sixty, his reward was to head the new Center for Vaccine Development, located at Salaya. Set back from the road in a stand of saplings, it looks from a distance like a low-rise ranch house. Up close, it has a shady central breezeway and three floors of labs, production areas, and offices. This is Dr. Natth's domain when he is not in Geneva, Washington, Paris, or some other international capital.

In the early 1990s, when Thailand first realized the severity of its AIDS problem, the country had no government or corporate capacity to invent or produce candidate HIV vaccines on its own. So the National AIDS Committee, or NAC, decided that Thailand's best bet was to become, in Dr. Natth's words, "a global partner in getting the vaccine out for public health use." The word "partner" was key to Dr. Natth and the NAC, which felt that in the past Thailand had not been properly rewarded for testing U.S.-made vaccines.

In the 1980s, thousands of Thai people had participated in huge field studies of experimental vaccines for hepatitis A, Japanese encephalitis, and malaria. As a result of these trials, the hepatitis A and Japanese encephalitis products were licensed for use in the United States and in Thailand. They were still manufactured exclusively in the United States, however, and were sold at full price in the country where they had been tested. In the future, Dr. Natth wanted to guarantee that Thailand would benefit when its people took risks that helped bring a vaccine to market.

Dr. Natth's long-term goal was to cultivate a Thai vaccine industry capable of everything from discovering candidate vaccines to manufacturing hundreds of thousands of doses. Obviously, this would take years. The first steps in that direction, however, were laid out in the National AIDS Vaccine Plan, which specifies what corporate or government sponsors must do in exchange for testing vaccines in Thailand. Most of the requirements involve sharing certain kinds of technical expertise. For example, the NAC wanted Thai physicians to be coinvestigators in clinical trials, working shoulder-to-shoulder with outside experts. They also wanted the sponsor to strengthen the country's infrastructure for carrying out trials, which could mean training laboratory scientists on virology techniques or teaching doctors and nurses how to conduct trials according to good clinical practices. Finally, the NAC wanted trial sponsors to set up data management facilities in Thailand and train local staff in how to collect, process, and analyze the millions of observations that are needed to determine whether a vaccine works or not.

When a company or government agency applied to conduct clinical trials in Thailand, these were some of the factors that the NAC and its subcommittees would weigh before reaching a decision. The NAC's wish list would increase the burden on vaccine sponsors, but it was worth it. In order to advance biotechnology in Thailand, the committee was willing to create an approval process that would be as restrictive and bureaucratic as U.S. requirements for drug testing.

In the early days, however, before the Thai system was really in place, it was still possible for a maverick to slip through.

On June 6, 1994, without benefit of approval by the NAC, a well-known Bangkok physician launched the country's first AIDS vaccine trial. Dr. Praphan Phanuphak was head of the Thai Red Cross, an organization with royal patronage. On his own, he had agreed to test an experimental vaccine made by United Biomedical, Inc., a small company on Long Island in New York. This was the outfit Wayne Koff joined when he left the DAIDS vaccine program.

Dr. Praphan recruited thirty volunteers simply by holding a televised press conference on opening day and telling people how to sign up. When the Ministry of Public Health tried to put a stop to the trial because it lacked proper approval, Dr. Praphan publicly accused the government of trying to stop him from protecting the Thai people against AIDS. His action was a savvy public-relations move, and the government backed down. After this, however, the NAC resolved that no trial would ever again be launched in Thailand until every possible official, committee, and subcommittee had formally signed off on the plan.

●

While all this was going on in Bangkok, the Chiang Mai researchers were exchanging increasingly anxious e-mails with John McNeil, who was back at WRAIR in Rockville. If ARAC voted against a gp120 efficacy trial on June 17, which was certainly possible with all this bad publicity, then what would happen in Thailand? Both Chiron and Genentech, with encouragement from the army, were making gp120 vaccines tailored to protect against the clade E HIV that was ravaging Chiang Mai and the surrounding countryside. But those vaccines might never be tested if Fauci—bolstered by a no-go vote from ARAC—decided to halt domestic trials of the clade B products originally designed for American use.

After much back-and-forth, John and his Chiang Mai collaborators decided that Thai scientists who wanted to see gp120 vaccines tested in Thailand should express their concerns directly to Fauci. Such a group, called THAIVEG (for Thai Vaccine Evaluation Group) Consortium was hastily pulled together by some of the army's Bangkok colleagues, notably Dr. Prasert Thongchoroen, the current president of Mahidol University.

Chris Beyrer and Joe Chiu, working in one of the small humid offices on the third floor at RIHES, wrote a rough draft of a letter. Chirasak Khamboonruang, the director of the Institute and a well-connected member of Thailand's science establishment, shepherded the draft through a lengthy editing process that involved the other THAIVEG participants. The final version of the letter, dated June 13, said that they expected trouble if Fauci decided not to proceed with efficacy trials in the United States, "especially if such a position statement is phrased in such a way as to cast in serious doubt the potential benefit or safety of proceeding with efficacy evaluation given any other set of circumstances than those which exist in the United States."

One concern was that manufacturers might turn their backs on AIDS vaccine development. As a consequence, products being developed by Chiron and Genentech expressly for Thailand would surely be abandoned. Even if the companies stayed in the game, a second worry was that developing countries might lose confidence and postpone or abandon vaccine testing. This "could have devastating effects on our population, as Thailand currently has very high rates of infection," the THAIVEG members wrote.

No matter what decision Fauci made about vaccine trials in the United States, the Thais urged him to make it clear that he was not specifying what any other country ought to do. "Given the explosive character of the epidemic in Thailand, as public health experts and scientists representing the interests of Thailand, we feel that the parameters for choosing whether or not to proceed with vaccine trials, including efficacy evaluation, are substantially different here."

Although the letter to Fauci bore the signatures of some of Thailand's most prominent immunology and virology researchers, the powerful Dr. Natth was not among them. "They did not ask me to sign. They knew that I would not sign," he said in a later interview. His objection was that the letter had been "engineered" by Americans; in his words, "I like Thais to be independent."

●

To keep an appointment with Tony Fauci, one takes the elevator to the seventh floor of Building 31, a centrally located but architecturally bland tower where the directors of the various institutes are stacked, one office above the other. Step off, turn right, and the view is a long, featureless, and highly polished hallway that leads to Fauci's office door. Inside the suite, four lavender-upholstered chairs are lined up facing the visitor. Behind the row of chairs is an open office where three administrative staff members are busy with calls and faxes and old-fashioned snail mail, when they're not staring into the monitors glowing on their desks.

People who come to see Fauci are asked to take a seat in the row of chairs. Visitors are at eye level with a copy machine and a small refrigerator, but as their gaze inevitably rises in this high-ceilinged anteroom, they behold dozens of awards and honorary degrees that Fauci has received from institutions around the world. This wall turns out to be just the tip of the honorary iceberg: Inside his spacious corner office is what might be the world's largest display of Perma Plaque technology, hundreds of official tributes annealed to dark wood and sealed for eternity. Not even Bob Gallo has more.

With an American flag standing at attention next to an expansive desk and a comfortable conversation area for meetings, Fauci's office as NIAID director is imperial in comparison to the "cramped little office" at the NIH Clinical Center where in 1981 he remembers reading about unusual cases of pneumonia among gay men in Los Angeles. For the next three years, he was one of many doctors who lost every patient that he treated to this new, mysterious type of immune suppression.

Fauci was also a laboratory researcher, and when he decided to devote his lab to this new scourge, he was cautioned that doing so could ruin his career. "Resources were not plentiful and there was no inducement for investigators to leave fields in which they were successful to pursue something with no guarantee of support or success. Young investigators followed the lead of their mentors and stayed away from AIDS," he said in a 1999 speech about the history of the epidemic.

When he was made director of NIAID in 1984, Fauci once again bucked advice from his elders. He fought for and secured a $60-million budget increase on top of the $300 million that had been allocated for AIDS in 1984. Fauci's single-minded focus on AIDS made him unpopular with NIAID researchers who feared that new AIDS spending would gut the budgets for other infectious diseases. They need not have worried. In fact, the non-AIDS portion of the NIAID budget kept pace as the new discipline grew. And the tremendous investment in AIDS research "gave birth to an entirely new field of medicine," in Fauci's view. Along the way, Fauci acquired a series of White House photographs that show his black hair becoming progressively more gray as he shakes hands with President Reagan, then Bush, then Clinton.

Fauci's actions and accomplishments during the first decade of the AIDS epidemic are a perfect illustration of what has been described in the *Harvard Business Review* as "productive narcissism." AIDS upended the conventional wisdom in medicine and public health, which held that infectious diseases had been tamed and there was nothing antibiotics couldn't cure. Socially, it brought the sexual revolution to a screeching halt and gave rise to widespread and often ugly mistrust of others. During chaotic times like these, "narcissists thrive," wrote anthropologist and psychoanalyst Michael Maccoby, an expert on leadership styles.

Tony Fauci was not afraid to take risks and try to shape the future of research on this new disease, and he was able to articulate his vision and motivate others to follow him. He was remarkably successful in persuading Congress to increase funding for a disease that was mainly striking homosexuals and IV drug users, populations that most legislators did not view as mainstream constituents. And he dared to bring AIDS activists, who were his sworn enemies at first, into the NIH tent. Fauci's personal ambitions and the public good were one, and the public benefited tremendously from the building of his AIDS empire.

Although a productive narcissist can accomplish amazing things, this style of leadership also has a darker aspect. In contrast to outer-directed personalities, who need to be loved, narcissists need to be admired and can be quite aggressive in pursuit of affirmation. The symbols of distinction that crowd the walls of Fauci's office are evidence for this, many having been gained through what a former staff member called "an active award-seeking strategy." Office staff are said to have spent time identifying honors that would be appropriate, putting together nomination packages, and lining up people who were positioned to submit Fauci's name. The one that mattered most to him, and which didn't happen overnight, was being voted into the National Academy of Sciences in 1992.

As a narcissistic leader becomes more successful, Maccoby writes, he also becomes more sensitive to slights or challenges to his vision. Instead of asking others to help him keep things in perspective, the stressed narcissist is more likely to withdraw into his bunker—alone save for the comforting presence of loyalists who believe he can do no wrong. Fauci's vision for AIDS research was repeatedly challenged in early 1994. Although Bernie Fields didn't mention him by name, there was no doubt that the federal research agenda that Fields criticized in *Nature* was Fauci's brainchild. And by creating the Office of Aids Research, Congress had given its director Bill Paul more control over AIDS spending than Fauci had at the peak of his influence. Adding insult was the fact that Paul been a lab chief at NIAID, where Fauci is the boss, until Hal Varmus tapped him to become director of OAR.

Paul was a famous immunologist, and like Fields had been chosen for the NAS earlier than Fauci. In short, he was the kind of person most likely to incite intensely competitive feelings in someone like Fauci. Paul's first task as OAR director would be to survey current AIDS programs throughout the NIH so that he could decide where changes should be made. The OAR would need to collect detailed information about activities in DAIDS, which managed the lion's share of the federal AIDS budget. But the word inside DAIDS, say scientists who were there at the time, was that when OAR asked for information, "you don't help them, you don't do anything they say."

Clearly, Fauci was juggling a lot of balls in the spring of 1994, when each passing day brought the efficacy trial decision one step closer. In early May, shortly after the VWG voted to expand vaccine testing, Fauci told Jon Cohen of *Science* that he didn't know whether he was leaning toward launching the big trial, or away from it. One month later, after Crewdson broke the story of the infected volunteers, Fauci had recast his message in a subtle way. Without saying what he personally thought should happen, he told *Science* that the bad press "absolutely tilts the political framework" against going forward with the efficacy trial.

Looking back, during a 1997 interview, Fauci acknowledged that during this period in 1994, his opinion was that the efficacy trial should not go forward. He wasn't enthusiastic about gp120 vaccines that induced antibodies but no cellular response. He also felt that because the spread of AIDS was slowing in the United States, an efficacy study would have to be so large and costly that it would doubtless take resources away from other types of research. Although he had an opinion, Fauci insisted, he had not made up his mind in advance. He wanted to hear what ARAC would have to say.

Did Fauci try to influence ARAC's vote by inciting public fear that the gp120 vaccines were dangerous? That is impossible to know. At any rate, it's clear that he was not professionally or personally invested in seeing the trial go forward. That was the domain of Pat Fast and the other program scientists at DAIDS, who had tremendous sweat equity in the proposed efficacy test. They had worked closely with the biotech companies for years, they had taken great pains to make sure that contract laboratories were ready to test patient samples, and they had doled out millions of tax-payer dollars to clinical investigators in the AVEG and HIVNET sites.

The DAIDS vaccine staff saw two main reasons for going ahead with a big trial: One was to test the efficacy of the product in the vials; the other was to discover whether they could successfully carry out a vaccine trial in high-risk populations. Could enough volunteers be recruited? Would participants keep coming back to the clinic for three years, first to be immunized and later to be tested for evidence of infection? The program scientists didn't know whether it was possible to pull off such a feat or not, and they thought it was imperative to find out.

Many of the most successful "productive narcissists" are known for their lack of empathy toward others in their organization. This is some-times a tremendous advantage, because it liberates them to make decisions that another type of leader might avoid, rather than taking the risk of making subordinates upset or angry. Narcissistic leaders do what they think is best, with no regrets.

The concerns of people several rungs down the administrative ladder were probably not on Fauci's mind at all.

9

DEATH IN THE AFTERNOON

F ARUK SINANGIL WAS FEELING ragged when he and Anne-Marie Duliege stepped out of the taxi that had brought them from Washington National Airport to the Hyatt Regency in downtown Bethesda. It was never easy for Faruk to sleep on a red-eye from San Francisco to Washington, in part because his legs were too long for the confines of economy class. But this flight had been worse than usual. Faruk's efforts to take a Zen attitude, to let the white-noise roar of the engines drown out his anxieties, had been only intermittently successful. I am a scientist who works with test tubes, he kept telling himself, and not a businessman or a politician. Anne-Marie has to make a presentation, not me. And whatever happens here is not going to be about science.

It was June 17, 1994, and Faruk and his colleagues at Chiron Biocine, the company's vaccine division, had good reason to be nervous about the meeting at the "NIH Hyatt"—a hotel so close to the southernmost edge of the National Institutes of Health that it might as well be on the campus. Kathy Steimer would ordinarily have been part of Chiron's delegation, but she had asked Faruk to go instead.

At stake was the future of gp120, the AIDS vaccine that had so far cost Chiron eight years of work and millions of dollars. Since 1990, this vaccine had been Faruk's livelihood and the center of his life as a virologist. He was one of a team of twenty researchers and technicians working on the gp120 project, and none of them knew whether they would still be with the company next year, or even next month. So much depended on what happened today.

In the Hyatt's garage, Pat Fast was glad to find a parking space after inching into Bethesda with all the other commuters from the Maryland and Virginia suburbs. It was hot and muggy and she did not have a good feeling about how the day would unfold. As head of the vaccine program for the Division of AIDS and the person responsible for overseeing research on gp120 and other candidate vaccines, her assignment for the meeting was to summarize the clinical trial results for the Chiron Biocine and Genentech products. Sensational press coverage that began on Memorial Day weekend had made these studies wildly controversial, and today's meeting had the potential to turn into a farce or a brawl. What Pat had to do was stay neutral, lay out the facts, and not make waves.

Inside, crowds were squeezing through the tall dark doors of the Crystal Ballroom. Three dozen members of two NIH advisory committees prowled around the tables that formed a large open square in the center of the ballroom, looking for the name card that would tell each where to sit. On a large platform at the end of the room, some fifteen television crews wrestled with their cables and tripods and jostled for space with still photographers. More than fifty print reporters fiddled with their tape recorders and notebooks, torn between claiming a good seat and button-holing government officials and committee members in the premeeting hubbub.

Faruk and Anne-Marie made their way to the front row of the spectator section, where seats were reserved for corporate representatives. They exchanged greetings with Biocine president Dino Dina, who had traveled on his own and arrived earlier. Next to him were Don Francis, Phil Berman, Tim Gregory, and some lesser-known people from Genentech. Reporters buzzed around Don Francis, the celebrity member of the group, while pretty much ignoring everyone else.

Out of the spotlight, Faruk and the Genentech scientists didn't have much to say to each other. The two biotechs had been rivals for years, and now they were jointly petitioning the NIH to put their vaccines into an efficacy trial together. Politics had once again made strange bedfellows. Kathy knew Phil and Tim pretty well, and if she'd been there, she probably would have made conversation with them. Faruk barely knew them, but he could tell they were not in the best of moods. Phil's hackles had risen the instant he saw the mob of reporters and TV cameras, and all he could think was, "This is a set-up. We're gonna get murdered." Tim was of the same mind.

The rest of the room was fast filling with people who develop, test, or regulate HIV vaccines. Standing out among the middle-aged people in suits were the AIDS activists who had traveled from New York, Boston, and San Francisco, as well as from nearby Washington. Six months earlier, most of them had been only dimly aware that vaccines that might prevent AIDS were being tested in numerous small trials. Recent reports that a few volunteers had become infected, however, coupled with the suggestion that the vaccines might have been responsible, roused the activists like a three-alarm fire. Although a few radicals thought that vaccines might be a genocidal attack on the gay community, cooler heads realized that the real impact would be economic: NIH money spent developing a preventive vaccine was money that wouldn't be available for treatment research.

Faruk, who was both a powerful believer in vaccines and a resident of one of the world's most politically conscious cities, understood where the activists in the Crystal Ballroom were coming from. He knew that even the ones who weren't infected with HIV saw themselves as advocates for a community of people who were. Unless better antiviral drugs were developed, and fast, people who already had the virus were headed for certain death. If the NIH approved a gp120 efficacy trial at the conclusion of this meeting, there was no denying that treatment research would take a hit.

Faruk was still eyeing the activists when the meeting got underway at 8:30 with an official update on DAIDS activities from its director, Jack Killen. For nearly thirty minutes he droned on about routine matters such as new committee appointments, internal reorganization, and changes in grant-making procedures. The thirty-six committee members seated around the big table were mildly inattentive as they sorted through the multicolored folders stacked before them, poured water, and settled in for what promised to be a long day.

The atmosphere changed abruptly when Tony Fauci swept in a few

minutes after 9:00. The room exploded with light as flash guns and camera lamps ricocheted off the tall narrow mirrors on the ballroom walls
and seemed to bounce off Fauci himself. He seemed to be made of tightly
wrapped wire, with salt-and-pepper hair cut close to his skull, shiny avi-
ator glasses, and a propensity for narrow suits the color of brushed alu-
minum. On the day of this meeting, Fauci wielded an annual AIDS
budget of $558 million and had more power over HIV research than any-
one else in the world. He moved through crowded rooms like a slender
column of laser light, and no one smart ever forgot that he was there.
Almost everyone referred to him as "Tony," and he was a gracious host.

Fauci's welcome to the committee members was so warm, his regard
for their counsel so serious, that they felt like honored guests. Which is, in
fact, what membership on a politically appointed advisory body like the
AIDS Research Advisory Committee boils down to. Every ARAC member
had a personal or professional connection with AIDS; some were experts
in their own right, but that wasn't the only reason they were chosen. NIH
has a formula for constituting committees so that women, minorities, a
spectrum of academic institutions, and different parts of the country are
represented. If a group already had too many Californians, for example, a
distinguished potential member could be passed over. So a committee
like this ended up being the best and the brightest that could be assembled according to government guidelines.

NIAID had a host of advisory groups, and although they operated
independently, their domains sometimes overlapped. HIV vaccines, for
example, fell under ARAC and the AIDS Subcommittee of the NIAID
Council. Having them meet together, to make a joint decision about efficacy testing, ruled out the possibility of disagreement down the road.

Unlike the Vaccine Working Group, whose members knew one
another well, neither of these two groups had the opportunity to become
a well-oiled machine. Both met infrequently, they hardly ever met jointly,
and three-year appointments meant constant turnover on both. On this
occasion, two members were attending their very first meeting and four
were finishing their terms and picking up certificates of appreciation. All
this churning left little opportunity to find common ground, learn each
other's passions and strengths, and figure out who asked good questions
that should be pursued.

So the members were houseguests at the NIH Hyatt. They knew that their views would be politely heard and their humor appreciated, but they also knew that they shouldn't presume too much. They should not discipline the children and they should eat what was on their plate.

Fauci told the group that they should listen to presentations about the candidate vaccines and make up their own minds about whether the vaccines made by Chiron and Genentech should advance to an efficacy trial. Although an earlier meeting of the VWG had endorsed the idea of doing a large trial, they had not had all the facts. Now there was new information, Fauci said, and the people in the Crystal Ballroom were about to hear it.

As they listened to Fauci read his remarks, individual committee members could not keep from glancing nervously around the ballroom. There were so many reporters and so many cameras. And the gallery was packed with activists, many of them severe young men with multiple piercings and black T-shirts. Even AIDS old-timers were not used to being put under a microscope this way. How sobering it was to hear Fauci say, "Your mission is to advise me as the director of NIAID concerning the next step in the process of vaccine trials." And what a relief to have him add, "My responsibility is to make a decision regarding these two vaccine candidates, taking your recommendations into very serious consideration."

Even if the committee recommended against an efficacy trial for Chiron's and Genentech's gp120 vaccines, Fauci assured them that NIH's commitment to vaccine research would be as strong as ever. "There may be a chilling effect on our industrial partners," he acknowledged, but that prospect shouldn't enter into the advisers' thinking. A shiver ran through the corporate representatives as they heard these words. Don Francis knew that if the government balked, there was no way the top brass at Genentech were going to pour millions of their own dollars into an efficacy trial. They saw the AIDS vaccine as one of many products in development, not as a crusade, and were more likely to invest in drug treatments with more earning potential.

To Pat Fast, Chiron and Genentech were only the beginning of a corporate avalanche that would hit if an efficacy trial wasn't approved. At DAIDS, she had run seventeen small clinical studies of thirteen different candidate vaccines; she was in constant touch with company scientists and medical directors, and their anxieties were heading off the charts. Stockholders and venture capitalists who had read sensational news about people being infected in HIV vaccine trials were on the verge of deciding that there must be easier ways to make money. If the efficacy trial was canceled today, Pat had a mental list of companies she thought would abandon HIV vaccine research.

Fauci wound up his remarks by saying that he planned to stay all day "to get a firsthand flavor of the discussions." Although this seemed unremarkable to many in the room, in fact it was extraordinary coming from a man who was so impatient that his own senior staff often felt as though they were wasting his time and whose idea of a half-hour appointment was twenty-three minutes. "Thank you and good luck to all of us" was his closing line.

Jack Killen came back to the microphone to explain the agenda and the ground rules for the meeting. There would be six short presentations on various aspects of vaccine research, and the committee members would be able to ask a few questions after each one. Following lunch, representatives of Genentech and Chiron Biocine would briefly give their views on future vaccine testing, Killen said; then forty-five minutes of public comment would be heard. Only people who put their names on an official list before 12:00 noon would be permitted to address the committee, and no one would be allotted more than five minutes. "The remainder of the day is open for discussion and the development of a recommendation," Killen said. This meant that people seated at the big table could talk, but only when recognized by the chairman.

The goal of the meeting, he emphasized, was to pass a specific recommendation about the future of the gp120 vaccines. "Knowing Dr. Haase's chairmanship talents as we do, we are confident that he will get you there before the day is through," Killen said. On that note, he turned the meeting over to Ashley Haase, who was the first speaker on the agenda as well as the meeting's chairman.

On first impression, Haase looked like Clark Kent: He was a square-jawed, square-shouldered fellow with horn-rimmed glasses and a low-key manner. But the more one knew about this self-described "shy guy from Minnesota," the more obvious it became that he was an NIH insider, whose many roles included being chairman of ARAC and serving on many NIH study sections that decide which researchers will get grant money. In April, he had been asked to pinch-hit as cochairman of the Vaccine Working Group, and now he was to tell the members of ARAC, many of whom were not vaccine experts, what had gone on there.

Some participants in that earlier meeting listened to Haase's report with a growing sense of amazement, because it bore little resemblance to their own recollections. What stood out for them was that Chiron and Genentech had relaxed their guard on proprietary information and allowed the scientists to present their rawest new findings. The young vaccine developers from California had swapped ideas with Merck's Maurice Hilleman and Mary Lou Clements from Johns Hopkins, giants of the field whose vaccines had defeated infectious diseases around the world. Everyone critiqued everyone else's experiments, speculated about the ornate chess game that goes on between HIV and the human immune system, and freely debated where to go next. In the end, the VWG decided that there was nothing more to be learned from laboratory experiments and animal studies. The only way to find out whether gp120 vaccines protected against AIDS was to test them in more people. So they asked DAIDS staffers to go back to the office and draft plans for two possible efficacy trials, a definitive Cadillac version and the more modest Chevy-style experiment.

For people who had been part of the give-and-take at the VWG meeting, Haase's summary was like listening to a tax lawyer read the lyrics to a love song. All the words were there, nothing was inaccurate, but all the sizzle was gone. On slide after slide, Haase showed two balance scales: One set tilted slightly toward doing an efficacy trial with dispatch, the other tilted toward putting it off. Haase chose the image because "for every positive thing you could say, you could counter with 'Well, but.'" Haase had worked and reworked these slides for the past two weeks, going over what had happened at the VWG in phone conversations with Tony Fauci. The more they talked, the grayer everything looked.

As a result, Haase's presentation was so scrupulously balanced, so larded with caveats, that some committee members probably concluded that members of the VWG hadn't really cared much—one way or the other—about expanding the clinical trials. Sitting around the ARAC table were several people who had also served on the VWG, including

Susan Zolla-Pazner, the antibody researcher from New York University. She grew increasingly impatient during Haase's account of the earlier meeting, raising her hand when he finished.

"Ashley's summary of the meeting is really excellent and very accurate," Zolla-Pazner began. But he had not told ARAC that "at the end of the second day of meetings, we went around the table and each individual was asked to give his or her impression and opinion about what we should do. The decision was really overwhelming. It was not quite unanimous, but almost, that we should proceed with these scaled-back trials," she said, her gaze traveling slowly around the table. "I would like to get that emphasis across, that it was a nearly unanimous decision. It was stronger than what sounds like lukewarm approval."

Did the vaccine experts vote for a clinical trial because they believed gp120 would protect people against HIV, one ARAC member asked, or because they wanted to gather scientific data that would be useful in the future?

"The consensus was that these probably are not the vaccines that we are going to end up using broadly ten or twenty years from now, but that these were products that were worth going ahead with, because they might be efficacious and because certainly we would learn more doing the trial," Zolla-Pazner answered.

A subset of the ARAC members were bona fide vaccine experts, and they came from two main camps. Some, like Zolla-Pazner, felt certain that an efficacy trial was the next logical step. Others were opposed to doing a trial with gp120 and wanted to hold off until canarypox, or possibly naked DNA, was ready for testing. But the majority of the committee members weren't directly involved in vaccine research and did not come to the Hyatt with strongly held views. Neither the companies nor Tony Fauci could predict how they would vote at the end of the day.

By this point it was a little after 10:00 A.M., and Faruk noticed that although some people were paying close attention, others were not. In the life of a meeting there is a time in midmorning when some participants, no matter how compelling the topic, begin slipping out to visit the rest room or make surreptitious phone calls to the office. Faruk didn't leave his seat but flagged a bit during the next talk, which summarized animal experiments related to HIV vaccines. He wished that he had gotten more sleep on the plane.

Pat Fast was next in the lineup of speakers from the Division of AIDS, and she started her update on clinical trials with the basics: DAIDS had tested thirteen different candidates in 1,400 HIV-negative volunteers since 1988, mostly in small Phase I trials but more recently in larger studies of the gp120 products. She told the group that the Chiron and Genentech vaccines appeared to be safe and to stimulate immune responses, although there was certainly debate about how protective those responses might be. That was the easy part of the talk, the part she had given dozens of times.

Then Pat tapped the remote control and a new slide came up: HIV Infections in Vaccine Trial Participants. She could hear the rustling of notepads as the reporters in the back of the room came to attention. This was what they had come for, the media and activists, and why the members of ARAC were conducting their business in full view of TV cameras.

"There has been a lot of interest recently in the small number of volunteers who become exposed to HIV and despite having received some doses of experimental vaccines have become infected. Unfortunately, there has been a public perception that the vaccines directly infected the volunteers," Pat said. Some of the people who had called her with this rumor during the past two weeks were probably in the room now, obscured by the glare of the lights.

"The members of this committee will certainly know that this is not possible. These vaccines are made by genetic engineering techniques. They do not and they never did include whole virus genomes or live viruses and they cannot be infectious," she said.

She aimed a laser pointer at the total shown on the slide—twelve HIV-infected participants in vaccine trials sponsored by NIAID or by corporations. This was the total a few days ago, Pat said, "but we have just in the past day turned up one additional case, which is in a gp120 trial." She went on to explain that when the infected volunteers had been interviewed, all admitted to having had contact with someone who was HIV positive, either sexually or by sharing needles.

These thirteen infections occurred among 1,450 volunteers in NIH trials and another few hundred in studies sponsored by corporations. Over-all, the incidence was low—less than 1 percent. One of the newly infected volunteers had received all the shots called for in a study of MicroGeneSys gp160; among gp120 volunteers, none had gotten the planned series of four immunizations. The informed consent forms and counseling sessions had always emphasized that experimental vaccines can't be viewed as protective and that people had to take precautions on their own. Now the Data and Safety Monitoring Board had decided to beef up these warnings and had asked trial sites to check more frequently for signs of infection in volunteers.

When Pat finished, hands shot up around the big table. Virologists wanted to know whether the volunteers had encountered a fierce or unusual strain of the virus. Immunologists wondered how the antibody responses of the infected few compared with vaccinees who remained healthy. And once vaccine recipients were infected, did they go downhill faster than other patients? The answers aren't in yet, Pat had to say; the work is in progress. And then Haase said that her time was up, and Pat headed back to her chair.

It was a point of pride for Pat that she was trusted by everyone she dealt with in the complicated world of vaccines, whether they were pinstriped executives or activists with Kool-Aid hair. Today she had told the truth and done it as dispassionately as she could. She had not been asked to sway the vote of the committee; her task was to provide them with some facts.

The next presentations by DAIDS staffers laid out a detailed picture of the choices ARAC faced. By the end of the day, committee members would have to vote on one of several choices. If they wished to go forward with efficacy testing, they would have to choose between a classic or a scaled-down version of a trial in which people would be randomly assigned either to one of the gp120 vaccines or to a placebo. A classic efficacy trial would require 9,000 volunteers, take three and a half years, and cost $9 million to $18 million per year. The up-front costs of recruiting and screening so many volunteers would be tremendous. On the plus side, a massive study like this doesn't miss much: It would certainly pick out a vaccine that worked more than 50 percent of the time, and it could probably tell if only one person in three was protected. Best of all, if approved at this meeting, this Cadillac of clinical trials could determine the value of gp120 vaccines by the year 1998.

A scaled-down, Chevy-type trial would enroll 4,500 volunteers and last only two years. For $4.5 million to $9 million per year, it could identify a completely useless vaccine or an effective one that protected people at least 60 percent of the time. It would cost less at the beginning and recruitment would be less daunting, but if test results fell in a large gray area, it would still be necessary to take the next step, which would be the Cadillac version. This trial could not get underway until 1997 at the earliest, and results would not be available for another three and a half years. Efficacy would be known after mid-2001.

The first people to shoot up their hands were statistically inclined committee members who asked technical questions about the two designs. This discussion of the proposed trials was as abstract as an exercise in a college statistics textbook until the focus shifted to the volunteers themselves. Uninfected gay men and IV drug users were the people most at risk and thus the ones where a vaccine's impact could best be seen, and the HIVNET sites had already identified 1,000 to 3,000 likely volunteers from these groups. Recruiting 6,000 to 8,000 more for a definitive efficacy trial might require 8,000 interviews, or it might mean screening 32,000 people. That was impossible to calculate.

Not every potential volunteer is enthusiastic about an experiment that pays nothing, requires lots of clinic visits, might make them test positive for HIV, and might inject them with a worthless placebo. And as ARAC member and long-time activist Martin Delaney pointed out, volunteers would be even harder to find if the AIDS community actively opposed the trial.

The next speaker on the agenda was Derek Hodel, a full-time AIDS activist and VWG member, who expanded on Delaney's comment. There is a highly organized constituency of HIV-positive people and their friends and loved ones, and they had become expert at navigating the federal system. Many of them were suspicious of experimental vaccines, he said, and they had the public's ear. The committee needed to realize that if the efficacy trial went forward, it would be vociferously opposed. No one would speak out on the other side, because there was no organized group of uninfected people to champion the vaccine cause.

Six presentations had rushed past in two and a half hours when Haase announced that it was time to adjourn for lunch. The committee members had been bombarded with thousands of details about the vaccines and the immune responses they elicit, laboratory tests of dubious value, imperfect animal models, clinical trials that sounded costly and complicated, and community activists who thought the vaccines might be a horrible government plot. It was enough to give anyone indigestion.

The Chiron and Genentech teams fidgeted through lunch together. They were eager to get their turn at the microphone. Back in California, they had agreed that Don would open, Dino Dina would follow, and Anne-Marie Duliege would close. Phil, Faruk, and the others were spear carriers, unless they needed to supply scientific details that one of the speakers had momentarily lost.

Even people who disagree with Don's views acknowledge that he can be a charismatic speaker, although a bit too preachy for some. His purpose at this meeting was to deliver a barn burner that would rouse the committee from its post-lunch torpor. He was determined to use words and pictures to bring the human carnage of the epidemic into the Crystal Ballroom: There were 5,000 new infections a day worldwide, and even if the epidemic magically stopped right now, it would still leave 750,000 dead Americans in its wake. Francis juxtaposed slides of the AIDS quilt laid out on the Washington Mall with images of the Vietnam Memorial, saying that it took ten years for 50,000 people to die in Vietnam, but it was taking only one year for the same number to die of AIDS in the United States. In other countries the situation was much worse, and without a vaccine the death toll would continue to climb.

The need for a vaccine was urgent, Don insisted, and even a partially protective one would slow the rate at which the virus was rampaging around the globe. Money, he suggested, should not stand in the way of doing an efficacy trial. The total cost of medical care for people with AIDS had reached $10 million per day in the United States, which made the price of even a full-scale efficacy trial appear trivial. Conducting one year of a definitive trial would cost no more than two days of treatments for Americans with AIDS.

Francis was a hard act to follow and Dino Dina knew it. So he used his status as president of Chiron Biocine to present himself as a model of executive reserve. The companies and the NIH had agreed on what it would take for a vaccine to advance to an efficacy trial, he said, and Chiron had honored its part of that pact. Dina turned the microphone over to Anne-Marie, the medical director for the gp120 project. Having worked on HIV vaccine trials at Genentech and Chiron, Anne-Marie had become passionate about the need for a large-scale study.

Although scientists disagreed about the technical merits of the gp120 vaccines and although bad publicity had recently prejudiced the public against them, "scientifically and ethically we should do a definitive trial," Anne-Marie said. Not a small trial that would yield uncertain results, but a full-scale study that would settle the protectiveness question. Chiron had new ideas about improving their vaccine formulation, and she was confident that a trial approved now would be able to test state-of-the-art technology.

For hours, committee members had listened to academics and government employees comment on the pros and cons of the gp120 vaccines. But if they had any questions for the people who actually made these products, they were out of luck. Without skipping a beat, Haase plowed ahead as soon as Anne-Marie uttered her closing words. "I am going to go now to the public comment portion, and the first person to speak will be Dr. Donald Burke," the chairman said. He held a list, prepared by ARAC's executive secretary, of people who had signed up with her that morning.

Burke, who was still in charge of WRAIR's Division of Retrovirology at this point, spoke on behalf of Thai scientists who had been testing HIV vaccines made by American companies. In his opening remarks, Tony Fauci said he had received a letter from Thai researchers. They did not want ARAC's recommendations to slow their progress toward efficacy trials in Thailand, where the epidemic was spinning out of control and where there was no money for treatments. Burke reiterated that message and urged the committee to explicitly limit its focus to the United States when it came time to actually write a recommendation.

Burke was followed by a series of gay men, emissaries from the front lines of the AIDS epidemic, who delivered the kinds of morally charged statements that make academicians squirm in their seats. An Ichabod Crane-like figure from Boston shook his finger at the committee and warned that the proposed trials would have serious enrollment problems unless their benefits, both to individuals and to society, were clearer. A Latino activist waved a letter from the New York chapter of ACT UP, which called the trials "not only premature, but extremely unethical and dangerous." An HIV-positive man painted a nightmare scenario in which people with AIDS would demonstrate in front of vaccine trial sites, protesting the shift of NIH research funds from treatment to vaccines.

These remarks struck an emotional chord in some committee members, who felt that they should support whatever people from the most hard-hit parts of society wanted them to. Faruk thought committee members might have other, more personal reasons, for voting against an efficacy trial. Under the white drape of the committee table, these people probably felt a hand groping for their pockets. Most of them got grants from NIH, and most of those grants were not for vaccine work but for basic science, treatments, or risk reduction. If a definitive efficacy trial ended up costing $80 million, which it might, some of that money was bound to come out of their research budgets. Faruk did not find this thought encouraging.

Bill Snow, a well-regarded activist who was an adviser to NIH's clinical trials, asked the committee to look at the big picture. He reminded them that in the morning, Haase had presented four possible recommendations: Stop all research on gp120, do a definitive efficacy trial, do a limited version, or hold off on efficacy testing until a second type of vaccine could be compared with gp120. Yet the formal presentations from DAIDS had focused on two possible efficacy trials, Snow observed, neither one of which might be ideal from a scientific or social point of view. Why must a decision be made today, he asked? An unspoken answer flashed through the brain of more than one person at the committee table: "Because Tony wants an answer, and he wants it now."

The final public comment came from a physician-epidemiologist who had just left DAIDS for an academic post. For six years he had designed HIV vaccine trials, so no one was surprised when he spoke in favor of doing a big one. On that note, Dino Dina and Anne-Marie Duliege quietly made their way out of the ballroom. Business demanded that they catch a plane to Paris, and they now left Faruk as Chiron's sole representative in the room.

The minute that Haase called for discussion, a dozen hands went up and he scribbled down names, then began working his way down the list. The result was a jumble. A statistician jumped on fine points of trial design, the next speaker mused about the benefits of safe-sex counseling for volunteers, and the next wanted an update on primate studies. People had their say without making reference to what had gone before.

In this atmosphere, highly questionable assertions went unchallenged. A famous primate researcher predicted that within six months, animal studies would reveal which laboratory results correlated with protection in humans. People who didn't know better could have seen this as a good reason for postponing an efficacy trial. Larry Corey, one of two "no" votes at the VWG, told ARAC that the prime-boost strategy might be ready for clinical testing in twelve to fourteen months, which subsequent speakers took to mean that it could enter an efficacy trial by 1996. Why go ahead with gp120, some members must have asked themselves, if exciting new discoveries are just over the horizon? But there was no time to talk about this at length.

Faruk and the other corporate representatives sat silent, because the rules of the meeting did not permit them to speak. If only they could respond to what was being said, they would help the committee get a better grip on the realities of vaccine development. Faruk did primate work, he kept up with what was happening, and he knew that no one was close to finding correlates of protection in animals. As for the prime-boost strategy, which Chiron was working on with Pasteur Mérieux Connaught, he knew it had a long way to go before an efficacy trial would make sense. A few seats away, Tim Gregory practically writhed in frustration. "Our hands were tied and we had tape over our mouths," he said.

During a short afternoon break, Clark Kent stepped into a phone booth and the Man of Steel emerged. Ashley Haase was freshly determined to get a decision before the scheduled adjournment at 5:30. "Please make your comments crisp," he said. "I want to hear concrete proposals, however flawed." But the committee members continued on a meandering course that did not flow clearly toward a decision of any kind. Some people were preoccupied with laboratory assays, some with animal studies. Others mused about doing an efficacy trial at some future time, when a type of vaccine other than gp120 could be included. And one member proposed a trial bigger than a Phase II and smaller than a Phase III, which Haase facetiously dubbed a Phase 2.76.

Finally, when the clock had passed 4:00 and Haase could feel the scheduled adjournment drawing near, he lost patience and lopped off the two most dramatic choices facing the committee. Unless somebody objected, he said, shelving the products was off the table and so was the 9,000-person efficacy trial. No one said a word. Haase's first efforts to draft a recommendation snagged on how big an efficacy trial should be, but he steered the focus away from size and toward the issue of timing. Several members felt that an efficacy trial should be postponed until gp120 and a second vaccine approach could be tested in tandem. There was much haggling about exactly how the recommendation should be worded, and finally a draft was projected on an overhead transparency.

"Do I hear a call to vote? A motion, please," Haase said.

He recognized a public-health professor from Maryland, but she disappointed him by not moving the vote. Instead, she haltingly said that she did not think the committee had enough time to formulate a recommendation. "I would like to suggest that what we do is develop a—some people may not like this—a subcommittee of ARAC members, the Council, the Vaccine Working Group, and really comb through this information some more and then come back."

Haase shook his head.

"You said no? You won't even put it up?"

"If you have a recommendation, a motion, we can discuss that," Haase said. And he got a motion from the next person he called on, which was then amended and tinkered with by other speakers. The most substantive suggestion came from Susan Zolla-Pazner, who wanted to make sure that the gp120 vaccines could be advanced to an efficacy trial on the basis of new scientific findings about them, rather than having to wait for prime-boost or some other strategy to mature.

In the end, the proposed vote was a restatement of the status quo: "The Institute should continue ongoing programs and current trials of the two gp120 vaccine candidates, as well as the development of other candidates. NIAID should proceed with expanded clinical trials when other concepts and/or compelling data from current studies are available." Fewer than

700 people had been injected with gp120 so far. If the recommendation passed, they were likely to remain members of a very exclusive club.

"What I am going to do now is go around the table and we are going to record everyone's votes. Your choices are yes, no, or abstain," Haase said. The room was tense and silent during the roll call, and pens moved swiftly to tally the count: twenty-three in favor of the recommendation and four abstentions. Several members moved swiftly to tack on a motion limiting the ARAC's recommendation to trials in the United States. It passed quickly, and Haase adjourned the meeting at 5:25.

As soon as it was over, Tony Fauci huddled briefly with Killen and a few others, then headed straight for the eager reporters. Ordinarily he would have gone to the industry representatives first, to shake hands and assure them of his continued goodwill and his desire to work together in the future. Instead, speaking just in time for the evening news, Fauci told reporters that he accepted the committee's recommendation and that it was now the official position of the NIAID. "Dr. Fauci denied that the recommendation was a setback to the development of an AIDS vaccine, though he said that others might view the recommendation as having a chilling effect on the drug industry," Lawrence Altman reported in the next day's *New York Times*. The article also quoted Fauci as saying that it would be another two or three years before any efficacy trials could be done.

The minute the meeting was adjourned, Don Francis had come out of his seat like a feral dog whose pup had been attacked, bearing down on luckless members of the committee. Later he would say, his eyes widening with amazement at the shortsightedness of others, "They had no idea that what they did was kill vaccines."

Faruk was stunned by the realization that the world was different now, changed by a one-day meeting that ended five minutes early. This was nothing like the afterglow of the VWG meeting, only two months earlier, when the future seemed boundless and bright. Now Faruk had been nearly sleepless for two days and was demoralized and exhausted, but he wasn't off-duty yet. Dino and Anne-Marie were on a plane over the Atlantic. Only Faruk remained to deliver the bad news to Chiron headquarters.

He made his way out of the room and across the ballroom lobby, taking a left toward the bathrooms, where he recalled seeing a bank of telephones. He arrived at exactly the same moment as all the reporters who had just finished talking with Fauci. Less than twenty-four hours ago he had been a key member of a team with a shot at beating AIDS. Now he was a rumpled, exhausted man clutching a corporate phone card, fighting to hold his place against people who had lots of experience winning the race for a phone.

Finally Faruk got through to Corey Dekker, the vice president for Chiron's clinical department, who was in her office on the edge of San Francisco Bay. He told her the outcome, read off the votes, and concluded, "We are stuck. We are not going anywhere." He could barely hear her reply over the bedlam in the hallway. Faruk hung up and headed upstairs to catch a cab to the airport. That westbound flight has remained the most depressing journey of his life.

Two levels up from the Crystal Ballroom, in the atrium of the Hyatt, committee members gathered at the cocktail lounge to unwind from a tense day under the television lights. But instead of seeing themselves on the big screen above the bar, they saw O. J. Simpson in his white Bronco, leading a dreamy parade of patrol cars. None of them could have predicted, on that infamous night in 1994, that O. J. would get two verdicts in the courts long before gp120—or any other AIDS vaccine—would get one in a clinical trial.

III

GOING TO TRIAL

July 1994–August 2000

IO

THE BIG CHILL

KATHY STEIMER WAS HAUNTED by insomnia during the summer of 1994. She would lie wide-eyed in the darkness, brain racing, while her husband Martin slept beside her. Eventually she would get up, wrap herself in a warm robe, and go downstairs to the living room, trailed by Leroy, her big black poodle. She would pick up a novel, perhaps something by Margaret Atwood or Louise Erdrich, and nestle into an oversized green leather chair. The poodle would wedge himself into the chair beside her.

The house was in Benicia, a small town an hour north of San Francisco. The room where Kathy sat was large, with a cathedral ceiling and a freestanding wood stove, and had a glass wall overlooking the Carquinez Strait. On clear nights she could see the lights of Port Costa shimmering on the opposite side; other times the fog blotted out everything beyond the giant rosemary hedge in the front yard. Kathy's view of her own life was much the same—sometimes dazzlingly clear, sometimes dismally obscured.

When Tony Fauci decided not to go forward with the efficacy trial, effectively stalling development of the gp120 vaccine she had designed a decade earlier, Kathy was not surprised. Her own experiments, after all, had cast doubt on the vaccine's power to protect. The media had sensationalized breakthrough infections in the Phase II trial, AIDS activists had come out against expanded testing, and NIH had reaffirmed its commitment to doing basic rather than clinical research.

Kathy had surveyed this dismal landscape and decided that she could not bring herself to attend the AIDS Research Advisory Committee meeting in June.

As a result, she missed hearing Fauci's prediction that not going forward with the gp120 efficacy trial might have a "chilling effect" on industry. But she certainly felt the temperature plunge at Chiron after the ARAC meeting. The NIH's willingness to pay for clinical trials had been a major incentive for all the biotech companies working on experimental HIV vaccines. With that incentive gone, the scientists and laboratory technicians who worked for Kathy were shell-shocked and afraid for their jobs. She felt obliged to protect them.

At the same time, Kathy was so burned out that she considered leaving Chiron entirely. She had given twelve years of her life to the company, working day and night, worrying all the time. And her work had been appreciated: She had gained an international reputation in AIDS research and had been rewarded with a series of promotions. Nevertheless, in the weeks following the ARAC meeting, the quieter world of academia seemed more alluring than the biotech pressure cooker. She had strong ties to the University of California-Davis, where the faculty included her husband Martin Wilson, her close friend Kathryn Radke, and her former colleague Paul Luciw, with whom she had done pioneering work on HIV a decade earlier. UC-Davis announced that an endowed research chair was available, and although it wasn't a perfect fit for her credentials, Kathy decided to apply.

Kathryn Radke was on the search committee and was asked to call people Kathy had listed as references. Years later, Kathryn remembered the horrified reaction of Pat Fast, head of the HIV vaccine program at DAIDS, upon being told that Kathy might leave vaccines for academic research. "We can't lose her. It would be a national disaster," Pat insisted to Kathryn. As it turned out, Pat need not have worried: The hiring committee offered the chair to someone else. Even if the UC-Davis job had come through, Kathryn wasn't sure her old friend could have abandoned the work that had obsessed her for so long.

Once Kathy knew she would remain at Chiron, she had to deal with the unfinished business of making a vaccine. The first step was to make sure that her carefully assembled HIV vaccine team would still be there if more funding became available later. She found slots for them on other projects she controlled, such as the analytical immunology department. There, scientists like Faruk Sinangil, who had helped her develop assays for measuring immune responses to gp120, switched gears and did lab work for experimental vaccines against herpes, flu, and other viruses.

Under the circumstances, it was a bold step when Kathy hired a new scientist, Susan Barnett, to do another experiment with gp120. Kathy had already shown that chimpanzees immunized with gp120 were protected against challenge with SF2, the HIV strain on which the vaccine was based. But so what? Kathy and other virologists now regarded SF2 as a tame, laboratory-adapted strain that might be far too easy to defeat. Before Kathy gave up on gp120, she wanted to know whether it could protect other animals against a more virulent type of HIV—a virus more like a tiger than a tabby.

Susan Barnett's scientific background was nearly as varied as Kathy's own. After getting a Ph.D. in molecular biology, Susan had done cancer research, worked with animal models, and learned virology as a postdoc in the UC-San Francisco lab of Jay Levy, who supplied the virus samples that Kathy had grown years earlier at the spooky Navy Biosciences Lab. Susan's diverse skills would be essential if Kathy could get support to move beyond first-generation vaccines like gp120 and tackle newer technologies like live vectors and naked DNA.

At the same time, Kathy continued to champion clinical trials. Even when she was deeply depressed and uncertain about her future at Chiron, she did everything possible to ensure that clinical testing of gp120 would go forward. Her main ally in this was John McNeil from the army, who had persuaded her to work on a clade E-based gp120 for Thailand. Right after the ARAC meeting, she had sent an SOS that brought John and Don Burke, his boss, to Chiron in early July.

Kathy had arranged for them to meet with Bill Rutter and Ed Penhoet, Chiron's founders, to sell the idea of army-sponsored clinical trials in Thailand. The plan was to begin with small-scale tests of SF2 gp120, followed by studies of the new clade E vaccine. These experiments would recruit heterosexual volunteers in Bangkok and the northern city of Chiang Mai, where HIV was spreading most rapidly. Because the U.S. armed services theoretically exclude male homosexuals and IV drug users, they were primarily interested in vaccines that could prevent the heterosexual spread of AIDS. This was how most people in Thailand became infected, so results gained from studying them could be generalized to soldiers.

The army would pay to conduct the clinical trials in Thailand. Chiron's part of the bargain would be to supply vials of the original gp120 product, which had already been manufactured, and to put the finishing touches on the clade E vaccine and produce enough of it for Phase I testing. This was a commitment that Rutter and Penhoet were willing to make after talking with John McNeil and Don Burke.

"Kathy was eager to do the trials, and we thought that we wouldn't be doing any harm to the subjects and we might learn something very valuable. There was at least some probability that it might save a few lives," Penhoet later reflected. He believed testing would be more beneficial in Thailand than in the United States, where some feared that gay male volunteers, assuming the experimental vaccine would keep them safe, would forget about safe sex and intentionally take more sexual risks. Penhoet didn't see this as a problem for a Thai trial. "In Thailand, there's a lot less individual choice in risky behavior. People are exposed because they are sex workers, or they are exposed because they are addicts," Penhoet said. "That was the primary human reason for pursuing this."

Despite the high-profile cancellation of the domestic efficacy trial, smaller gp120 trials were still being conducted at U.S. government expense. In late 1992, NIH officials had brokered a collaboration between Chiron and Pasteur Mérieux Connaught, which coupled gp120 with PMC's canarypox vector in a prime-boost immunization scheme. Ordinarily the two companies would have been competitors, not allies. But with NIH footing the bill for all the prime-boost studies, including elaborate and expensive immunology testing, executives at Chiron and PMC would have been fools to say no. Besides, everyone would gain if the prime-boost approach proved successful.

By October, Kathy had reason to sleep better. Although her HIV vaccine program had been scaled back, it was still alive, and Bill Rutter reassured her that she was squarely in charge. Chiron had also acquired Via-gene, a small biotech company in San Diego that designed live vectors for gene therapy—vectors that Kathy and Rutter agreed had promise as vac-cines. She spoke up in favor of clinical testing in Thailand and traveled to Bangkok to address Thai researchers at a conference organized by the powerful Dr. Natth Bhamarapravati. Although the NIH decision had def-initely cooled HIV vaccine development at Chiron, Kathy was not out of the game.

●

The situation was worse at Genentech, where Tony Fauci's predicted "chilling effect" hit like a freak ice storm in July. Tim Gregory, who had manufactured the company's gp120, came home from the ARAC meeting hopping mad. "We were politically naive, because we thought that win-ning the scientific case in front of the Vaccine Working Group the month before was enough. We thought that science would talk and bullshit would walk, but that's not the way it works at NIH," fumed Tim.

The internal committee that set Genentech's research priorities now regarded gp120 as a loser. They had a potentially hot drug for breast can-cer in development, and they didn't want to spend another penny of their research budget on gp120. Phil Berman, notorious for his inability to take "no" for an answer, had a hard time wrapping his head around this. "We were in denial until September or October," he said. After all, corporate executives had told Phil to shelve HIV vaccines eight years earlier, then reneged when they found out the vaccine protected chimpanzees in an experiment Phil and Tim did on the sly. This time, however, the official word was that stealth vaccine activity was out of the question. "I wasn't supposed to work on this at all," Phil said.

His lab was filled with clones of HIV strains from the United States and Thailand, which he had expected to use in making new, improved ver-sions of gp120. But the hammer fell with such force that Phil's only option was to store them in freezers and shut down his lab. He was transferred to another part of the company to work on anti-inflammatory drugs, which he accepted because, as he said, "I just wanted to do something else."

Meanwhile, in the clinical affairs department at Genentech, Don Francis was having an equally difficult adjustment. "I kept thinking that some-one in the government would say, 'Oh, come on, this is ridiculous,'" he recalled. Don fired off letters to friends in high places at the Department of Health and Human Services, urging them to override Fauci's decision and push for an efficacy trial, but to no avail. "Pretty soon it became clear the government wasn't going to change." Nor was anyone on Capitol Hill willing to help: Members of Congress had appropriated $20 million for the MicroGeneSys trial, only to have it metamorphose into a giant, rolling dung-ball that fouled everyone it touched. No way would they stick their necks out for another AIDS vaccine.

Nor could Don rally support on the Genentech campus. Although the company had spent upward of $50 million on gp120, senior management had never thought through what would happen if NIH support faltered before the vaccine was fully tested. The company had charged ahead on the assumption that if it complied with NIH's every request, such as per-forming specific lab tests and supplying certain data, the trial would be approved and paid for. Obviously, they had been wrong. With no Plan B, Genentech now wanted to extricate itself from HIV vaccines as fast as possible.

Don was incensed. "I didn't know who I was going to get the money from, but an efficacy trial was such an obvious thing to do that somebody was going to have to support it. It was not an option to stop." Phil thought salvation was most likely to come from one of the large pharmaceutical companies, which could codevelop gp120 or else license the entire tech-nology from Genentech. Don and Phil, along with Tim Gregory and a friend from Genentech's business development office, spent several evenings drafting a proposal for out-licensing the vaccine.

Don, Tim, and their business adviser made pilgrimages to major drug companies in Switzerland, France, and elsewhere in Europe, desperately seeking someone willing to help with gp120. Time and again they struck out. Sometimes the rebuffs were brutal, as when a Pasteur Mérieux Con-naught representative told Don that "the only collaboration would be that your facility is used to make our gp160," referring to a protein subunit vac-cine that PMC has just begun to develop. After the NIH decision, gp120 was as appealing to drug company executives as a bouquet of poison ivy.

In mid-October, the World Health Organization tried to lift the gloom. WHO convened vaccine experts as an ad hoc advisory group on scientific and public-health reasons for going forward with a gp120 efficacy trial. Invited to meet in Geneva were not just the usual cast of characters from the United States and Europe but also scientists and public-health officials from Asia, Africa, and Latin America, where most of the world's 17 million HIV-infected people lived at that time.

After two days of discussion, the advisory group urged WHO to spearhead Phase III testing of the gp120 vaccines and identified Thailand as the country most likely to host such a study. Thai officials were alarmed by the wildfire spread of subtype B virus among Bangkok's large population of IV drug users and were willing to recruit them as volunteers for a gp120 study. But there were serious obstacles. Even if the government was willing, such a trial could not happen overnight. It would take at least two years for approvals and logistic arrangements, and even then WHO would probably not have the money to pay for such an undertaking.

Still, the enthusiasm of WHO's advisory group helped prolong the life of Genentech's gp120 project, which had shrunk from forty people to one full-time scientist, Don Francis, and a couple of part-time workers. "At least we were alive," Don said after the Geneva meeting. "We weren't kicking, but at least we were alive." The plan was to get started as soon as possible with a Phase I study in Bangkok, funded jointly by the Thai government, WHO, and Genentech.

Genentech had some 300,000 doses of vaccine stored in South San Francisco, and shipping the amount needed for a fifty-person trial to Bangkok would cost little. Beyond that, the company would need to kick in only $30,000 for the Phase I study—peanuts compared with the more than $50 million that it had already invested in gp120. Still, the corporate head of medical affairs, who oversaw all of Genentech's clinical trials, made Don practically beg for this small sum. And when the medical affairs head later discovered that he had signed up to spend $30,000 per year for a two-year study, he was angry because "he thought he had been sandbagged for $30,000," Don recalled.

Genentech's total revenues for 1994 were nearly $800 million; $30,000 was about what the company would pay a lab technician for a year's work.

When Don had to go to the mat for $30,000, he knew that the vaccine was doomed at Genentech. His only hope was to come up with millions of dollars from someplace else, and fast.

●

The chill that ARAC cast on Genentech and Chiron didn't reach Pasteur Mérieux Connaught, even though the company wanted to boost its canarypox vaccine with Chiron's gp120. In the executive suite in Paris, PMC medical and scientific director Stanley Plotkin was comfortable with Tony Fauci's decision. He thought Fauci was right not to spend millions of dollars testing two nearly identical products, both designed to elicit antibodies but neither capable of arousing a cellular immune response. "My opinion was that if you could set up a trial to test antibodies and cellular immunity comparatively, that would have been worth doing," Plotkin said. "Had the canarypox been ready I would have argued strongly for a comparative trial. It would have been worthwhile." PMC was still struggling to manufacture canarypox in large quantities, however, and Plotkin thought these vectors needed other improvements as well. But he was confident that when PMC was ready, NIH would surely pay for an efficacy study.

Sitting in his lab at Virogenetics, the tiny Troy, New York, outpost of the PMC empire, Enzo Paoletti's initial reaction was that Fauci's decision "had put a damper on the whole field." Like Plotkin, however, he thought it was irrelevant to canarypox's chances for an efficacy trial down the road. He worried less about large-scale trials in the distant future than about the incessant demands made on him by PMC executives in Paris. "Improve the vector, improve the vector," that was the message Enzo heard over and over again. Phase I studies had been going on since 1993, and it was obvious that the corporate guys were not satisfied with the level of cytotoxic T cell activity stimulated by vCP125, the prototype HIV vaccine that Enzo had made. In some trials as few as 15 percent of volunteers developed CTLs against HIV; in others, as many as 40 percent did. Plotkin and the other top executives wanted to see more.

The only antigen delivered by vCP125 was the gene for gp160, the full-length version of HIV's envelope protein. If other antigens could be added to the payload, perhaps more vaccinees would make CTLs and maybe those T cells would recognize and destroy more strains of HIV. Enzo and Jim Tartaglia, his right-hand man in the laboratory, packaged three additional HIV genes into their original canarypox vector and renamed it vCP205. By May 1995, the NIH was testing this version in a Phase I trial. Leading the study was Larry Corey, the University of Washington researcher who was a cheerleader for the prime-boost approach during the ARAC meeting.

In addition to wanting more HIV genes in the mix, PMC was pressuring Enzo to reengineer the vector itself. The French production team complained that canarypox was difficult to grow and that the yield was too low to permit large-scale manufacture. Enzo still seethed over PMC's refusal to set up a manufacturing facility in Troy, insisting that low yields were the fault of human laziness and lack of skill rather than flaws in his vector. So instead of reengineering the delivery system, Enzo inserted pieces of two more HIV genes into the same old canarypox, bringing the total to six antigens, and dubbed it vCP300. For reasons that he never understood, this version would prove even harder for the French to make than the earlier vectors. And this was not a good thing.

●

"Make a new plan, Stan," Paul Simon advises in "Fifty Ways to Leave Your Lover." This was generally Kathy Steimer's philosophy when something in her life didn't go right: Instead of moping endlessly over what had gone wrong, she went after the next big thing. In January 1995, however, she hesitated when offered the chance to become vice president of Chiron Biocine Research, part of the international vaccine operation owned jointly by Chiron and Ciba-Geigy. Instead of supervising thirty people, in the new job she and the scientific director of Biocine in Italy would share oversight of 180 researchers. In addition to research and development of new products, Biocine marketed adult and pediatric vaccines in Europe, Scandinavia, the United States, Canada, and Australia. It was a big business.

Kathy told Ed Penhoet and Bill Rutter that instead of taking on the title of vice president, she would like to try doing the job. She would be promoted to senior director and would do the work of the vice president for one year. If she liked it and performed well, they would name her vice president the following January.

Once Kathy took on her new responsibilities, she became a global player no matter what it said on her business card. She was also in demand as a conference speaker and a member of national and international review panels and advisory groups. Her horizons had expanded far beyond the confines of the laboratories where she had forged her reputation as an HIV researcher.

Still, even after Kathy was promoted, "she would sit down with technicians and go over data herself, and do troubleshooting. She would spend extra time and weekends doing that. She liked the scientific detail," Susan Barnett recalled. Most scientists-turned-executives, in contrast, get rusty so fast that technicians bar the door if they come near the lab.

No matter what else was on her plate, Kathy did not ignore gp120. NIH was testing it as a boost for PMC's vCP205, and Kathy threw her support behind the army's August 1995 launch of a Phase I study in Thailand.

Even though her job responsibilities had expanded dramatically, Kathy remained 100-percent committed to the making of an AIDS vaccine. Looking to the future, she and Susan had especially high hopes for the hot new naked-DNA technology.

●

Don Francis and biotech entrepreneur Robert C. Nowinski shook hands for the first time in the early summer of 1995, on the steps of a beautiful Tudor house outside Seattle. They strolled through exquisitely landscaped grounds to a brick terrace on the edge of a bluff overlooking Puget Sound. Four Roman columns stood sentinel, and there were snowcapped mountains in the distance. The men spent the day talking about their childhoods and families, about where they came from and what mattered in their lives so far.

By the end of the day, these two strangers recognized in each other something surprising and essential and familiar.

Don was fifty-three, Bob three years younger. Don was still boyish, with a shock of tawny hair falling over a forehead made only marginally higher by the passing years, and looking at him now it was easy to envision him during his hippie years. Bob had the calculated simplicity of a man who does not need to advertise his status with a Rolex, expensive jewelry, or electronic gizmos hitched to his belt. His long face was set off by modishly small eyeglasses with metal frames, his salt-and-pepper hair and beard were shaved into a burr. He could have been from anywhere, except for the Brooklyn accent that persisted after more than two decades in Seattle.

Don had spent twenty-one years of his professional career in the U.S. Public Health Service, and Genentech was the only company he had ever worked for. Bob had founded and sold three biotech companies before he turned fifty. The stately home was his, of course, bought after the sale of his first business.

The catalyst for this meeting was George Baxter, a New Jersey attorney for whom Don and Bob had each served as expert witnesses in product liability cases. In separate trials, they had testified on behalf of people who were infected with HIV after being transfused with contaminated blood. Don's crusade to force blood banks to screen for the AIDS virus made him famous in the early 1980s, inspired Randy Shilts to beatify him in his book *And the Band Played On*, and made him too controversial to be promoted within the CDC. Bob's first biotech company, Genetic Systems, developed one of the original HIV test kits used by blood banks, a test that was slow to be approved because it was based on the virus discovered in France, not on Bob Gallo's version.

Knowing that Don wanted to start a company and that Bob had the experience Don needed, George Baxter brokered the introduction that led to this meeting. Before flying up to Seattle, Don did an on-line search on Bob "to find out if he was on the up-and-up." Originally trained in New York as a retrovirologist, Bob had been a thirty-six-year-old full professor at the University of Washington when he left academia in 1981 to found Genetic Systems. Soon afterward, he teamed up with Syntex and Bristol-Myers to start Oncogen, where Shiu-Lok Hu created the first live-vector HIV vaccine ever tested in humans in the developed world.

By the time that landmark trial took place in 1988, Bob had already sold Genetic Systems and Oncogen to Bristol-Myers. This 1986 transaction was said to be a Borgia-like drama filled with back stabbing and intrigue. According to the articles that Don found on-line, Bob Nowinski had pissed off everyone involved in the deal, alienated his strongest supporters, and walked away with $6 million for himself and a spot as vice president of Bristol-Myers. His enemies dubbed him "No-lose-ski." Three years later, Bob left Bristol-Myers under a cloud, returned to Seattle, and started another biotech in 1989. By 1991, he was no longer part of that arrangement, reportedly forced out by his partners. He had started yet another biotech in 1992, which he had just sold his interest in when he and Don met in 1995.

"I saw all of his problems, how it had come down to war with every company he started," Don said. "I knew all about him before I went up and talked to him."

Bob Nowinski, for his part, had done no research on Don Francis at all. He knew Don's name because they had both started out in retrovirology. But he had never read *And the Band Played On,* nor had he seen the HBO movie. During their preliminary phone conversation, Bob learned that Genentech was eager to get rid of gp120. He knew Don was determined to start a company to conduct efficacy trials and, assuming that the vaccine worked, take it all the way to market. He also figured Don hadn't a clue about how to make this happen.

Once the two of them had settled on the terrace with the panoramic view, Bob asked Don "to open up and tell me about yourself." Take several hours if you want, he invited, and then I'll do the same. Don talked about growing up in Marin County as the child of two doctors, and the battle with dyslexia that plagued his childhood. He had attended UC-Berkeley in the prerevolutionary era when it was a repressive powder keg about to explode into the 1964 Free Speech Movement. In medical school he had become an activist for civil rights and against war, traveled to India before starting his internship, and signed on with the Centers for Disease Control as an alternative to being drafted.

There, Don forgot all about becoming a regular pediatrician as CDC transformed him into a warrior against "dangerous bugs." He was dispatched over the years to hot zones like Africa, where he investigated outbreaks of cholera and Ebola, and to India where he worked to control smallpox. Of all the bugs he fought, HIV was the one that caught and held his attention for twenty years.

AIDS and Randy Shilts had made him famous, and his fame kept Genentech from showing him the door after the NIH trial fell through. Don had extraordinary access to reporters, and Genentech's top executives did not want to open the morning paper and read "Famed AIDS Research Says Greed Caused Genentech to Ditch AIDS Vaccine."

Company executives were relieved when Don did not trash Genentech in a high-profile story titled "Who Put the Lid on gp120?" that ran in the *New York Times Magazine* in late March. But writer Jesse Green treated Don as an icon, making his bulldog-like devotion to the vaccine sound so heroic that the top brass were reminded why they wanted to stay on his good side. Don knew his celebrity bought time and gave him leverage to spin off gp120, but so far he'd been thwarted at every turn. None of his political contacts in San Francisco, including rich people who had backed his public-health campaigns when he worked for CDC, would give Don a dime toward a start-up company.

Bob learned all this about Don during that first long meeting, and he reciprocated by revealing aspects of his life story that weren't reflected in the newspaper and magazine stories Don found on-line.

Although Bob probably stopped short of saying he was experiencing a midlife crisis when Don turned up on his doorstep, he admitted he was uncertain about exactly where he was heading just now. He had been highly successful as a biotech entrepreneur, yet his only business enterprise now was a high-end art gallery that handled a mix of contemporary artists and works by modern masters like Picasso. He was fifty years old, with three young children and a shaky marriage.

Thirty-five years earlier, when he was a geeky high-school student, Bob landed a part-time job at Sloan-Kettering's research facility in Rye, New York. He got so excited about retrovirus research that he skipped classes to rush to the lab. Bob barely graduated from high school and scraped through college because the only place he really wanted to be was the lab. He was the despair of his parents, who wanted him to make good grades and become a doctor. His lab-rat habits served him well, of course, in graduate school and in his years as an academic researcher.

Both he and Don knew what it was like to be gripped by what Bob called "the divine obsession," although years later he inscribed quotes around the term with an ironic laugh. This capacity for throwing themselves headlong into something, putting everything else on hold, drew the two men together.

When they finally did get around to talking about gp120, Don asked Bob what would motivate him to work toward a vaccine against AIDS. "And he said, 'I've got three small kids.' And that was it. Bob was the person. I never looked at another person or explored anything else."

●

The two executives from Pasteur Mérieux Connaught arrived in Troy, New York, on Friday, October 13, 1995. One was Philip Kourilsky, Paris-based director of corporate research and development for PMC, and the other was a lower-ranking U.S. executive. Troy had fallen on such hard times that the city was $50 million in debt and there was a "for sale" sign on City Hall. They passed blocks of forlorn and empty storefronts on their way to pick up Enzo Paoletti at Virogenetics. The plan was to have lunch together, but because there was no place in Troy where anyone would go for an expense-account meal, especially not anyone accustomed to eating in Paris, they crossed the Hudson River into Albany.

Over lunch, Kourilsky told Enzo that Virogenetics's payroll was about to be cut by 70 percent. If downsized employees were willing to relocate, they would be offered jobs at other PMC facilities in North America. The remaining 30 percent would remain in Troy and work on the vaccine program, which would continue on a smaller scale. And then it happened. "He told me that I, a person of my stature, would not want to be involved any further with such a reduced entity and that I should go back to academia," Enzo said. "I was fired. And after that, they went out of their way to let the scientific community know that they had fired me."

Jim Tartaglia, who had been working with Enzo off and on since he was a graduate student in the early 1980s, was not surprised "Kourilsky and Enzo never got along, from the time that Kourilsky took over," he said. One wedge between them was that Kourilsky was a scientific administrator who thrived in complex hierarchies.

Enzo was at heart a loner, someone not constitutionally suited to function as a cog in an industrial machine. He had understood from the beginning that he could not make an AIDS vaccine on his own; and he and the late David Axelrod had worked hard to secure corporate backing for the project. Even though he knew PMC's partnership was essential, Enzo railed against the slow pace of canarypox development, complied grudgingly with demands that he change the vector, and generally didn't bother to conceal his disdain for how the big company operated. Enzo's passionate conviction—that he had discovered the key to a successful AIDS vaccine—probably blinded him to the realities of life at PMC, where "canarypox was not the only horse in the field," in the words of Stanley Plotkin, the company's scientific and medical director.

Six months before Enzo was fired, PMC had entered into a new agreement with Agence Nationale de Recherches sur le SIDA, the French equivalent of the NIH Division of AIDS. Half of all the AIDS research done by the company was underwritten by contracts and grants from ANRS, and that money, like all government funding, had strings attached. The agreement obligated PMC to pursue four approaches to AIDS vaccines: recombinant poxviruses, noninfectious viral particles, a gp160 protein subunit, and synthetic peptides. In addition, PMC agreed to develop new antigens for clade A and E viruses, which are common in Africa and Asia, in addition to B-based vaccines like the ones Enzo had made.

Plotkin, who was responsible for overseeing PMC's entire scientific portfolio, was an American who had mastered the Gallic shrug. "The history of Virogenetics is a typical history of a biotech company in this era. It started out with a good idea, the scientists tried to make something commercial out of their discovery, it eventually got bought up by a larger company. This is what biotechs hope will happen," he said. If the canarypox vectors had stimulated killer T cell activity against HIV in a majority of volunteers and if the vectors had been cheap and easy to manufacture in large quantities, Virogenetics would have grown and prospered.

Instead, the concept fell out of favor at PMC when canarypox vectors produced disappointing immune results and proved devilishly hard to make. Given this situation, it was probably inevitable that Enzo would be unhappy and his divorce from the company would be ugly. Negotiations for a severance agreement lasted for two full years after his dismissal, and loose ends remained for twice that long. Neither Enzo nor Plotkin would ever say exactly what the sticking points were.

●

Two days before Kathy Steimer was scheduled to leave for a Thanksgiving vacation in Mexico with her family, something very odd happened. The events are engraved in her husband Martin's memory. "She developed a strange symptom that alarmed me enormously. The left half of her tongue was paralyzed; the right-hand side was fine. She had sensation, but it became paralyzed. She could speak okay, but she would bite her tongue by mistake. When you looked at it, it was clearly deviated on that side and she couldn't move the muscles," recalled Martin, who is a neuroscientist by profession. "I knew instantly that it was a cranial nerve problem and my immediate suspicion was that it was a brain tumor at the base of her skull."

And he was right. What he could not have guessed was that the tiny tumor pressing on the cranial nerve was insignificant compared with the large malignant mass in Kathy's mediastinum, the middle of her chest where the heart is packed together with the esophagus, lymph nodes, and other essential parts. After weeks of inconclusive answers from neurological workups, blood tests, X-rays, and CAT scans, doctors used a special endoscope to snip a bit of tissue from the mass. They expected the tissue to show that the tumor was some type of lymphoma, a cancer that arises from the lymphatic system.

Although hospital pathologists would be scrutinizing the specimen, that wasn't enough for Kathy. Like many scientists, she believed that her own laboratory did better work than anyone else's. She authorized Alta Bates Hospital in Berkeley to give a bit of the biopsy sample to Susan Barnett and another Chiron molecular biologist. Soon the two young scientists found themselves running lab tests on a piece of flesh from their boss, who was only a decade older than they were, looking for specific cells that would tell them whether Kathy had a fast- or slow-moving type of lymphoma. To their astonishment, they found no lymphocytes at all.

It was nearly Christmas when all the tests were done and Kathy's doctors told her she had non-small-cell lung cancer. This was a shock to someone who had never smoked. Although the best treatment for such a tumor would be to cut it out, this one was already too large and invasive to be surgically removed. CAT scans also showed the cancer had spread to several parts of Kathy's skeleton, including her spine and pelvis. Kathy and Martin searched the medical literature, and what they read was bleak. Radiation could be used to try to slow tumor growth, and chemotherapy sometimes reduced symptoms and helped people live longer. But cure was out of the question. "We thought we might get some relief from treatment, but it was clear that it would only be a temporary thing," Martin said. "We looked at the statistics and figured that she might have a year."

Kathy brought a stack of articles about non-small-cell lung cancer to the office and asked Susan Barnett and the rest of the lab to read them "so we wouldn't be scared." Susan recalls that scared was hardly the word—they estimated she would be dead in six months and they were terrified. Once the diagnosis was made, Kathy and everyone around her realized she hadn't been well for some time. She was always tired and had lost weight, which they had attributed to a brutal travel schedule that had her constantly en route to the Biocine operation in Italy or to Washington for committee meetings. She had suffered persistent pain in one shoulder, but so do other people who always carry a laptop.

It had never occurred to Chiron CEO Ed Penhoet that anything could be seriously wrong with Kathy, who in the past had been a bit of a hypochondriac. He remembered a time in the early 1980s when she was sure she had AIDS, infected by some of the virus she'd grown in the lab. So he was stunned when Kathy told him she had lung cancer. Once the reality sank in, he and others went to work locating top doctors and state-of-the-art treatments. Emotionally, these efforts were as futile as trying to close a sucking chest wound with a Band-Aid. "Kathy was integral to the place," Penhoet said. "We had a natural response when she was sick, to care for one of our own who was in trouble. The news that she had this illness was devastating to everyone." Biotechnology was still a young industry and Chiron a young company, and this was the first life-threatening illness to hit one of its principal players.

"We sit here with all this technology, surrounded by the best molecular biology in the world, and one of our own comes down with lung cancer and there's not a thing we can do about it. It was frustrating beyond imagination," Penhoet said.

●

While Kathy struggled to come to terms with her illness, Don Francis spent several weeks during the fall of 1995 hunched over a laptop in a spare office at Heller, Ehrman, White & McAuliffe, a law firm perched in a glass-and-steel aerie on Fifth Avenue in downtown Seattle. This was the second time in less than six months that Don had been what amounted to the firm's writer-in-residence. Bob Nowinski had generally been right beside him as the two worked to get their new company off the ground. On this occasion, however, Bob was on the phone, calling from the dumpy little house where he'd been exiled since his marriage had spiraled toward a divorce. Despite being laid low by a severe case of pneumonia, Bob was trying to dictate revisions to the prospectus for the new company. He would utter a few hoarse words between coughing fits, and on the other end of the line, Don, who was not world's greatest typist, would painstakingly enter them into the draft.

Bob would hear: Click click click click "Oh SHIT!" Click click click click click "Oh SHIT."

"Don't say that, you're scaring me," Bob would say in exasperation. But Don would keep typing and cursing.

Earlier that summer, after the men bonded while overlooking Puget Sound, Bob began limbering up for the launch of his fourth biotech company in fourteen years. The first thing he did was fly down to South San Francisco to meet with Phil Berman. They sat together in Phil's orderly office, where raw data, results, and publications are neatly shelved in binders, and reviewed the entire history of gp120. Because Bob was a retrovirologist, he was interested in details most executives would have ignored. For example, he looked at the genetic sequences of the viruses that "broke through" to infect a handful of volunteers during the Phase I and II studies. Satisfied after this visit that the vaccine idea was scientifically sound, Bob was ready to start on the prospectus.

Bob and Don began their first stint at Heller Ehrman, working with two of the firm's attorneys to draft a prospectus for spinning off gp120. This document had to inform potential investors about every detail of the licensing agreement between Genentech and the new company, as well as give them a clear picture of HIV vaccine research in general and this product in particular. Genentech had the right to approve everything in the prospectus that pertained to them, and their lawyers and executives had scribbled all over the first draft. All these details had to be squared away before Don and Bob could start to raise capital.

Meanwhile, Genentech was in a state of upheaval. A few months earlier, controversial CEO Kirk Raab, a staunch supporter of Don's, had been ousted after it became known that he had gotten a large personal loan from Roche, the Swiss company that held the majority interest in Genentech. His successor was Arthur D. Levinson, one of the original "clone or die" guys from the early days, and more recently czar of the company's scientific agenda. When Levinson became CEO, investors weren't happy about a scientist taking command of such a large enterprise, so Levinson set out to win their trust by focusing resources on a few likely winners and ditching everything else. The gp120 vaccine fell squarely into the "if we're not going to do it, let's kill it" category.

As a result, Don and Bob had a new urgency about launching the company they dubbed Genenvax, in tribute to its origins. In November 1995, with the revised prospectus in hand, they completed all the legal steps needed to make it an official California corporation. Although the paperwork was finally done, the new company wasn't much to look at.

At Genentech, Don and his sole assistant took over some unused space in Building 7, home to lots of administrative offices and core facilities like the library. Phones, computers, and other necessities were provided by Genentech as part of the spin-off deal, but Don and his assistant were bumped whenever somebody more important needed the space where they were squatting. "People were awfully nice to us," Don recalled, "but when they had to decide who got space, we always got hind tit."

Nor was there a ticker-tape parade in February 1996, when Genentech officially announced the spin-off. A short news item in *Science* bore the headline "Investors Sought for AIDS Vaccine Trials" and identified Don Francis as "president and sole employee of Genenvax."[17] A later article in *Nature Medicine* misspelled the name of the company as "Genevax," but otherwise gave a fairly accurate account of the agreement that Don and Bob had negotiated. Genentech was putting up $1 million in seed money and would put in $1 million more if Don and Bob could raise at least $18 million from other sources. Only after they had secured funding would Genentech hand over exclusive rights to the gp120 technology.

In the gossipy world of HIV vaccines, the betting was that Don would never, ever be able to raise that kind of money.

●

Kathy seemed to be deteriorating so fast in January 1996 and suffering so mightily from the side effects of chemotherapy and radiation, that Martin feared she would be dead in a matter of weeks. Yet she went straight from treatments at the hospital to Chiron, hardly missing a day of work. She had a small pallet in her office where she would rest when overcome by pain or exhaustion.

Ironically, the one-year anniversary of her provisional promotion came during this miserable period. She was often too sick to get out of bed, and yet Penhoet and Rutter pressed her to accept the title of vice president of Chiron Biocine Research. It took all of Bill Rutter's persuasive charm, which is abundant, to convince Kathy she had earned the title, and there was nothing wrong with relishing the promotion and working only as much as she was able.

By early spring, when the hills of the San Francisco Bay area turn emerald green and the acacia trees are as bright as goldfinches, the cancer had backed off a bit and Kathy felt better. She and Martin were able to enjoy a reasonably good quality of life for a few months, even though she was never free from pain. Not surprisingly, she also spent more time at the office. Kathy had become increasingly well-dressed as she moved up the ladder at work, and during this period her outfits bordered on the flamboyant, as she chose colors that were more vibrant than the subdued tones she'd favored before. She covered her chemo-induced baldness with bright scarves and exotic hats from Mexico. Her back hurt when she drove her old stick-shift Honda, so Ed Penhoet loaned her a Mercedes with an automatic shift. She cut quite a figure on the expressway, commuting to work.

Everyone knew, of course, that this was only a temporary respite. And indeed, as the hills began drying out and fading to brown, the cancer was back with a vengeance. The bone metastases multiplied, spreading up and down Kathy's spine, into her hips, and into the bones of her legs and shoulders. The pain was unremitting and she tried every form of morphine available, though she disliked the dullness it brought. Still, she wanted to come to work, and Chiron hired a driver for days when she couldn't manage on her own. And then, inevitably, there came a time when even being a passenger hurt too much. Now Kathy's administrator and the senior scientists started coming to her home in Benicia, and senior staff meetings were often conducted by phone. For most of the ninety people she supervised, Kathy became a wraith seen less and less.

●

During 1996, 3.1 million previously healthy adults and children were newly infected with HIV, bringing to 23 million the number of people worldwide carrying the virus. A distressing 400,000 of the year's new cases were in children, most born to infected women in African, Latin American, and Asian countries where there was little hope of health care for mothers or their babies. So far, the AIDS pandemic had claimed 8.4 million lives. For 1996 alone, the death toll would reach 1.5 million by year's end.

As grim as these numbers were, the Eleventh International Conference on AIDS in July 1996 will always be remembered as one of the most optimistic moments in the history of the AIDS pandemic. Reading media coverage of the meeting, it is as though a golden shaft of sunlight split the overcast skies of Vancouver and illuminated the podium when David Ho stepped up to speak. Born in Taiwan and trained at Harvard, this forty-three-year-old physician was head of the Aaron Diamond AIDS Research Center in New York.

With his boyish face projected on giant screens that dwarfed the stage, Ho told a story that hundreds of thousands of AIDS patients were eager to hear. He described new findings about an experimental "cocktail" of three anti-HIV drugs: two were standard agents and the third was a new protease inhibitor, quite similar to the one that Merck was developing. Ho and his colleagues at ADARC, as the Diamond Center is usually known, had identified two dozen gay men who had been infected for less than ninety days. They began treatment immediately, and soon the amount of virus in their blood fell so low that it could not be measured in the lab. Not only that, but if a mathematical model of how HIV copies itself in the body turned out to be correct, then this regimen might eventually wipe out the virus completely. People could stop taking drugs and, for the first time, doctors could use the word "cure" in talking about AIDS. And even if the virus couldn't be eradicated and a true cure wasn't possible, the cocktail approach might let AIDS patients live normally for years, much like people with successfully treated diabetes or hypertension.

Ho's presentation touched off a rising storm of hype that culminated just before Christmas, when Ho was named *Time* magazine's 1996 Man of the Year. Along the way, hundreds of newspaper and magazine stories glorified not just Ho but the other scientists at ADARC, a small, privately endowed institution founded only seven years earlier. "The AIDS Dream Team" was the title of one especially adoring article. Eventually the publicity got so out of control that some of the irreverent gay men who volunteered for studies at ADARC nicknamed the director "Media Ho." Although the Vancouver AIDS conference was just the beginning, Ho and his colleagues knew they were destined for greatness.

At the Vancouver conference, the drug cocktail was such an obvious page-one story that many reporters wrote nothing about vaccine research. People who were naive about how epidemics spread and who did not understand that it is always better to prevent an infectious disease than to try to cure it may even have thought that this wonderful new treatment meant it was no longer so important to search for a vaccine.

Most scientists, of course, knew better. Some came to the vaccine sessions on the program, including one with Phil Berman of Genentech and John Moore from ADARC. Both presented studies of volunteers infected during the Phase I and II gp120 trials. These were the "breakthrough" infections that had helped torpedo the proposed Phase III study two years earlier, in June 1994, and the views of these two speakers could not have been more different.

Phil and John Moore used the same approach: They both scrutinized the "bad guys," those individual strains of HIV that escaped the antibody "street cops" and infected a small number of volunteers. Yet they reached entirely different conclusions.

When Phil analyzed samples from seven HIV-infected vaccinees, he found that three were carrying typical, MN-like viruses—ordinary thugs that the vaccine supposedly trained the street cops to recognize. So why didn't they? Medical records showed that individual volunteers had been exposed to HIV when their antibody levels were low, either because they hadn't gotten all their shots or had gotten them so long ago that levels had fallen. In other words, if not enough cops are on the beat, crime happens—that's easy enough to understand.

But the more controversial part of Phil's analysis concerned the remaining four infected vacinees. He attributed their infection to wise guys from out of town—strains of HIV that were genetically different from typical MN viruses. These variations changed the shape of the V3 loop, a prominent physical feature that the vaccine trained the immune system to recognize. It was as though the cops saw unfamiliar guys in the neighborhood but didn't recognize them as dangerous. By analyzing these breakthrough strains, Phil could figure out how to improve gp120 vaccines. The idea was to construct a vaccine that would train police to recognize all criminals, regardless of where they were from. This was exactly the sort of vaccine that Phil envisioned as the flagship product for the new spin-off company.

John Moore had heard in advance of the Vancouver meeting about Phil's analysis and thought he was dead wrong. In fact, Moore had already sent e-mail to other scientists characterizing the findings of "some corporate scientists" as "hogwash." He gave his competing version of the story at the AIDS conference. Instead of focusing only on breakthrough infections in volunteers who got the Genentech vaccine, he also looked at those who received Chiron Biocine's gp120 before becoming infected. His conclusion, although he didn't use these exact words, was that all the criminals who eluded detection were ordinary MN-like HIV that the antibody cops should have recognized. The variations in the V3 region changed their appearance in trivial ways that did not set them apart from common strains. Moore's bottom line was that if the gp120 vaccines couldn't teach cops to protect against these viruses, then these products were useless and would not protect against anything. In essence, these vaccines were incompetent instructors who had taught the cops nothing new and had cost the taxpayers a bundle. So far as John Moore was concerned, gp120 had been a moribund concept for two years, and Phil was "clutching at straws" in an attempt to justify testing that Genenvax hoped to carry out.

Who was right—Phil Berman or John Moore? Some say that it's impossible to tell because they chose different sets of viruses as controls for the breakthrough strains. For example, a bald criminal might be difficult for an eyewitness to pick from a row of other bald men but easy to identify if the other guys in the lineup have hair.

"In each case, the control set of viruses was supposed to represent what participants in the trial would actually be exposed to, and you would look at what they were exposed to versus what actually infected them and ask whether there is anything peculiar about that subset," explained Peggy Johnston of NIAID, two years after the Vancouver conference. "But what are they exposed to and how do you define that? The best way is to take people in the same community, with the same risk factors, matched as much as possible, who aren't in the vaccine trial and see what infects them. Neither [Berman nor Moore] had an appropriate control group."

When Phil got home from the Vancouver meeting in July 1996, he returned to his well-equipped lab in Genentech's Building 20, perched on a hilltop with a great view of San Francisco Bay. The nascent Genenvax, however, was still moving from empty office to empty office in the bowels of Building 7, where there was no view to speak of. Bob Nowinski's desk was a rolling office chair that he used to ferry paperwork from place to place. Although the spin-off had been announced back in February, it was taking forever to work out the final details with Genentech. Executives who were called in for some of these meetings say that an oversupply of ego made the negotiations difficult. Bob and Genentech's chief representative "each liked to be the biggest person in a room," said one observer.

●

Jim Tartaglia was the antithesis of Enzo Paoletti. Except for being virologists of Italian extraction, they could be from different planets. Enzo is lean, wiry, and watchful. Jim is large and stocky and turns an open countenance to the world. So perhaps it was not surprising that Pasteur Mérieux Connaught, having had a thorny relationship with Enzo, picked Jim to head the downsized Virogenetics. In August 1996, ten months after Enzo was fired, PMC officially named Jim research director. The thirty-seven-year-old molecular biologist had been doing the job all along, and he was happy to have the title.

Although Jim admired Enzo's passion and intelligence as a scientist, it was also obvious that his former boss had made enemies. Enzo's attitude toward some of the French vaccine developers bordered on the contemptuous, and when disputes arose, Enzo's stance was often "my way or no way." One of the first tasks Jim faced was to smooth some of the feathers Enzo had ruffled, and he didn't have a problem with that. "In an industrial setting, one needs to really work with individuals within the company to push things along," Jim said. He also knew that considerable patience would be needed to keep his vaccines moving within PMC, where many other products were competing for resources and the business structure might change at any time.

Fortunately, there was outside pressure to keep going. Six months earlier, Tony Fauci, speaking to a large HIV vaccine meeting at NIH, identified the prime-boost strategy as the leader in the field. Fauci not only said that this approach was further along in development than competing vaccines, but "he strongly hinted that the combination might be the first AIDS vaccine to make it to full-scale effectiveness testing in the United States," according to reporter Lawrence K. Altman, who covered the meeting for the *New York Times*.

If PMC was leading the vaccine race at the turn, it was not because canarypox was the best horse but because so many competitors had been scratched, had stumbled in the gate, or had faltered early. Top executives in France still had doubts about the canarypox vectors and were pushing Jim and his small team, just as they had pushed Enzo before him, to improve the constructs. After the disappointing results with vCP125, Enzo's original vector, the company ditched it. Now development focused mainly on a revised vector, vCP205, even though in most studies it stimulated cytotoxic T cell responses in only about one-third of volunteers. This was like having detectives who only show up to investigate one case in three.

Before PMC spent millions supplying vaccine for a clinical trial, the company wanted to see CTL responses in a greater proportion of vaccinees, according to Michel Klein, the company's vice president for vaccines. Jim was pushed to make vectors that delivered more antigen for longer periods, which might cause more people to respond. Two additional, and challenging, assignments were to insert as many HIV antigens as possible into canarypox, and to alter the virus so that it would be easier to grow. None of this would be easy to accomplish in the sparsely staffed lab at Virogenetics.

In the Paris-based medical department of PMC, Jean-Louis Excler was worried that endless tinkering with the vector could sabotage clinical testing. He viewed the quest for a "perfect" version of canarypox as an impossible dream. "You cannot endlessly postpone, postpone, postpone until you have reached your final dream," he said. "You have to build from these first steps, to learn. Otherwise you will never know whether the next dream is better than the previous one." In other words, if PMC dragged its feet, canarypox might lose its front-runner status with the French government and the NIH. Jean-Louis needed to reassure these agencies that canarypox vaccines would be available, in a timely manner, for efficacy testing. He was also worried that Chiron might back out of the prime-boost deal at any time. The company had gotten involved in the first place only because NIH insisted; now Chiron had cut back on HIV vaccine development.

Although Fauci said publicly that the prime-boost concept was the leading contender for a tax-supported efficacy trial, some Division of AIDS scientists weren't sure how likely it was to protect against AIDS. None of the canarypox constructs had protected chimps against HIV challenge, for example, and only some protection had been observed in monkeys immunized with both canarypox and gp120. In early human trials, the gp120 booster shots generated antibody levels similar to those seen using gp120 alone—and the government had decided in 1994 that this wasn't good enough. Canarypox produced CTL responses in some volunteers, it was true, but lab tests rated this as "strong CTL activity" in only a few individuals. As a result, there was no real passion for prime-boost within DAIDS. It was the leader by default.

●

By the autumn of 1996, a year after they formed a partnership, Don Francis and Bob Nowinski were poised to raise money for their new company. Although nearly all biotech or high-tech start-ups rely on financing from venture capitalists, Bob shunned VCs because eventually they would want more control than he was willing to cede. Instead, he planned to rely on the retail approach to financing that he had used to launch his earlier companies. This meant working with a small number of "trusted broker-dealers who bring their clients to the table, and then we make the presentations, and these broker-dealers assist us in legally closing the transaction."

This is a time-consuming, labor-intensive process not unlike a political campaign. For accounting reasons of its own, Genentech insisted that fund-raising begin before the end of 1996. The first meetings could not be scheduled until December, which Bob saw as the least desirable time of year because the Christmas and New Year's holidays disrupt the flow. "If you halt a financing, to begin it again is like jump-starting a dead heart," he said.

Even as they scrambled to set up meetings with potential investors, Don and Bob had another messy situation to confront: They had to change the new company's name. Shortly after the spin-off of Genenvax was officially announced, Don was contacted by a law firm representing Apollon, the Pennsylvania biotech that was developing Dave Weiner's DNA vaccine against HIV. Apollon had trademarked the name "Genevax™" and said that the word "Genenvax" was too close for legal comfort. Don threw away the letter and went about his business.

More recently, Apollon had moved to sue Genenvax, a matter Don now had to settle or else disclose in the prospectus for the new company. This was not something he and Bob wanted to try explaining to prospective shareholders. Fortunately, a few thousand dollars and a promise to change the company's name made the lawsuit disappear. But this left the enterprise nameless and it was time to print the prospectus, not to mention letterhead, business cards, and all the other recyclable trappings that a business requires.

Don gathered a small group around a table, legal pads at the ready, to brainstorm about what the company might be called. They wrote down everything. One of the giddiest suggestions was Rolling Pin Vaccines, a tribute to Rolling Pin Donuts, a tiny shop on the edge of the Genentech campus that sent sugary aromas wafting into the labs every time they baked. Finally, Don, who was impatient with the naming exercise, declared that the company would be called VaxGen. When a search showed that the name wasn't taken, the issue was settled. "We didn't have time to worry about this sort of thing," Don said impatiently, gesturing as though brushing away a gnat.

●

Kathy and Martin's daughter Casey was five, an age when "surprise" is a magical and exciting concept. So she was very involved in the surprise birthday party that she and her father held for her mother in August 1996, when Kathy turned forty-eight. Kathy was taking high doses of steroids at the time, and the drugs sparked a weird energy that was almost like her old mania. So Kathy felt good enough to walk to a nearby park with her husband, child, and Leroy the poodle. By the time they returned, a gang of friends had slipped into the house and laid out a lavish spread of food and gifts.

"When she came in, she was just so happy," recalled her friend Kathryn Radke. "It was wonderful." During the party, Kathryn was astonished to hear Kathy talking about building an addition to the house and swimming pool—fantasies most likely induced by the drugs she was taking. Martin took it all in stride. "She's just trying to live the rest of her life in the rest of her life," he told Kathryn. And it did seem as though Kathy was intensely engaged with her husband, her daughter, and the dog who seldom left her side.

At the same time, she remained passionate about Chiron. "Work has a different meaning for people here, or at least it did in those days," recalled CEO Ed Penhoet. "The experience is very intense. It has a familylike connection. She did have strong feelings for her family, and this doesn't take anything away from them. But she might have argued about using the term 'work' for what she did here. Because for most people, work is associated with a job, and work is something that you have to do. Kathy was driven by wanting to understand this virus. It's a battle of wits between you and nature, in a way, and it's a commitment that is more like people in the arts. If you asked Picasso, 'You're not feeling well today, would you rather paint or put your feet up?' He'd probably rather paint. It's that kind of dedication to the process."

Chiron also needed to have Kathy on the job, even if she was working fewer hours. She was an idea person who also did "beautiful work" in the laboratory, and she remained a major scientific contributor until the end of her life.

John McNeil traveled to Chiron in October to talk about the gp120 trials that the army was sponsoring in Thailand. A Phase I study of the original clade B vaccine was underway, with a Phase II trial expected to start in a few months. These trials would pave the way for a much larger Phase I/II test of the clade E version that Kathy had designed after her unforgettable visit to Chiang Mai Hospital. "She was very positive about what Chiron was doing with us in Thailand and saw that as a viable avenue to advance testing," John remembered.

Much of their conversation took place in a car, as John drove her to and from a radiation therapy session at a nearby hospital. Under these circumstances, it was impossible to avoid the topic of Kathy's illness, and her decision to devote so much time to Chiron. "She loved her work, and I think it was also something to occupy her mind, so that she wouldn't just think about her cancer. I talked with her a lot about doing that versus being at home with her daughter. This was a choice that she made because it was best for her," he said.

Kathy's health worsened during October and November, and she moved from her bedroom upstairs to a hospital bed in a study on the main floor, so that she would not need to climb stairs. Martin took care of her with assistance from a part-time housekeeper and neighbors who helped with Casey. Kathy was in and out of the hospital, and Kathryn organized teams of friends to bring dinner to the house, stay overnight, and leave in the morning.

Kathryn Radke tried to pay special attention to Leroy, who began looking unkempt, now that Kathy could no longer take him to regular grooming appointments. "Leroy was always with her when she was sick, and he was very, very attentive," Kathryn remembered. As primary caregiver, Martin had a million things on his mind besides the big black poodle. So when Kathryn came to help out, she made a point of taking Leroy for a long walk.

As the twelve-month anniversary of Kathy's diagnosis approached, it was obvious to Martin and everyone else that she would not live much longer. The disease and drugs had ravaged her body so that she looked seventy-eight, not forty-eight. One Thursday evening in November, Kathryn and a couple who also lived in Davis drove to Benicia to fix dinner for Kathy's family and spend the evening.

Kathy had just come home from the hospital and was in the thick of things as the guests cooked and drank wine. "We got pretty rowdy, and I kept thinking that we shouldn't be wearing her out. Finally she had to go to bed, and Martin helped her and we went in and kissed her good night. And she said, 'I haven't had this much fun in months,'" Kathryn recalled. "Although the purpose of our going was to say good-bye to her, I just couldn't say those words."

The next day she began to fail so fast that Martin called her father, Harry Steimer, and asked him to come from Sacramento. Together the two of them tended Kathy with help from hospice nurses, who came every few hours. There was also Casey to think about, as she shuttled between her mother's sickroom and close friends who lived around the corner.

On Saturday, November 16, Kathy died at home in Benicia. Her family was at her bedside. And when she was gone, Leroy raised his muzzle and howled.

II

THE VIRUS MUST BE LAUGHING AT US

L ONG AGO, BEFORE THERE WERE such things as hook-and-ladder trucks or other modern fire-fighting equipment, a beautiful hotel near the shore of a lake caught fire. People with rooms on the lower floors were lucky enough to escape, but many others remained trapped in the lovely old building. Men whose families fled the fire seized basins and buckets and formed a line to scoop water from the lake, pass containers hand-to-hand, and douse the flames. But the men began quarreling among themselves about which containers were best and whether it was better to fill them completely, which made them heavier and slower to pass, or fill them halfway so they could be handed along more rapidly. As heat and exhaustion made the group increasingly fractious, some men walked off the job or dumped their water on the ground. Although the remaining volunteers worked as hard as they could to contain the fire, it overpowered their efforts and destroyed the hotel, killing its occupants.

The moral of the story? Fighting feeds the flames.

●

The NIH's decision not to go forward with efficacy trials caused so much stir that the news media stopped paying attention to HIV vaccine research sponsored by the Department of Defense. That was fine with Debbi Birx, John McNeil, and the other researchers at Walter Reed Army Institute of Research, who had suffered enough notoriety during the fire-fight of 1992. In the early 1990s, WRAIR was split between the camp of Colonel Don Burke, who made preventive vaccines his top priority, and Colonel Bob Redfield's clinical research group, which was testing Micro-GeneSys's gp160 vaccine in HIV-infected patients.

This dispute came to a head in September 1992, when heavy lobbying by MicroGeneSys moved Congress to approve $20 million for a Phase III trial of the gp160 vaccine made by the Connecticut-based biotech. The timing could not have been worse, as the military had just begun investigating charges that Redfield had exaggerated the benefits of gp160 in an earlier clinical trial. The ensuing media frenzy dragged on for more than a year.

When the spotlight shifted to the NIH in mid-1994, army researchers heaved a sigh of relief and went about their business in relative peace. Not in harmony, necessarily, but at least shots were no longer being fired across the moat, as WRAIR staffers called the parking lot situated between the buildings housing the Redfield and Burke laboratories. The Phase III trial for gp160 had been dropped, and Burke now had an additional $20 million in his budget for the Division of Retrovirology. Most of this would be spent developing vaccines to prevent AIDS, not treat it.

Officially, Redfield was still chief of retroviral research in Burke's division; in fact he hardly came to WRAIR at all. He had gone back to being a doctor, spending his days looking after AIDS patients at Walter Reed Hospital down in Washington. As Redfield's second in command, Debbi Birx's duty was to finish the Phase II study of gp160. Hundreds of AIDS patients at seventeen centers had volunteered for this experiment in good faith, and lab work and data analysis were needed to wrap it up. The work went slowly, because Debbi had only a skeleton staff and no money to hire outside experts. Aside from her small group, no one else at WRAIR still worked on—or cared about—therapeutic vaccines.

Don Burke had been disappointed by the NIH's decision not to mount a Phase III study of the two gp120 vaccines, and he moved quickly to portray WRAIR as the leader in the march toward efficacy testing. In August 1994, while the California biotechs were reeling from the NIH decision,

Burke wrote an editorial on the topic for the *Journal of the American Medical Association.* "In the simplest terms, the choice is between a cautious strategy of more basic research vs. an approach based on 'thoughtful empiricism.' The history of vaccine development bears strong witness to the value of thoughtful empiricism. Smallpox was eradicated from the face of the earth, yet no one can say (with certainty) how the vaccine works," Burke wrote. The editorial was coauthored by John McNeil and John Mascola, an antibody expert at WRAIR.

Burke gave frequent lectures about the importance of moving ahead with large field trials. One place he delivered his impassioned message was at a World Health Organization workshop in Geneva, which in October 1994 recommended that WHO design and carry out efficacy trials. This group advised that studies be conducted in countries where HIV was spreading fast, and where some clinics and lab facilities were already in place. Using these criteria, Thailand was a logical choice for the world's first efficacy trial, followed by Brazil and Uganda. The only trouble with these plans for international efficacy testing was that WHO had hardly any money and no corporate partners prepared to supply products.

WRAIR, on the other hand, was working with several companies and had about $15 million to spend on HIV vaccine research. Burke had allocated nearly half of this to clinical trial preparation in Thailand. John McNeil shuttled back and forth between the United States and Thailand, navigating a labyrinth of government committees and agencies in Bangkok and making sure that future vaccine test sites were equipped with everything from nitrogen freezers to latex gloves. What remained of his energy was spent negotiating with executives at Pasteur Mérieux Connaught, Chiron Biocine, and other companies whose products the army wanted to test.

Rumors about WRAIR's free-spending ways on the opposite side of the globe did not play well at 13 Taft Court, where Debbi Birx and her people were slogging away in dingy labs with malfunctioning phones, still analyzing data from Redfield's ill-fated therapeutic study. "All I knew was that John McNeil was taking a bunch of money and putting it in Thailand, and that's why there wasn't money for the gp160 trial," Debbi recalled. "We had no idea who he was, but we knew we didn't like him."

In late 1995, John McNeil and Francine McCutchan, the civilian virologist who was the military's leading expert on global variations in the AIDS virus, reached out to Debbi and asked if they could get together on her side of the moat. Debbi was wary during that initial meeting. "They said, 'We need the immunology piece to move forward with vaccine development.' And I looked at them like 'Yeah, right, I'm gonna work with you two?'" Fortunately, they continued to talk. Over a period of several months, Debbi came to see John's solo mission in Thailand and Francine's accomplishments in the lab as extraordinary scientific undertakings. Because Burke's management style did not encourage researchers in different programs to interact, this was a revelation to her. "We honestly didn't know," she said. "All the groups were kept separate."

As she and John got better acquainted, "I realized that he really didn't have horns," Debbi said. He wanted her to set up a laboratory program for analyzing the immune responses of Thai vaccine volunteers, which would enable her to pick up scientific inquiries she had dropped when financing for the gp160 trial fell apart. This was the type of research that interested Debbi as an immunologist. John was even willing to help lift the gp160 albatross from her neck. Knowing that her bare-bones department didn't have the right people to finish analyzing the trial data, he sent statistical experts from his group to lend a hand.

In early 1996, WRAIR and MicroGeneSys announced, with minimal fanfare, that AIDS patients treated with gp160 got just as sick, just as quickly, as those given a placebo. Although the treatment was a failure, Debbi Birx succeeded in getting a clear answer for the patients who had volunteered. Redfield made good on his promise to retire from the military after this study was laid to rest. As one door closed, another opened. His old friend Bob Gallo was leaving NIH to head the newly created Institute of Human Virology at the University of Maryland, and Redfield was brought in to head treatment research.

"It was clear to me that if given a choice in the AIDS epidemic, to spend my energy working on prevention or treatment, the immediate need I see is treatment," Redfield said. After twenty-three years in the army, where he had never been a particularly good fit, Bob Redfield landed on his feet in the civilian world.

●

Despite considerable federal spending on robotics, scientists have so far been stumped by the challenge of designing robots that can reproduce themselves.

In contrast, tax-supported researchers have had no trouble forming committees that reproduce themselves ad infinitum. Consider the NIH Office of AIDS Research, which was set up in early 1994 with the distinguished immunologist William Paul as its director. Paul's first mandate at OAR was to examine how the NIH's $1.4 billion AIDS budget was being spent and to figure out how it might be more effectively used.

Paul was a true believer in NIH's traditional emphasis on investigator-initiated research. In this system, academic scientists write proposals telling what they want to study in their labs. These proposals compete for NIH support, and the ones selected by peer-review committees get the money. In most NIH programs, this process is used to allocate 50 percent of the extramural budget; for AIDS, the figure was only 20 percent. The bulk of NIH's AIDS spending was distributed through contracts dreamed up not by university professors, but by program administrators at NIH. These government scientists decided what research needed to be done and awarded contracts to university scientists who would carry out laboratory experiments, clinical trials, or data analysis.

This centralized approach may have been valid a decade earlier, when the field of AIDS research was created from scratch, but by 1994, Paul believed that contracts "had become shackling, rather than liberating, and we had to move away from that." Academic investigators had flocked to AIDS-related research, and he was eager to see them set their own scientific agendas, not execute projects devised by NIH desk jockeys. In addition to reversing the balance of contract and investigator-initiated research, there was another budget problem Paul wanted to fix: "We were spending dreadfully little money on vaccine development."

In order to change the status quo, Bill Paul would need a committee, or two, or six, or maybe even more. The crusade to revamp spending began with the OAR's Advisory Council, a group of outside scientists leavened with a few AIDS activists. In late 1994, this group endorsed Paul's idea of establishing a huge committee to review how every institute and center and office at NIH was spending its AIDS money. This new entity was saddled with a ponderous name: the NIH AIDS Research Program Evaluation Task Force of the Office of AIDS Research Advisory Council. No wonder it immediately became known as the "Levine committee," after its chairman, famed Princeton microbiologist Arnold Levine.

More than 100 scientists and advocates were recruited for the Levine committee, which quickly spawned six "area review panels," or ARPs. One of these ARPs focused on vaccine research and development. This fifteen-member panel morphed into three subpanels devoted to major aspects of HIV vaccine development: basic science, targeted research using animal models, and clinical trials. These small groups were clearly where the real horse-trading would be done, and everybody brought a horse.

John Moore, for example, who chaired the basic-science subpanel, believed that the whole HIV vaccine field had rushed in the wrong direction, chasing after antibody protection, and he was determined to halt the charge. As one of the self-anointed "next generation" of AIDS experts, affiliated with the vigorous young Aaron Diamond AIDS Research Center in New York, Moore didn't doubt that he could help straighten things out.

The targeted-research group was led by Harriet Robinson, a pioneering DNA vaccine researcher whose work had been poorly supported at the University of Massachusetts and largely ignored by NIH study sections. If anyone knew specific steps the NIH could take to help inventors develop their vaccines, she did.

The clinical-trials subpanel was led by Bill Snow, an HIV-positive AIDS activist from San Francisco who had spent so much time on NIH committees that he now felt quite at home among the elite academic scientists who dominated them. He and other advocates had already revolutionized how treatments were tested, and vaccines were the next challenge.

For nine months, from May 1995 through February 1996, various configurations of the vaccine ARP listened to presentations from NIH officials, military vaccine researchers, academic scientists, and corporate representatives, including Don Francis. They met and teleconferenced and e-mailed and finally produced a document that boldly stated the obvious: "The major theme of this report is that HIV vaccine research and development is in crisis."

The vaccine ARP echoed Bill Paul's claim that too much was being spent on contracts and not enough on investigator-initiated research.

Besides advocating for more money, Moore's basic-science group said a cultural shift would be needed to "entice leading immunologists and virologists from within and outside the AIDS field to contribute their expertise" to HIV vaccine research. World-class scientists were staying away, the subpanel implied, because vaccine work was perceived as a low-prestige, low-pay backwater populated by second-rate researchers. The "culture" of vaccine research needed to change, and this would require that NIH create a new committee of outside experts.

The propagation of new committees did not stop there. Harriet Robinson's subpanel complained that animal models had been used in a hit-or-miss fashion and had cost a great deal while yielding little. Her group recommended that NIH create another new committee to oversee pre-clinical vaccine tests and come up with more systematic evaluations. Bill Snow's clinical-trials subpanel also saw problems that would require attention from an outside committee of experts. This group should reassess the status of HIVNET, the network that had been set up to conduct Phase III vaccine trials but had so far been used for modest tests of antimicrobial contraceptives and other prevention strategies.

The vaccine panel's recommendations, along with those from five other ARPs, were funneled into the overall report of the Levine committee's working group. While the panel had cast doubt on the ability of NIH employees to set the agenda for HIV vaccine research, the final version of the Levine report stated outright that they were not up to the task. "The entire vaccine research effort should be restructured. A trans-NIH vaccine program should be established with leadership and oversight provided by distinguished, non-government scientists." The Levine report proposed an AIDS Vaccine Research Committee, or AVRC, which would consist of elite scientists and be led by an academic investigator with credentials so stellar that he could walk across the Potomac with dry shoes. A few NIH scientists should be invited to the table, but not many.

The mammoth Levine report landed on Tony Fauci's desk on March 6, 1996, and was quickly circulated to the Division of AIDS as well. For Pat Fast and the rest of the DAIDS vaccine program staff, this was like being kicked while they were down. Two years earlier, they had slaved to devise efficacy trials that ARAC might endorse, only to be gravely disappointed.

Morale had since sagged lower and lower. Even Jack Killen, who never doubted for an instant that Tony Fauci had been right to nix the Phase III study, could not help but notice that some staff scientists had left DAIDS rather than live with Fauci's choice. Others had stayed, but their attitudes toward top NIH officials had become so cynical that they would have fit right in at Genentech or Chiron.

People who were passionate about the need for a vaccine had reason to be depressed, even angry. There were now fewer candidates in the pipeline than at any time during the past decade. In a memo to Killen, Pat Fast listed fifteen companies and cataloged every HIV vaccine concept they had worked on. The current status of these products was a depressing litany: development stopped, plans dropped, no longer available for trials, doubtful that this will be pursued, uncertain when available, timeline unknown, development halted, no plans for clinical development.

Less than one month before the Levine report hit his desk, Fauci had tried to put a good face on this situation when he addressed a large HIV vaccine meeting on the NIH campus. He told a skeptical audience that NIH was going to forge strong new partnerships with industry and lure companies back into the field. His idea was that companies would once again invest in HIV vaccines if NIH could specify, in advance, exactly what a vaccine would have to accomplish to advance from animals to humans and from small safety trials to larger studies. But lots of people in the auditorium thought it would be impossible to establish rational hurdles. Even if this could be done, there was no guarantee that companies would trust the NIH.

When Tony Fauci ruminates aloud about his career in AIDS, he portrays himself as a man bold enough to make the tough decisions, regardless of the consequences. But experienced Fauci-watchers say he is often hesitant to take decisive action, especially if doing so would risk criticism from A-list scientists. It was humiliating when activists persuaded Congress to take budget oversight away from Fauci and give it to the Office of AIDS Research, whose head reports only to the NIH director. And it was not a good thing when OAR released the Levine report, in which a large group of outsiders implicitly questioned Fauci's ability to command NIH's war against AIDS.

The Levine report "was not intended to say that NIH leadership had done a bad job," demurred John Moore. The point of the vaccine recommendations was simply to "highlight the inadequacy of vaccine research," not to insult Fauci, Moore said. "It was an exercise in helping the NIH improve its performance. And sure, a lot of the top NIH officials resented it."

Although many academic scientists didn't view Fauci as a world-class researcher, they nevertheless respected his longevity as an administrator. He had stayed alive in the shark-infested waters of Washington for a dozen years, after all. Far more vulnerable than Fauci or other institute directors were midlevel administrators like Pat Fast, as well as the Ph.D.s who worked for her, who had been making decisions about what sorts of science NIH should fund. This was the power that the Levine report said rightfully belonged to high-level academic investigators, people like Larry Corey at the University of Washington and David Ho at the Aaron Diamond Center. These people were accustomed to telling NIH what they intended to study, not the other way around.

"The Levine committee report was very difficult for a lot of people here," recalled microbiologist Carole Heilman, who came to DAIDS to implement some of the committee's recommendations. "The remarks of a lot of non-government scientists hurt a lot of people deeply who really tried very hard to make a difference, or who really felt they had contributed quite a bit to [vaccine research] activity." Pat Fast put it more bluntly: The Levine report told DAIDS program scientists that "we were all cretins."

John Moore, for one, makes no apology for the message sent to NIH staff. As he put it, midlevel DAIDS scientists "are not the caliber of the top academic scientists in the extramural community, almost by definition. Nobody goes to work for the NIH by choice. It's not the kind of thing where you're a twenty-four-year-old college graduate and you say, 'Gosh, I want to be an NIH bureaucrat.' You say, 'I want to be a leading academic scientist.' I'm not trying to be insulting, but there are certain decisions that should not be taken by intramural officials; they should be taken by the leading scientists in the nation." Prominent academics, in his view, possess sounder judgment and are more likely to make objective, scientific decisions than government employees, who may lack judgment and "abuse their power and prerogatives."

•

During spring 1995, while the Levine committee was scrutinizing AIDS research at NIH, thirty-six-year-old physician Chris Beyrer had one of the most exhilarating moments of his public-health career. He was alone in a former animal research room on the top floor of RIHES, the Research Institute for Health Sciences at Chiang Mai University. This was a tile-walled space that now held desks, telephones, and a computer. Chris was head of the local AIDS prevention and vaccine evaluation project, which had first been called PAVE but now was one of nine international HIVNET sites.

Most Western doctors in his position would have left data entry to their office staff, but not Chris. He was hunkered down at the computer, painstakingly entering the latest raw data from an ongoing study of conscripts into the Royal Thai Army. About 800 of these young men were stationed at a large RTA base just outside Chiang Mai, with 400 more at smaller camps farther from the city. When the study began in 1991, blood tests showed 12 percent of the conscripts were already carrying HIV when they entered military service, with an additional 2.4 percent becoming infected each year. In an attempt to slow the spread of the virus, Chris's program and the RTA worked together on an educational program that emphasized using condoms, cutting back on alcohol consumption, and reducing contact with prostitutes. Over time, this intervention reduced the rate of new infections among participants by about 50 percent, compared with soldiers given no special instruction.

"We had been having roughly fifteen new infections every six months" prior to this particular spring day, Chris said. "Suddenly, we had a zero. I remember charging down the hallway to Chirasak's office and saying, 'It worked! The intervention is working! The HIV rate is coming down!' That doesn't happen often in life. It was really thrilling." Chris grinned at the memory. He believes the goal of any public-health effort is "to put ourselves out of a job," and if nobody is getting infected, then that is the definition of success.

The trouble with success, of course, is that it's not universal and it doesn't last. Even as young soldiers demonstrated that they could change their sexual behavior, Chris knew that there were plenty of male civilians in Chiang Mai and elsewhere who didn't always use condoms, continued to visit brothels, and would marry young women who had no idea what danger they were in. For these people, a vaccine could make the difference between life and death.

Chris's friend and colleague Dr. Chirasak Khamboonruang had been visiting some of the small villages outside Chiang Mai, recruiting volunteers for the first HIV vaccine trial in northern Thailand. After long negotiations with Ministry of Public Health officials in Bangkok, John McNeil and his Thai collaborators had finally secured approval for a Phase I study of Chiron's gp120 vaccine based on SF2. This would be a small study aimed at demonstrating safety and would help pave the way for testing the clade E vaccine that Kathy Steimer had designed for Thailand.

A native of the hill country outside Chiang Mai, Dr. Chirasak knew firsthand the toll that AIDS was taking in these areas. He went to villages where Chris Beyrer's program had conducted vaccine-preparedness studies, encouraging participants to take the next step and volunteer for an actual clinical trial. The goal was to enroll healthy, twenty- to fifty-year-old adults who were at "low to no" risk for infection, who could come to RIHES for immunizations and follow-up appointments spread over forty weeks.

Dr. Chirasak's efforts soon rounded up twenty-seven qualified volunteers in the Chiang Mai area, while AFRIMS, the Army research facility in Bangkok, enrolled another twenty-seven. Two-thirds of the people who signed up said they volunteered because they wanted to "help society." Their average age was thirty, about half had been to university, and in their ranks were business owners, medical professionals, monks, laborers, and factory workers. The first injection was given on August 29, 1995, more than four years after John McNeil first stepped off an airliner and into the cacophony and grit of Bangkok.

Thirteen months later, this groundbreaking trial would be over, marking the first time that the U.S. government and a host country had worked together to successfully test an American-made HIV vaccine in an international setting. When the results were in, no one had dropped out of the study, the most common post-immunization reaction was pain at the injection site, and no severe adverse events were reported. It was a good first step on the long journey toward an efficacy trial in Thailand.

•

Meanwhile, Colonel Don Burke, who admitted that he was "not afraid to step in front of a god-damned freight train," was stripped of his command as director of military AIDS research in May 1996.

Trouble had been brewing for years between the Pentagon and the maverick Burke. In an organization where "chain of command" is a sacred concept, Burke was an atheist. In September 1992, for example, he asked no one before colluding with friendly Capitol Hill staffers to slow Congress's plan to spend $20 million testing MicroGeneSys gp160. As a result of this freelance effort, "I got a reputation in the army for messing in things that I shouldn't with Congress," Burke acknowledged with no trace of remorse. Nor were top brass necessarily impressed in 1993, when Burke's revisions to the bill eventually caused the $20 million to end up in a budget that he controlled. After a hastily arranged competition, the money went for newer vaccine strategies like naked DNA and live vectors.

By February 1995, Burke was in hot water again. Under fire from Republicans in Congress to eliminate "non-defense" programs from the military budget, the Pentagon announced that it would say "thanks but no thanks" to $33 million for AIDS research and $150 million for breast-cancer studies. In a controversial move, these sums had been added to the DOD's initial budget request by Democrats who wanted to see more aggressive government responses to these diseases.

Breast-cancer research wasn't Burke's concern, but HIV certainly was. The fiscal year was underway and Burke had committed to spending $47 million on AIDS research—$14 million that the Pentagon had originally requested and the $33 million "plus-up" from Congress. Burke warned his commanding officers that if the Pentagon turned down the plus-up, then key research contracts would be canceled and pink slips handed out at WRAIR. Especially hard hit would be the Henry M. Jackson Foundation, where civilian scientists like Francine McCutchan had done ground-breaking work on global variations in HIV. If the Pentagon snatched back the supplement, "I told people they should be prepared for some unfavorable publicity," Burke said.

Although Burke says he didn't reach out to Capitol Hill or to reporters, others surely did: A front-page story about DOD's plan to turn down funding for AIDS and breast-cancer research appeared in the *Washington Post* on February 10, 1995, with similar articles on the wire services and in other major newspapers. That same day, White House Chief of Staff Leon Panetta wrote a letter to Defense Secretary William Perry, saying that President Clinton had read the *Post* story and regarded research on both diseases as "a high priority for this Administration." The letter left no doubt about what the White House expected: "As you continue to carry out this important program, please keep the President advised of your progress," Panetta wrote.

The Pentagon accepted the AIDS and breast-cancer money, a reversal that embarrassed the chain of command. Coming on the heels of the gp160 mess, "it didn't do my own reputation much good. I was already seen as being too concerned with my own program and not concerned enough with the larger issues that were important to the DOD," Burke recalled.

Burke's third strike came early in 1996, when WRAIR and Micro-GeneSys were preparing to announce that gp160 had bombed in the Phase II trial. Burke's program called together investigators from the seventeen sites where the trial had been done and handed them a summary of the results. Although Burke insists that this summary was an internal document and that his superiors knew about it, he said DOD construed it as "another of these cowboy activities where there was going to be a press release on an important trial without having it properly cleared."

Burke was relieved of his command in May and given the rest of 1996 to find another job. Until then, he was appointed WRAIR's associate director for emerging threats and biotechnology. Although this looked like a golden parachute, Burke felt he was regarded warily as "the mad uncle in the attic." Finally, he decamped for a post at Johns Hopkins University School of Public Health. Like Bob Redfield, he had spent twenty-three years on active duty, then retired with the rank of colonel and went to an academic job in Baltimore.

Burke's military career self-destructed because "he forgot who his constituency was," said Ed Tramont, who had once commanded both Burke and Redfield and was now Redfield's colleague at the University of Maryland. Grandiosity may be more of an occupational hazard for AIDS researchers than for others. Everyone in HIV research harbors the desire "to make the world safe from AIDS," and Don Burke was more enamored of this goal than most, according to an army scientist who worked at WRAIR when Burke was in charge. "He had this dream and the army said that's all well and good, but that is not your mission. Your dream is not your mission. You're in the army."

Once Don Burke had been edged out of the Division of Retrovirology, WRAIR needed a new commander for the outfit. One contender was a navy captain who studied HIV's resistance to antiviral drugs and who wasn't taken seriously because he was not senior enough and not focused on prevention, which was the military's main concern. The other two contenders were Debbi Birx and John McNeil, both lieutenant colonels in the army, which traditionally spearheads infectious-disease research.

Debbi had more seniority than John, but she several things working against her. For one thing, she was an immunologist, not a traditional infectious-disease physician. For another, she had worked for Bob Redfield, who had been a major source of embarrassment and irritation to the Pentagon. And finally, she was a woman: a tall blond with a wide smile who resembles Julia Roberts and is glamorous in the same quirky, slightly abashed way.

Nevertheless, the commander of WRAIR picked Debbi to head the U.S. military's research efforts against AIDS. When the navy contested her promotion, she was paraded through the corridors of civilian and military power. Although Debbi did not enjoy being scrutinized by so many people, the vetting turned out fine. "I didn't go to defend myself, but to talk about the program. And it was really well received. So without having to lobby, which I would never do, people in the House and Senate and the White House got to know about the program again." One thing about being only the second female division chief in WRAIR's history was that she stood out, and people remembered who she was.

Back in Rockville, she and John agreed to work together and make their campus a neutral, no-fire zone. "We come at this from very complementary perspectives; she is very basic science and lab-oriented, and I am very field and public-health oriented," John said. "But we do have a structure. Debbi is the boss. She's the division director. And I'm chief of the Department of Vaccine Development." As Debbi and John figured out how to pull in tandem, the atmosphere in the division relaxed so much that scientists and staff were able to joke about the era of the moat, when the Redfield and Burke camps had been split by hostility.

People who worked at WRAIR during the Redfield-Burke era were like "members of a dysfunctional family who were bonded by shared trauma," Debbi said. "We would never have been as strong or as dedicated, or as goal oriented, if we hadn't gone through all that together." She was awed by the toughness and determination of researchers who stayed focused on their mission, which was learning how to prevent HIV infection among military personnel, no matter what went on around them. She did not want to disappoint the good soldiers she now led.

In addition to the challenges that anyone would face on a demanding new job, Debbi had to confront her fear of dying on an airplane. Since 1988, when a severe allergic reaction on a cross-country flight had nearly killed her, she had refused to board any plane scheduled to be aloft for more than two hours. Shortly after her promotion, she was invited to give a talk at the 1996 International AIDS Conference in Vancouver. She was going to turn it down rather than face a long, coast-to-coast flight.

However, "the guys in the lab ganged up on me and said, 'Look, you're now our department chief. It's your job to represent us. And this will make us look good, so you have to do it,'" Debbi recalled. "So I had to go." This trip was a huge breakthrough for Debbi, who has since logged hundreds of thousands of air miles on military business. Everywhere she goes, she hauls boxes and coolers of safe, nonallergenic foods.

She still doesn't like traveling but doesn't see an alternative. "If I want WRAIR to seriously consider another female director ten or fifteen years from now, I don't want them to be able to say [about me], 'Yeah, she did the job, but she wasn't willing to do the whole job.' I didn't want them to have an excuse not to pick the next woman."

●

The presidential Christmas decorations were in place when a small group of well-known scientists arrived at the White House on December 3, 1996. From nearby Bethesda came the NIH delegation: Director Hal Varmus, OAR chief Bill Paul, and NIAID head Tony Fauci. Helene Gayle, head of HIV/AIDS prevention at the Centers for Disease Control, had come from Atlanta. Secretary of Health and Human Services Donna Shalala was on hand, along with Chief of Staff Leon Panetta and assorted White House aides. The purpose was to brief President Clinton and Vice President Gore on progress in AIDS research and to give them ideas about what should be done next.

Although nothing stronger than coffee was served, this White House meeting was all about cocktails—drug "cocktails" built around protease inhibitors that had given many AIDS patients a new lease on life. This had been a major news story during the summer, when David Ho made his now-famous presentation at the Vancouver AIDS conference. Drug cocktails had since become feature material for the likes of the *New York Times Magazine* and the *Wall Street Journal,* both of which had recently published testimonials from high-profile, HIV-infected journalists who marveled that these miracle medicines had snatched them from the brink of death. For AIDS patients like them, with adequate incomes or health insurance, this was going to be the most festive holiday season in years.

The president and vice president, like other readers of the national press, knew this was a genuine breakthrough in AIDS care. They were probably less familiar with what was happening in vaccines, such as the Levine committee's demand that HIV vaccine research at NIH be completely reorganized. Although the Levine report created a huge stir in Bethesda, it got little ink except in magazines read mainly by scientists.

Bill Paul used the December 3 briefing to update Clinton and Gore on why a vaccine was needed. His central argument was that "if you had a really good vaccine, you might eradicate this infection. I mean the way smallpox has been eradicated." He talked about the imperative to invest more resources in HIV vaccines without robbing other research areas, about the long-term benefits of creating a state-of-the-art vaccine research center at NIH, and about the importance of giving the vaccine effort a higher public profile.

"If we were going to win, it had to be this way," Paul remembers saying. "If there was ever a moment we should start, it was now. That was the pitch." The president and vice president listened, asked questions, and seemed willing to help. Balls started to roll.

Like many key meetings in Washington, this one took place behind closed doors. Five months later it surfaced, almost as an aside, in a newspaper story. In contrast, there was intense media coverage on December 13, when NIH announced that David Baltimore would chair the new AIDS Vaccine Research Committee. Baltimore was one of the few American scientists whose name was known to general assignment reporters.

At the precocious age of thirty-seven, David Baltimore had shared a Nobel Prize for discovering reverse transcriptase, the enzyme that HIV and other retroviruses use to copy themselves in host cells. At MIT, where he was a faculty superstar, Baltimore had founded the Whitehead Institute, a clubby laboratory blazing with the brightest young lights in molecular biology. Despite those achievements, it took a scandal to make him really famous. For ten years, Baltimore had been dogged by accusations of scientific fraud, caught up in an unseemly mess that had cost him the presidency of Rockefeller University. He had left MIT to take this prestigious post in New York, only to be forced out after one year in office. Baltimore had since returned to MIT, the last misconduct charges had been dropped only six months earlier, and now he was being made a kind of federal AIDS vaccine czar.

When Baltimore accepted chairmanship of the new committee, Bill Paul told reporters that the Nobel Prize winner was going to "reinvigorate" a research program that had been disappointing. "David Baltimore will make a difference," NIH Director Hal Varmus declared to the *New York Times*. The press could not resist the idea of Baltimore being restored to grace as the savior of a troubled enterprise.

The AIDS Vaccine Research Committee instantly became known as the "Baltimore committee." It was the *uber mensch* of committees spawned by the Levine report, the only one that attracted widespread attention while other bodies soldiered on in obscurity. Its official charge was sweeping: "Advise the vaccine research programs at NIH with regard to scientific opportunities, gaps in knowledge, and future direction in research in order to accomplish the goal of the discovery and development of a safe and effective HIV vaccine."

The Levine report recommended that most members be "outstanding non-government scientists with appropriate expertise," plus representatives from NIH's major HIV vaccine programs and one from OAR. In actuality, Baltimore was free to pick whomever he wanted. And he did. He chose nine academic scientists, all full professors at major institutions and only one of them female. The tenth member was Bill Snow, the San Francisco activist who had served on the Levine committee, whom Baltimore had never met but who came highly recommended by NIH. Government vaccine researchers were not among the anointed. Corporate vaccine makers were also excluded, so that possible conflicts of interest would not be an issue. As a result, Harvard primate expert Norm Letvin was as close as the committee came to having an active HIV vaccine researcher on board.

●

There is a star system in science that is as powerful as anything in Hollywood. In the entertainment industry, it's safe to assume that actors as a group are better looking than most people; in science, one can figure that researchers are generally smarter than the average Joe. Yet in both industries, some become stars, secure in their A-list status, while others who are equally attractive, smart, or talented are never accepted into the elite, even though they work hard and perform well. Connections, pedigree, and ambition may explain what differences in ability cannot.

David Baltimore was definitely on the A-list. He brought both intellectual gravitas and celebrity to the HIV vaccine effort, and Hal Varmus and Bill Paul, A-list guys themselves, sang his praises at every opportunity. This must have been difficult for Tony Fauci to witness. Although he aspired to walk among the superstars as an equal, Fauci had not quite made the grade. In comparison to the lavishly praised Baltimore, Fauci looked like an able-enough administrator, but not a scientific leader. He was like an actor who works steadily in television but never lands the role of leading man in a feature film.

Although the A-list scientists believed that NIH had shortchanged basic science on Fauci's watch and gone overboard on clinical trials, a less glittering group contended that the opposite was true. In the history of the AIDS epidemic, the NIH had supported only two Phase II vaccine trials. The first, of course, involved the gp120 products made by Chiron Biocine and Genentech. The second began shortly after Baltimore's appointment, in April 1997, testing PMC's canarypox vector with a Chiron gp120 boost. It would enroll 435 volunteers at fifteen sites and marked the first time that HIVNET had been used for its charter purpose—evaluating AIDS vaccines. Starting this trial was Pat Fast's proudest accomplishment so far.

Some NIH critics said this was a good start but believed the agency should pour lots more money into testing vaccines that might, regardless of how they performed in test tubes, protect people against this dreadful disease. This was the only conceivable response to the urgency of the epidemic. Most people with this view came from a public-health background and had worked in developing countries, rather than spending their careers in laboratories and classrooms.

Although Don Francis's celebrity made him stand out among critics of NIH's vaccine policies, many A-list scientists didn't take his complaints seriously. Don could play the crusader when he worked for CDC; now that his employer was a biotech with a financial stake in government-sponsored vaccine trials, the old role didn't fit. The WHO advisory group, which endorsed international efficacy trials in late 1994, had more legitimacy. In reality, though, its recommendation had little impact. For a time, it seemed as though there was no point going out on a limb to advocate for efficacy trials.

That changed when Baltimore was appointed. "A newcomer to vaccine research, he will become part-time chairman of yet another committee of outside advisers. This is unlikely to overcome the handicaps of the N.I.H. in promptly developing a vaccine," an op-ed piece in the *New York Times* said of Baltimore on January 4, 1997. The authors of the piece were identified as Bruce G. Weniger, a member of the Presidential Advisory Council on HIV and AIDS, and Max Essex, professor of virology at Harvard and chairman of the Harvard AIDS Institute. They were an odd couple.

Weniger drafted the opinion piece and then recruited Essex as coauthor, believing that a more famous name would lend credibility to the message. Weniger was impassioned but not very well known. For twenty years, he had been a physician and epidemiologist with the Centers for Disease Control, and in the late 1980s, he was stationed in Bangkok when AIDS hit Thailand. He and several Thai collaborators published a landmark description of the epidemic there, and when he came back to CDC in the early 1990s, he was convinced that AIDS had the potential to devastate Asia as well as Africa. Weniger's interest in HIV vaccines deepened after his 1995 appointment to the president's AIDS council, but his survey of the field led him to conclusions opposite those of the Levine committee.

Max Essex was a retrovirologist who collaborated with Bob Gallo during the early hunt for the AIDS virus, and he had since focused on genetic variations in HIV and related monkey viruses, mainly in West Africa. Many young African scientists had trained in his lab at Harvard, as Don Francis had done back in the 1970s. Essex's contribution to vaccine research was his discovery of the gp120 protrusion on HIV's surface. Despite his seniority at Harvard, Essex was not on the A-list with Varmus, Baltimore, and their cronies. His reputation had been tarnished, on several occasions, when findings from his laboratory could not be reproduced by other investigators. Still, NIH continued to fund work in his lab, and Essex remained a big name in international AIDS circles.

Although AIDS vaccine researchers had been fighting among themselves for years, their squabbling had been kept relatively quiet. The article by Weniger and Essex blew the lid off the split between the rational and the empirical camps. Even if *New York Times* readers didn't understand the subtleties, they might sense that infighting was slowing the search for an AIDS vaccine. The authors' empiricist leanings were clear as they revisited the history of polio vaccines. In the late 1940s, they credited an expedited, empirical approach to polio vaccines with keeping tens of thousands of children from being paralyzed, which they might have been if the government's more cautious, scientifically orthodox methods had prevailed. In their view, the contemporary search for an AIDS vaccine recapitulated the earlier power struggle between "the theorists of academic science and the empiricists of applied research."

"The theorists leisurely pursue new knowledge to build models to explain the complexity of nature and perhaps offer elegant solutions. The empiricists apply existing knowledge to seek pragmatic answers to urgent public health problems," Weniger and Essex wrote. They urged NIH to set up an organization for the sole purpose of developing an AIDS vaccine and to hire a senior scientist or research manager—ideally someone with an industry background—to lead the effort. In short, they were not in sympathy with Bill Paul's plan to channel millions of dollars into basic science, and David Baltimore was definitely not the leader they were looking for.

NIH Director Varmus, not surprisingly, wrote a letter to the *Times* calling Weniger and Essex's criticisms "cynical, misplaced and incorrect." He denied that NIH favored theory over applied science and said the agency had contributed to the development of several important vaccines. A Baltimore supporter wrote to say that the Nobelist from Boston was splendidly qualified to revamp the vaccine effort, adding, "Scientists already owe him a debt of gratitude for his scientific integrity."

Weniger and Essex had labeled Baltimore a "part-time chairman" with no experience in vaccinology. And in early 1997, intentionally or not, Baltimore often came across as a big star who didn't need to cultivate the supporting players. He skipped the first major AIDS conference held after his appointment, which a man with more of a common touch might have seized as a chance to rub shoulders with researchers in the field. In a January 22 interview on National Public Radio, he was confronted with Weniger and Essex's criticisms of NIH and waved them off. The obvious approaches to making an AIDS vaccine have been tried, he insisted, Weniger and Essex just don't like the results. He characterized NIH's approach to vaccines as being too empirical and urged more government support for virology research, his own area of expertise, "because that's where the action is."

●

May 4, 1997, was a beautiful spring day in Bethesda. All morning, scientists from the United States and abroad had been arriving at the Natcher Building on the NIH campus. This pale-colored stone-and-glass structure, situated on a rolling green rise, houses the large modern conference facility where the country's premier scientific conference on HIV vaccines was about to begin. The Ninth Annual Meeting of the National Cooperative Vaccine Development Groups for AIDS was universally referred to as NCVDG, for obvious reasons of convenience, and on this occasion about 500 people were expected to attend.

Scientific meetings such as this often start on Sunday afternoon or evening, which allows participants to spend part of the weekend at home before setting out. Not much typically happens on this first day—people have ample time to arrive, pick up their name tags and programs at the registration desk, and schmooze with friends. Often the only thing on the program is an opening-night cocktail reception.

This NCVDG meeting was different because the opening plenary featured back-to-back lectures by Tony Fauci and David Baltimore, together on the big stage for the first time since Baltimore was tapped to lead the AIDS Vaccine Research Committee. Hundreds of people, including many of the best-known names in vaccine research, were already in their seats when the opening bell sounded at 1:00 P.M.

When Tony Fauci stepped up to the lectern and adjusted the microphone, he looked as he always did: an intense, trim man in a gray suit, scrupulously groomed, delivering the official welcome to a conference organized by the Division of AIDS. He faced an auditorium filled mainly with people who were getting NIH money, either through grants or contracts, to work on HIV vaccines. They couldn't be sure, now that the Baltimore committee had started meeting, how their own projects might be affected. Whatever Fauci and Baltimore said, it would have as many different meanings as there were people in the audience.

The Clinton years were in full swing, pollsters were ascendant, and Fauci seemed to be figuring out which way the wind was blowing. He showed a familiar slide, which listed challenges faced by traditional vaccines and explained why each would pose an even greater biological problem for an AIDS vaccine. Then he veered off in a new direction, saying, "as you may hear from David in a few minutes," it might be time to reconsider live attenuated HIV vaccines, long shunned by many as too dangerous. That Fauci, a man not known as a daredevil, would even mention such a possibility came as a surprise.

A standard feature of Fauci's speeches is to highlight funding increases that have occurred during his reign at NIAID. He told the NCVDG meeting that for fiscal year 1998, 17 percent of NIAID's $678.2 million budget for HIV would be spent studying vaccines. He did not mention that this increase was due mostly to Bill Paul and the Office of AIDS Research. "Fundamental basic research" would be NIAID's top priority, as the

Levine committee had recommended, but clinical trials were also on the agenda. Fauci singled out canarypox and Dave Weiner's DNA vaccine as promising candidates for future testing and called gp120 and other protein subunit vaccines an approach "we elected not to pursue here in this country."

Finally, the screen showed the image of a balance scale, and Fauci turned to "the understandable tension between basic science and empiricism." Here he steered a middle ground, saying that what's needed is "a back and forth phenomenon," in which clinical trials help plug holes in basic knowledge and laboratory experiments help determine which clinical trials happen next. As part of this feedback loop, NIH must be a "good faith partner" to corporations and should "embrace them and get involved in what they do."

So far, NIH had bestowed hugs mainly on Pasteur Mérieux Connaught. In an interview after his speech, Fauci talked about all the time and effort he had invested in NIH's relationship with the giant French company, working "side by side, right from the very beginning." Ultimately, NIH might not fund an efficacy trial for canarypox. But if that was the case, the point was for the company not to be blindsided. Fauci did not want "to give industry a signal that all of a sudden some committee of wise people somewhere are gonna decide at any moment that oops, we need more basic science and to hell with our plan."

Fauci went on to describe himself as a "fundamental, basic scientist" whose job is to bridge the gap between his own field and the practical needs of government's private-sector partners. At some point, he said he would have to "bite the bullet" and decide that it makes scientific sense to proceed with an efficacy trial.

When David Baltimore stepped up to speak at the NCVDG meeting, the contrast between him and Tony Fauci was pronounced. Fauci has sometimes been described as "science in a suit." Baltimore looked exactly like someone who had spent most of the past thirty-five years at MIT, where the intellectual atmosphere is so rugged that students and faculty routinely describe it as "drinking from a fire hose." At fifty-nine, he was solidly built, his hair and beard more gray than brown, and he was wearing one of his many blue shirts and a tweed jacket. He had a strong profile, a direct gaze behind glasses with tortoiseshell frames, and a deep voice. He did not fidget and seemed laid back compared with the tightly wound and highly polished Fauci.

Vaccine researchers who expected Baltimore to declare that everything they knew was wrong were pleasantly surprised. His committee's philosophy was "let a thousand flowers bloom. We want to support every idea, we want to bring to clinical trials ideas that seem at all likely, to see if they will work in a clinical setting." Everything was still on the table so far as he was concerned. In fact, maybe live attenuated and killed virus approaches, which have protected against so many other diseases, deserve more serious consideration as vaccines against AIDS. Baltimore made an effort to come across as open-minded.

He said that his committee, the AVRC, was taking steps to "bring together people who have not historically focused their attention on vaccine research." They had already solicited proposals for the first batch of "Innovation Grants," which would be awarded for research on basic-science questions that interested the committee. These small grants, no more than $150,000 per year for a maximum of two years, were intended to lure bright young investigators into certain areas of research that might pave the way to new vaccines.

Baltimore then shifted gears to describe research in his own MIT lab that might relate to vaccines. An experimental assay might show whether HIV alters infected cells in ways that make it harder for killer T cells to sniff out the virus's hiding place. So far the results from this assay were preliminary, the kind of provocative finding that is usually presented by a postdoc in a ten-minute talk, not by a very senior scientist making his public debut as head of a powerful government committee. Baltimore's decision to talk about specific experiments in his academic lab sent an odd message about his priorities: Was he mainly a policymaker? A laboratory researcher? Or something else entirely?

Ten days later, headlines made it clear that Baltimore's most important new identity was as president of the California Institute of Technology, a private research university that is a smaller, more densely packed version of MIT. Although Caltech is tiny, with a total enrollment of only 2,000 undergraduate and graduate students, its faculty and alumni have won twenty-five Nobel Prizes. Despite having a new, full-time, and highly demanding job in California, Baltimore showed no inclination to resign as chairman of the AVRC. When he was based in Boston, he made it to Bethesda roughly one day a week. Now that he was going to a new post in California, critics thought it was even less realistic to expect him to "reinvigorate" the government effort to find an AIDS vaccine.

●

On the morning of May 18, 1997, President Bill Clinton did his part to raise the public profile of AIDS vaccines. He was onstage in the Hurt Gymnasium at Morgan State University, a century-old, historically black institution in northeast Baltimore. Hooded and gowned, flanked by faculty and administrators in full academic regalia, Clinton swung into a speech about the future of science and technology. Seated before him were 850 members of the Class of 1997, along with a throng of families and friends.

He invoked the spirit of President Kennedy's 1961 challenge to U.S. scientists, when he asked them to beat the Soviet Union in the race to the moon. It was a goal not only met but achieved ahead of schedule. Today it is global health, not space exploration, that is the great challenge of our times, Clinton said. Despite effective new treatments, AIDS is gaining on tuberculosis and malaria as the leading infectious killer in the world: 29 million people are infected, 3 million of them during the past year alone, and 95 percent of people with HIV live in the developing world.

"Only a truly effective, preventive HIV vaccine can limit and eventually eliminate the threat of AIDS," the president said, reflecting what he had heard from Bill Paul and others at the NIH, from Bruce Weniger and fellow members of his own AIDS advisory council, and from leaders of the newly launched vaccine advocacy movement. "Today, let us commit ourselves to developing an AIDS vaccine within the next decade," he said to applause. This would not be easy, he acknowledged, "but with the strides of recent years it is no longer a question of whether we can develop an AIDS vaccine, it is simply a question of when."

The president hailed scientists at the NIH and research universities as leaders of the vaccine effort and announced that NIH would establish "a new AIDS vaccine research center dedicated to this crusade." He also

challenged the pharmaceutical industry to make AIDS vaccine development a top priority, promising to enlist help from other industrialized
nations during an upcoming economic summit.

Critics were standing by, of course, ready to tell reporters what was
wrong with this presidential call to arms. Many wanted to talk about the
new Vaccine Research Center, which the president had proposed without
promising an infusion of new money to get it underway. As one vaccine
researcher put it, Clinton was getting on the vaccine bandwagon, but "he
didn't bring any fuel with him." HIV-infected AIDS activists warned that
money might be shifted out of treatment research and into vaccines, and
they opposed the VRC much as they had argued against efficacy testing in
1994.

Administration spokesmen said that the center would begin by bringing together NIH researchers who were already working on vaccine-
related projects, and would later have about fifty full-time scientists. This
plan also drew fire. "All he's doing is reshuffling a couple dozen employees," an ACT UP spokesman said of Clinton's new center. Tony Fauci
assured reporters that this was just a start, and with the president's strong
support, more resources would be poured into vaccine research in future
years.

One week after the Morgan State speech, the *Los Angeles Times* ran a
long, interview-rich feature about the impact of the president's
announcement on the vaccine field. This article identified Fauci as "the
man most responsible for implementing Clinton's vision" and David Baltimore as "overseer of the National Institutes of Health's AIDS vaccine
program." It laid out the differences in their views of the scientific challenge and the ten-year target date. Fauci expressed confidence that a vaccine would be developed, but declined to predict when. Baltimore said,
"Ten years of intense effort could really make a difference," but cautioned
that if no "strong candidates" emerged after a decade, "then we will have
to wonder whether it is possible to make a vaccine at all."

On balance, however, vaccine researchers appreciated their fifteen
minutes of fame. Having toiled mainly in obscurity, with none of the
kudos showered on treatment pioneers like David Ho, they were glad that
the president had finally gotten prevention into the public spotlight. An
editorial in the *San Francisco Chronicle* summed up the Morgan State

speech as "a dramatic gesture from the bully pulpit, and a positive step forward in the campaign against the deadly disease." A separate article in that newspaper pointed out that overall increases in NIH funding, largely the unsung work of Bill Paul and the OAR, meant more than Clinton's speech. "It was a rhetorical frosting on a vaccine program that already had been beefed up significantly," the *Chronicle* said, using a dubious culinary metaphor.

●

The Westin Chiangmai Hotel is a posh modern establishment on the eastern bank of the Ping River, a sludgy brown stream that snakes its way south from the infamous Golden Triangle. Visible on the other side of the river is the original Chiang Mai, a walled city that dates back to the thirteenth century, which is as noisy and crowded, albeit in a charming way, as the Westin is spacious and quiet. On a Monday morning in October 1997, 250 people assembled in the lobby of the hotel conference center, where huge arrangements of tropical flowers graced the registration desk and the air was spicy with the aroma of sandalwood.

They had come for a workshop on cellular and humoral immunity, organized by scientists from WRAIR and Thailand and paid for by the U.S. Department of Defense. The workshop's purpose was to prepare for a Phase II trial, set to begin in a few months, which the military hoped would be the final step toward the efficacy trial that John McNeil had been working toward for so long. Two-thirds of those in the lobby were from the host country, the men in suits and the women in jewel-colored dresses sewn from Thailand's famous silk. The Americans looked jet-lagged and rumpled by comparison, having recently survived the brutal, twenty-three-hour flight from the United States to Bangkok, followed by the commuter plane to Chiang Mai. The military officers were dressed in civilian clothes, because the DOD has no presence here except for AFRIMS, the medical research facility in Bangkok.

Pomp and ceremony dominated the opening session, as formal welcomes were extended by officials from Thai universities, the Thai and U.S. militaries, the city of Chiang Mai, and the U.S. consulate. The Thai scientists, who all speak English, were amused when the consul's representative delivered his remarks in English and halting Thai. All the dignitaries bowed to one another with the *wai*, pressing their fingertips together and bowing from the waist as a gesture of greeting and respect.

The festive atmosphere changed, however, as pleasantries were replaced with sadder stuff. A series of talks by U.S. and Thai epidemiologists traced the country's AIDS epidemic from its beginnings in 1984 to the present, when an estimated 800,000 Thais were infected. This works out to about one person in sixty. In northern Thailand, a professor from Chiang Mai said, "everyone knows someone who has died of AIDS."

By the end of the day, the cool, carpeted hotel ballroom felt like the staging ground for an impending battle. Over dinner, Thai doctors shared war stories about women who come to them for routine prenatal care and leave devastated by the discovery that they have HIV and that their baby has a 50-50 chance of being infected. The people on the front lines had every reason to want a vaccine.

Most Thai participants were not doctors who treat sick people, but immunologists, virologists, and molecular biologists. Many attended grad school or did postdocs at universities in the United States or Western Europe. They came home and were hired by research facilities such as RIHES, where the government maintains the physical facility and pays their basic salaries but cannot afford to support actual experiments. If they relied exclusively on the Thai government for support, these highly trained scientists would collect their meager salaries and sit watching their lab equipment decay into obsolescence. Fortunately, the ones who hustle can keep their labs going with money from institutions such as NIH and WRAIR, the World Health Organization and UNAIDS, the Rockefeller and Henry M. Jackson Foundations, and international family-planning agencies.

Like their U.S. counterparts, Thai immunologists wanted to discover what the body must do to fight off HIV. Although some were already performing antibody testing and some of the complicated T cell assays, others had not had an opportunity to learn. During this meeting, they signed up to conduct experiments with U.S. scientists who would teach them new immunology techniques. In addition to advancing the DOD's vaccine trial, Thai labs can use most of these techniques for other purposes as well. Technology transfer that makes indigenous labs stronger,

Dr. Natth Bhamarapravati and his National AIDS Committee have said all along, increases the likelihood that the Thai authorities will approve an efficacy trial when the time comes.

John McNeil had been working toward an efficacy trial for many years, and this workshop was an important step toward the Goal 2000 study. Four years earlier, at a different hotel in Chiang Mai, the late Kathy Steimer stepped forward as the first person willing to design a vaccine especially for Thailand. Other companies had followed suit, and the Goal 2000 trial would test three vaccines designed for Thailand: Chiron's clade E gp120 used alone, PMC's clade E canarypox with the Chiron vaccine as a boost, and—if Dave Weiner and Apollon came through in time—a naked DNA construct carrying clade E antigens.

John didn't really know how many volunteers Goal 2000 would have to recruit. Public education and condom campaigns had slowed the spread of HIV not only among military conscripts but also in parts of civilian society where the virus is transmitted via heterosexual contact. The rule of thumb in clinical trials is that the less frequent an event becomes, such as a healthy person becoming infected with HIV, the larger the study must be to detect it. Looking at the trends in Thailand, John and WRAIR statisticians estimated that 15,000 to 20,000 volunteers would be needed to show whether experimental vaccines keep people from becoming infected.

The precursor to this huge effort would be a small Phase I/II study starting one month after the Chiang Mai workshop. Twelve volunteers would participate in an "open-label" trial of two gp120 products from Chiron—half receiving the clade E gp120 alone, with the others getting a bivalent formulation that combined gp120E with the company's original gp120 SF2. Unlike a blind study, everyone involved in an open-label trial knows who is being injected with what. The point here would be to confirm that in Thais, as in American volunteers, a temporarily sore arm is the vaccine's most serious adverse effect.

John expected a Phase II study of the same two products to begin in January 1998. In this trial, Thai researchers at RIHES and three Bangkok sites would recruit 380 healthy, low-risk volunteers. Their immune responses would be measured, so that scientists could figure out whether the monovalent clade E vaccine or the bivalent B/E version generates more antibodies against Thai E viruses. The better of the two would advance into the Goal 2000 efficacy trial.

In these upcoming trials, John and Debbi have decided that gp120 should be tested on its own, even though NIH abandoned this approach. They fault the NIH for being fickle. "Every year something new comes up, and we still haven't evaluated the first generation of HIV-specific vaccines. People are writing things off without having tested them," John said. Even snooty A-list scientists believe that antibodies help the body resist HIV infection, and gp120 puts more of those immunologic cops on the street than any other type of vaccine. To John, it's a no-brainer to test gp120 before deciding that it doesn't work.

Former NIH administrator Peggy Johnston, who had left NIAID during the bleak first days of 1996, was a strong supporter of the army's efforts to mount an efficacy trial in Thailand. She believed that an AIDS vaccine should be a top international priority, yet she worked for an institution that seemed in no particular rush to get there. Private companies had mostly turned their backs on vaccine development in general, and when it came to the developing world, the U.S. military and tiny VaxGen were the only ones displaying any real interest. So after making her career in the belly of the bureaucracy, Peggy left NIH to become scientific director, and sole employee, of the fledgling International AIDS Vaccine Initiative.

IAVI had been launched with backing from the Rockefeller Foundation, the World Bank, and UNAIDS—making it a blue-blooded newcomer to the advocacy world. IAVI's grand plan was to promote development and testing of HIV vaccines for the poorest nations on earth and to make sure that any successful vaccine was available to the people who needed it most. What the organization did not have, at least not yet, was the financial or political muscle needed to make this happen.

Peggy had been with IAVI for eighteen months and had spent most of that time on the road. A poised and articulate public speaker, she had delivered IAVI's "international call to action" to scientific conferences, government meetings, and corporate boardrooms on nearly every continent. In her remarks during the Chiang Mai workshop, she praised Thailand as an international leader in HIV vaccines, and said the Thai-U.S. military collaboration was a model for future development efforts.

From Thailand, Peggy would fly to Manila for a conference on AIDS in

Asia and the Pacific, then to Paris for meetings with corporate and government officials before returning to Washington. A schedule such as this could make anyone haggard, but Peggy looked bad for other reasons as well. Back home in the Maryland suburbs, her partner of many years was dying of cancer. Peggy was dealing with the slow and agonizing loss of a loved one, while at the same time trying to excel in a hugely demanding new job. She never knew what a phone call from home would bring.

Neither, as it turned out, could other Americans at the meeting predict what might be beamed from the opposite side of the globe. Early one morning, before the workshop sessions began, calls from Washington brought news that Pat Fast was no longer head of the vaccine program at the Division of AIDS. Pat reported to Jack Killen, director of DAIDS, who in turn reported to Tony Fauci, a setup that distanced Pat from Fauci's inner circle. Removed as she was from the seat of power, Pat was the highest-ranking person whose job description specified that she was accountable for managing HIV vaccine research.

Pat viewed Killen's reluctance to push people or make decisions with distaste—sometimes so openly that colleagues thought she verged on insubordination. It seemed to her that decisions stalled in Killen's hands, and it was impossible to tell whether he was holding things up or was merely following orders. At any rate, Killen was often aggravated when Pat seemed to badger academic investigators or company executives to move faster.

After the Levine committee singled out vaccine research as the weakest link in NIH's AIDS programs, it was obvious that someone would have to pay. All things considered, it was no surprise that Pat Fast was the one voted off the island.

●

On May 18, 1998, the AIDS Vaccine Advocacy Coalition, an activist group, released a report called "9 Years and Counting: Will We Have an HIV Vaccine by 2007?" It began: "One year ago, the President of the United States invoked America's mission to the moon in challenging this country and the world to develop an HIV vaccine within a decade. That ten years is now nine. At the current level of effort, we will not have an

HIV vaccine in nine years. Unless more is done, the President's challenge will not be met."

The nine activists who comprised AVAC were not convinced that the strong correctives proposed by the Levine report had made much of a difference at NIH. Although the Baltimore committee was up and running, it was not at all clear that an advisory committee, whose members had many other professional responsibilities, had the time or energy to coordinate the government's vaccine efforts. Institute directors like Fauci continued to rule their fiefdoms as before.

The president had also announced that a new Vaccine Research Center would be created at NIH and that HIV vaccines would be its first task. In the ensuing year, Congress had voted $26 million to construct a new building for the VRC—but twelve months had passed and no director had been hired. Not only was the search not complete, but it had purportedly caused the Office of AIDS Research to lose the services of immunologist Bill Paul. Supposedly, Paul had stepped down from his OAR job in hopes of being named director of the VRC, only to find that NIH head Hal Varmus was determined not to fill the post with an NIH insider.

Soon after the AVAC "9 Years" report was released, Jack Killen began giving a stump speech to all the NIH administrative and advisory committees on AIDS research. His illustrated lecture laid out a plan for completely reorganizing the federal infrastructure for testing HIV vaccines and nonvaccine prevention methods, such as microbicides. Although Killen insisted that NIH was committed to moving toward efficacy trials, the proposed restructuring was massive. Anyone who had ever organized a bake sale could see that this would take years to accomplish. Many new committees would also be required.

The proposed HIV Vaccine Trials Network, or HVTN, would be led by a team of academic investigators who won the job by competing against other similar teams. The winning group would be chosen by a special committee. A second committee would evaluate applications from universities that wanted to be vaccine test sites, and the winners of this competition would be carrying out experiments designed by the leadership "core." The model for this elaborate setup was the AIDS Clinical Trials Group (ACTG), a system for testing AIDS drugs that NIAID had created in the late 1980s.

This NIH-sponsored network became notorious for its single-minded focus on AZT, which originated in a government lab, and its lack of interest in testing many medicines discovered elsewhere. The ACTG was also infamous for spending millions of dollars to create the infrastructure for huge trials, then letting most of this sit idle while conducting mostly small studies. Many old-timers looked on Killen's new vaccine plan with great dismay. On the other hand, there had been protest marches and street demonstrations about the urgent need for effective treatments. Vaccines stirred no such activism, so Killen would have plenty of time to tinker with the setup of the new system for testing vaccines.

Speed was certainly not of the essence for David Baltimore. In January 1997, shortly after being tapped to lead the AVRC, he had skipped the Fourth Conference on Retroviruses and Opportunistic Infections, an important annual event for AIDS researchers. In 1998, Baltimore not only braved February in Chicago for the Fifth Retro, as the gathering is familiarly known, but delivered one of the main addresses. In a press conference before his talk, he made his expectations clear: "I would be satisfied that we met the challenge if ten years from now we have candidate vaccines that we are confident we want to proceed to take to efficacy testing," he told journalists. "It is unlikely that in that time we will have a vaccine that we really know to be safe, effective and cheap."

In the meantime, HIV was reducing the number of healthy people on the planet by 16,000 every day.

12

THE NEXT GENERATION

ALTHOUGH THE 1994 ARAC decision froze HIV vaccine development at Chiron and Genentech and chilled the business climate for companies with similar products, it boosted the stock of some "second-generation" vaccines. The vaccines that fell out of favor were meant to protect by generating antibodies against the AIDS virus. When antibodies induced by the gp120 vaccines failed to neutralize primary isolates of HIV, however, most A-list scientists in academia and at NIH gave up on antibody-oriented vaccines and shifted their allegiance to some newer approaches, such as naked DNA and live vectors.

Naked DNA and live-vector vaccines were designed to activate the cellular arm of the immune system, in theory programming cytotoxic T lymphocytes, or CTLs, to seek out and destroy HIV that had weaseled its way inside human cells. Animal experiments and observations of HIV patients whose immune systems were unusually good at fighting off the virus indicated that CTLs might be the key to a successful vaccine.

As scientific opinion leaders promoted CTLs over antibodies, researchers like Margaret Liu, David Weiner, and Bob Johnston and Nancy Davis found their work suddenly in vogue. The disappointments suffered by scientists at Chiron and Genentech were like Weather Channel reports of snowstorms in a distant part of the country: the viewer may feel sympathy for the people who live there, but local meteorologists forecast mild weather.

At Merck, Margaret Liu appeared to be in an especially advantageous position. She worked for one of the world's largest health-care companies, famous not only for discovering hugely successful new drugs but also for having deep enough pockets to test what its scientists invented. When Merck wanted to put a drug or vaccine into clinical testing, it rarely relied on the NIH or anyone else to pay. The company could afford to carry out its own human studies, and it generally did.

As the leader of Merck's research on DNA vaccines, Margaret's first big job was to make sure that the DNA concept was safe and immunogenic in animals. The second hurdle was to demonstrate protection in an animal model. If these results were sufficiently convincing, then the company might consider moving toward clinical trials. Business realities force drug companies to discover as rapidly as possible whether a potential product is likely to work. This had proved notoriously difficult for gp120 and dozens of earlier HIV vaccines, both because there was no ideal animal model and because scientists disagreed about the best way to assess immune responses. Witness the debate over whether chimp protection studies were credible, and the bitter battles over neutralizing antibody assays. If speed was of the essence   and it was to a pharmaceutical company—then HIV vaccines were not the way to go.

Even though Margaret's burning ambition was to make an AIDS vaccine, influenza was a better choice for Merck's "proof of concept" experiments. Both mice and ferrets provide excellent models for studying flu, because if immunization fails, it's obvious: The animals develop the same fever and miseries as people with flu. There were also established lab tests for assessing immune responses to experimental flu shots. So Margaret could still work on HIV vaccines, but flu had to be tested first. In March 1993, she and her Vical collaborators had published evidence that a DNA vaccine protected mice against flu and that it did so by activating CTLs that killed flu virus.

In the four years since Merck licensed naked-DNA technology from Vical, Margaret's group had refined the original plasmid and used it to formulate potential vaccines against influenza, herpes, human papilloma virus, and, of course, AIDS. At this point, scientists from labs near Margaret's had finally stopped deriding naked DNA as "weird science" or "cold fusion."

Still, there was a great deal more work to be done. In addition to the scientific challenges of showing that DNA vaccines could prevent disease in larger animals, and ultimately in humans, Margaret also had to navigate the political and organizational complexities that are the warp and weft of any huge organization. Merck had nearly 50,000 employees, more than 7,000 of them at Merck Research Laboratories, where Margaret and her handful of scientists and lab techs were based. Although the flu vaccine was a hot topic in the larger world of vaccines, within Merck it was one vaccine project among many. And Merck's substantial vaccine program, in the context of the whole company, was dwarfed by the mammoth research program on therapeutic drugs. The reasons for this disparity were easy to see: Annual sales for a single cholesterol-lowering drug topped $1 billion, roughly equal to the combined revenues for all Merck's vaccines.

In 1994, the hottest item in Merck's viral-disease portfolio was indinavir, one of the protease inhibitors that would soon revolutionize AIDS care. Top executives thought that anti-HIV drugs "were doable and they were important," recalled R. Gordon Douglas, an infectious-disease physician and president of Merck Vaccines at the time. Patients were clamoring for better treatments, the FDA was anxious to approve such products quickly, and these drugs would surely generate huge revenues. The choice was obvious.

In the shadow of indinavir, Margaret worked hard to keep the company leadership excited about DNA vaccines. And she did this in a corporate setting where women who talked too much about their families or took too much time away from work were likely to be written off and passed over. It was not that Merck was especially insensitive; it was simply a company like any other. And Margaret was not a feminist revolutionary who went out of her way to buck the system; she was an ambitious scientist with a powerful distaste for the "mommy track."

In April 1994, for example, Margaret flew to Geneva, carrying not only her usual briefcase filled with paperwork and slides but also a breast pump and a small ice chest. She had been invited to speak at the World Health Organization's first conference on DNA vaccines, a must-attend meeting even though she was breast feeding her two-week-old daughter. Margaret crossed the Atlantic overnight, gave her talk, participated in the conference, and left the next morning. "Didn't you just come over with us?" airline crew members asked, eyeing Margaret and her little ice chest. "I felt as though I was leaving one baby to go take care of my other baby," she said.

●

Only a short drive from Merck Research Laboratories, where Margaret was wending her way through the corporate maze, the outlook for David Weiner's DNA project improved within months of the ARAC decision. For years, peer-review committees at the National Institutes of Health had shunned his requests for vaccine-related funding. After Apollon licensed his vaccine technology from the University of Pennsylvania, however, Dave could go after different types of NIH money. He and Apollon were now eligible for a program that bankrolled academic-industry collaborations on new AIDS treatments, and in September 1994, Penn and Apollon won a four-year, $4.2-million grant. Although the money was earmarked for testing the DNA vaccine as a treatment for HIV-infected people, not as a preventive vaccine, this was still a step in the right direction.

Dave's ultimate goal was to make a vaccine that was both safe and protective against AIDS. It would be exactly like the pink, green, and black vaccine his little daughter Rebecca had drawn, which she explained "has all of the good things that you need and none of the bad things that would hurt you." The vaccine wouldn't be as colorful as Rebecca's version, of course, but it would be safe enough for his own children and it would work.

But first things first. With the grant money now in place, Apollon's initial task was to make larger quantities of plasmids with various HIV genes stitched into them. These "cassettes," as Dave called them, could be tested for prevention later—after the therapeutic trial was underway.

Once the cassettes were ready, Apollon had yet one more hurdle: obtaining permission from the Food and Drug Administration to begin testing in HIV-infected people. Physicians at the University of Pennsylvania Medical Center could begin injecting volunteers only after the FDA approved an Investigational New Drug application, or IND, for the vaccine.

In early 1995, the FDA approved the trial, marking the first time that a DNA vaccine would be given to human volunteers. When television crews came to interview Dave about the upcoming experiment, they did not have to shoehorn themselves into the ancient lab in the Maloney Building, where snow insinuated itself through ill-fitting windows. Instead, they hauled their gear through the soaring lobby of Penn's newly constructed research showplace, the ten-story Stellar-Chance Laboratory. An elevator whisked them to the fifth floor, where Dave's new lab stretched along an entire side of the building, with offices at one end, a containment facility for handling HIV, and an open lab with bench space for a dozen researchers.

Dave had come a long way in a short amount of time. His work had been picked up by a biotech, he had secured his first major NIH grant, and in June 1995 Penn promoted him to associate professor. But what confirmed his ascension of the academic pecking order was the capacious lab, which his new funding made possible. In most academic medical centers, space is harder to obtain than a promotion or a bigger paycheck. Full professors have been known to connive like Medicis to secure a few hundred square feet of unglamorous space with linoleum floors and fluorescent lights.

By the summer of 1995, when sixteen HIV-positive volunteers were inoculated at Penn, tiny Apollon surged ahead of Merck and every other developer of DNA vaccines. As euphoric as they were at such a moment, Dave's corporate partners worried constantly about money. It cost a fortune to refine the vaccine cassettes, work out the technical requirements of manufacturing, satisfy government red tape, and test patient samples from the clinical trial. The work was going fine, but Apollon needed to make a deal with a larger, wealthier company to keep things going.

In the final months of the year, Apollon signed a $100-million licensing agreement with American Home Products, parent of Wyeth-Ayerst and its subsidiary, Wyeth-Lederle Vaccines. This was a real windfall, even though the money would be doled out slowly over five years. The trade-off was that Wyeth-Lederle now owned the rights to the three experimental vaccines Dave had made so far: products to fight HIV, herpes, and human papilloma virus. These licenses made Wyeth-Lederle a leader in DNA vaccines.

While the Wyeth-Lederle deal was being negotiated, Dave stuck as close to the laboratory and as far from the boardroom as he could manage. Although he had to be trotted out as the inventor of the vaccines, he was not like many scientists who thrill to the idea of becoming a captain of industry. On the subject of the licensing agreement, he grows testy and says, "What does that have to do with the AIDS vaccine, anyway? That wouldn't affect any of the real work; that would be something negotiated in some office by a bunch of lawyers." This attitude probably explains why he was not an Apollon founder, or a principal in the company, or even a member of the board of directors. All he cared about was the vaccines.

●

Dave Weiner wasn't the only one who suffered through a long funding drought, only to have money fall from the sky in late 1994. Bob Johnston and Nancy Davis had made an experimental AIDS vaccine by putting HIV genes into an attenuated version of VEE, the Venezuelan equine encephalitis virus. They had also been working on an influenza vaccine using the same vectors. Although the NIH helped support their basic investigations of the biology of VEE and related alphaviruses, the two University of North Carolina scientists had been rejected every time they asked for money expressly for vaccine development. As the NIH Levine committee would acknowledge the following year, vaccines were the kind of applied research that did not fare well in grant-making committees composed of academic scientists.

Frustrated by the NIH peer-review system, Bob and Nancy appealed to the military for help. The UNC team collaborated with army virologist Jonathan Smith to make the VEE vectors and had done some of key experiments at Fort Detrich in Maryland. The end of the MicroGeneSys debacle gave WRAIR $20 million to invest in developing novel AIDS vaccines, and Don Burke quickly set up a process and a committee for handing it out. Bob and Nancy had a track record, they were known to the committee, and they were awarded a four-year grant for $1.88 million in September 1994.

Bob and Nancy promised WRAIR that they would identify a desirable vaccine candidate by the end of 1999. The game plan was to create monkey versions of the human vaccines they were working on, compare the efficacy of these SIV vaccines in macaques, and use the results to determine which of their two VEE vectors would be more likely to provide safe protection against HIV. Once they knew what to shoot for, the remaining work would be more technical than conceptual. "If you can make the SIV version of a VEE construct, you can make the HIV version," said Nancy, who knew because she still did hands-on molecular biology.

The UNC plan made sense to the military. "The army is used to putting out contracts to buy a tank," Bob said of the ease with which they reached an agreement. "This kind of straightforward approach, of listing what we were going to do, appealed to them." At NIH, researchers were seldom pressed to state their goals so plainly.

The NIH's decision not to move forward with the gp120 efficacy trials gave a real boost to the VEE team, even though it didn't send any funding their way. "We were hearing that the immunologists were more and more convinced that CTLs were important, whereas the vaccinologists, who had made the first subunit candidates, were really focused on the antibodies," Nancy recalled. Based on what she knew about how viruses cause disease and how the body fights back, this made sense to her. "When you recover from an acute viral infection, it's largely CTLs that kick in."

The beauty of VEE was that it appeared to deliver antigens straight to the lymph nodes, little knots of tissue along the lymphatic vessels, which parallel blood vessels. One of the lymphatic system's roles is to filter out toxins and dead cells and to return viable cells to the bloodstream. In addition, lymph nodes are like military boot camps, where the immune system programs B cells to make antibodies and prepares CTLs to attack and kill virus-infected cells. In theory, no matter which arm of the immune system was needed to ward off HIV, a VEE-based vaccine should have it covered. But which VEE vector would best activate the immune system against the virus? That was the question Bob and Nancy hoped to answer with the upcoming monkey experiments.

They had made two different VEE vectors. One was a weakened but genetically complete version of the virus, which might cause illness if it made too many copies of itself in the body. They called this the "double-promoter vector," and it was an updated, refined version of the full-length VEE clone that Nancy first assembled during that 1988 heat wave at Fort Detrich. The second was the "VEE replicon particle," or VRP, a genetically engineered form of the virus that was too wimpy to reproduce in human cells. The double-promoter vector was more likely to stimulate a powerful immune response to the viral genes in its payload, but there was the possibility that it might revert to a wild and dangerous form and make people sick. Although VRPs were certain to be safe, they might fizzle out before the immune system had time to generate a protective response. Until monkey results helped them judge which was the better candidate, Bob and Nancy had to keep working on both.

During 1994 and 1995, life was frenetic in the eighth-floor lab of the Mary Ellen Jones Research Building at UNC. It was a typical grungy academic setting, with drab linoleum floors and scuffed walls that were mostly concealed by chunky pieces of equipment and shelves crammed with bottles and boxes of supplies. Nancy and a postdoc engineered a flu vaccine that could be tested in mice, an easy and affordable animal model. Ian Caley, the group's cloning ace, stuffed bits of HIV into double-promoter VEE, tinkering with the vectors to stabilize them and increase their ability to crank out antigens. All this happened in a room with barely enough space for four people.

In May 1994, Nancy's flu experiments were the basis for a patent application for the double-promoter VEE expressing a foreign antigen; one year later, they filed a similar application for the replicon technology. Both documents were broadly worded, to encompass vaccines against more than flu and HIV, and the intellectual property rights were held by the University of North Carolina. Scientists chafe at patent filings because they involve blizzards of paper and legal meetings that strain the patience of people who would rather be doing experiments. The data emerging from Bob and Nancy's lab, however, was so encouraging that it made up for the hassle.

By April 1995, Ian knew that his HIV double-promoter vector was eliciting HIV-specific antibodies in mice. It took much longer to set up an assay that could measure CTL responses, but by December, Ian and collaboratories in UNC's immunology department had a test up and running. No one had ever measured a cellular immune response to a VEE vector before, so it was a big deal when they found vigorous CTLs against HIV.

There was no time to kick back and savor these results. While Nancy and Ian kept refining their double-promoter vectors, they were also engineering replicons that contained HIV, SIV, and flu. Like Merck, the UNC team saw flu—with its readily available animal models and established immunologic assays—as an excellent way to show "proof of concept" for novel vaccines. This strategy began to pay off when a mouse experiment showed that replicons generated an antibody response to flu that was ten times more powerful than the double-promoter vector.

No one could predict, of course, whether the replicons would pack the same punch in the SIV experiments with monkeys. But there was no doubt that in the race for an AIDS vaccine, the dark horse in North Carolina was gaining on more pedigreed entries from big pharmaceutical companies like Merck and Pasteur Mérieux Connaught. By 1996, Bob and Nancy's primate experiments were underway; they weren't rich, but they had enough money to keep going, and UNC's newly opened technology transfer office was looking for a company to license VEE vaccines. Life was good.

●

To outsiders, Merck appeared to be going all-out to develop DNA vaccines. Four decades of innovative vaccine research ensured that the company would automatically be regarded as a heavyweight; beyond that, Margaret Liu and her group were gaining respect with each new publication about their successful experiments with DNA immunization.

Her team made a tremendous splash with an article in the June 1995 issue of *Nature Medicine*. They described inoculating ferrets with a DNA vaccine that delivered genes for a highly stable part of flu virus as well as rapidly evolving parts of its protein coat. The animals were challenged with a flu strain expected to hit that year and with another that struck unexpectedly and caused many human deaths. The DNA-inoculated ferrets were better protected against the rogue strain than animals immunized with that year's standard vaccine. Seeing these results, reporters marveled at the possibility that someday people might not have to line up for a reformulated flu shot every fall. The *Harvard Health Letter* named this discovery one of the top ten medical advances for the year.

These accolades, however, seemed to bounce off the front door of Building 16 at Merck Research Laboratories. Although Merck's culture was less nakedly competitive than Genentech's in the 1980s, when executives set teams of testosterone-crazed cloners at each other's throats, Merck scientists still jockeyed for attention and resources. So much attention was being showered on indinavir, and on project leader Emilio Emini, that everything Margaret's team accomplished was overshadowed. Emini's decision to work on AIDS drugs, instead of vaccines, was very savvy indeed.

Although Emini was not actively engaged in HIV vaccine research, he didn't hesitate to express his opinions about the quest for a vaccine. While Margaret's article about the ferret experiment was in press, Emini soberly cataloged barriers to HIV vaccine development in *Science and Medicine*, a journal that popularizes research topics. Much of the article focused on what he perceived as the failure of protein subunit vaccines, and he devoted only a single paragraph to each of several new vaccine technologies, among them naked DNA. Emini opined that an effective vaccine might be impossible to develop but that scientists should not abandon the quest because the AIDS pandemic was such a severe public-health emergency. He said nothing insulting about Margaret's efforts, and she made no rebuttal. But it wasn't the most supportive gesture from someone supposedly on the same corporate team.

Margaret and her colleagues, however, saw plenty of reasons to keep going. If immunizing ferrets with DNA from one flu subtype protected the animals against unrelated strains of virus, then perhaps it would be possible to design a vaccine that protected people against genetically diverse types of HIV. They thought this could be done, but with so many resources devoted to indinavir, HIV vaccine work was a struggle. When Margaret finally did get authorization to test an experimental DNA vaccine in chimps, for example, blood samples had to be shipped to outside laboratories for analysis. Merck had immunology labs that could have performed neutralizing antibody and CTL assays needed for the chimp study, but they were assigned to work exclusively on indinavir trials.

Margaret had resources at her disposal, of course, but these were supposed to go mainly toward flu. This was the flagship DNA construct that Merck wanted to move into clinical trials, and everything else would have to wait until that was accomplished. Margaret chafed at this. "Once you have a lead compound, you start working on backups," she said, emphasizing that Merck routinely takes this approach to therapeutic drug development. Although the DNA technology looked very promising, "you don't necessarily have to stick with what you have when you're trying to make a vaccine against a disease that's as wily as HIV. So I wanted to work on things that weren't just naked DNA, to start looking at ways to make this a more potent technology," she said.

As it turned out, Margaret's wishes would become decreasingly important as time passed.

●

Life was very exciting and more than a little nerve-wracking for Dave Weiner. In June 1996, only one year after the first HIV-infected patient had been inoculated with his DNA vaccine against AIDS, a doctor at Penn pushed the plunger on a syringe and injected a dose of clear vaccine into the arm of a healthy volunteer. This was a milestone for the entire field, because it was the first time that the FDA had ever permitted testing of a DNA vaccine against any disease in healthy people. And it was not Merck which had gotten here first, but Dave and his colleagues at upstart Apollon.

FDA approval had not been easy to come by because, as Dave readily admitted, "we don't really know the risks in people yet." Dozens of tubes of blood would be drawn from volunteers at every clinic visit, and twenty-three different assays and procedures would be used to look for any possible adverse effects. Among other things, the FDA wanted assurance that the DNA in the vaccine would not incorporate itself into the human genetic code. One of the final hurdles for Apollon was coming up with an assay that could tell whether the vaccine integrated itself into the nuclear DNA of one in 1 million cells. There was no evidence from animal experiments that this ever happened, but the Phase I study was meant to show safety and immunogenicity, and the FDA was being cautious.

Soon after the FDA approved the trial in February 1996, Dave got an additional vote of confidence from the NIH Clinical Center, the same giant research hospital where Tony Fauci still cared for some AIDS patients. The Clinical Center wanted to use Dave's vaccine for a Phase I study of its own, which would begin immediately. For a man whose vaccine had repeatedly been turned down for extramural grants, there was no doubt some satisfaction in having it chosen for intramural testing at NIH expense.

At times, it seemed that Dave was being transformed from an outsider into one of NIH's rising favorites. At the Institute's vaccine meeting in May 1997, when everyone in the field came to see David Baltimore and Tony Fauci on the same stage, Fauci gave Dave's DNA vaccine a favorable mention in his speech. In particular, he cited a chimpanzee study that appeared in *Nature Medicine* that very month, identifying Dave's vaccine as one of several likely candidates for future clinical trials.

The *Nature Medicine* article described an experiment where chimps had been inoculated with a DNA vaccine carrying partial genes from HIV_{MN}, then challenged with 250 times more HIV_{SF2} than it ordinarily takes to infect these animals. Immunized chimps were protected, whereas a control animal rapidly became infected. Despite the positive notice the study had gotten from Fauci and in the press, Dave had mixed feelings about it.

Staff scientists at DAIDS pushed him to do the chimp experiment, advising that "if we got responses in chimps, and protection in chimps, our vaccine would be much more accepted," Dave recalled. But it took two years to set up the study, nearly two to conduct it, and still more time to analyze the results. By the time all this was done, the chimpanzee model "had fallen out of favor, and as soon as we had the chimp protection, the reaction was 'Why did you do that study?'" he said.

While Dave's chimp experiment was in progress, NIH's view of this model changed after top administrators wrote off gp120. Don Francis argued that Genentech's version deserved an efficacy trial because Phil Berman had shown, back in 1989, that it protected chimps against what Don liked to call "a whopping dose" of HIV. Many of the A-list scientists in academia and the NIH dismissed this finding, because they had come to believe that the chimp model could not predict what might happen in humans. Although no one would really know until results from a human efficacy trial could be compared with findings from chimp studies, the prevailing notion was that what happened in chimps didn't count.

As a result, Dave's chimp results didn't carry nearly the weight they would have a few years earlier. Fauci's comments reflected this when the *New York Times* asked him for perspective on the *Nature Medicine* report. The good news, Fauci said, was that DNA vaccines could be added to the list of concepts that might eventually protect people; the bad news was "that we have seen protection in chimps before with other concepts for an AIDS vaccine and still do not have an effective vaccine for humans."

Given the uncertainty about the predictive value of animal models, Dave and many other vaccine developers looked for vaccine constructs that protected in as many models as possible, "to give us confidence that we're on the right track." Still, scientists knew that a vaccine might protect mice, chimps, and monkeys yet fail utterly in humans and, conversely, that one might fail in animals but be highly successful in humans.

For vaccine researchers, who still did not know what it would take to repel HIV, the lesson was to stay loose and humble. "The person who finds an AIDS vaccine will never win a Nobel Prize and will never be as well known as a mediocre second baseman for the Toronto Blue Jays," Dave mused.

●

Meanwhile, on the West Coast, the DNA vaccine effort that Kathy Steimer had launched before she died was one of the pieces moving on Chiron's business chessboard. Chiron Biocine had become a big player in the international vaccine market in 1992, when it bought into an Italian vaccine maker, and it later acquired the biggest supplier in Germany. Kathy's research program was considered part of global vaccine operations.

A corporate reshuffling moved vaccine research from the international division to a big technology department headquartered in Emeryville. Whoever led the vaccine effort would report to Lewis "Rusty" Williams, the physician-researcher who was president of Chiron Technologies. Ideally, putting all the lab groups under one administrative roof would inspire them to interact, share ideas, and come up with exciting new ways to prevent, diagnose, and treat the ills of mankind.

This was a fine-sounding vision that fell short in one key regard. At the head of Chiron's vaccine research program was a spectral black horse, with boots turned backward in its stirrups and an empty saddle. Kathy Steimer was gone, and the saddle needed to be filled.

At the pinnacle of Chiron's organizational chart, founder and chairman Bill Rutter still wanted to make an AIDS vaccine and thought that naked DNA had real promise. Following Kathy's death, he acknowledged that "there certainly was not a leader." Not only that, but the company's herpes vaccine had been abandoned after bombing in clinical trials. Like gp120, the herpes vaccine was constructed from a protein subunit designed to elicit protective antibodies. Coupled with the loss of Kathy, Rutter said, "this was a double death. We truly expected herpes to work. It was a super-big blow to the company, to vaccinology, and to our HIV program." Dino Dina, president of Chiron's vaccine business also resigned after the herpes vaccine failed.

●

The University of North Carolina's intellectual property office hired attorneys to pull together patent applications for VEE vectors invented by Bob Johnston, Nancy Davis, and their army collaborator, Jonathan Smith. Once this was done, in 1994 and 1995, UNC had only modest hopes for the earning power of those patents. "The idea was that they would recoup their application costs and get a little extra to put in their pot, so this could be used to apply for other patents. That was their mandate, to license and keep their little pot going," Nancy explained.

For two years, not much happened on the licensing front. Bob and Nancy had plenty to do in the lab, so they kept working and didn't give much thought to patents. In March 1997, however, the head of UNC's tech transfer office called to say that the university had gotten a very exciting offer for the vaccine rights. Thus began a seemingly endless series of meetings between lawyers in suits and the vaccine inventors, who were considerably more informal.

UNC's tech transfer folks were impressed that the offer came from giant Wyeth-Lederle Vaccines; so impressed, it seemed, that their critical faculties were on hold. "The offer on the table was $60,000, [for which] the university was going to give them worldwide, exclusive rights to all uses of this technology. And *give* is the operative word here," Bob said. In 1995, in a transaction widely reported in the business news, Wyeth had paid $100 million to license three of Dave Weiner's naked-DNA vaccines from Penn. But perhaps Wyeth thought that technology, like real estate, should be cheaper in the South.

Nancy and Bob knew that the offer was outrageously low for a platform technology like the VEE vectors, which could conceivably be used to make vaccines against many different diseases of humans and animals. "Vaccines could be big money makers," Nancy said. "They weren't always, but they could be. And what we had, with the right handling and the right opportunity, could be big."

The scientists' worse fear was that Wyeth-Lederle, which already had naked DNA and several other high-tech vaccine approaches in its portfolio, might be engaging in the business strategy of defensive licensing. "If you view this as a superior technology to the one you're already using, then you can buy up the licenses. And even if you never use it, you won't have to face it as a competitor. We were fearful that Lederle would do this," Bob said.

Bob hammered away at the transfer office, arguing that they should say no to Wyeth. There were other ways to commercialize VEE-based vaccines, he had ideas about how to do this, and a different approach could make a lot more money for UNC. Eventually the tech transfer staff came to agree with Bob, which meant that the suitor had to be turned away.

"I remember a very tense meeting with the Wyeth people, who thought they had the deal. For all I know, UNC told them they had the deal. So we sat in a room with them and said, 'You have not got a deal,'" Nancy recalled.

The Wyeth acquisition team did not give up easily. They tried to shake the resolve of the scientists and lawyers, but the UNC side stood firm. Although it was clear by the end of the meeting that Wyeth's licensing proposal was dead, Nancy said, "We didn't say you guys are out of it. We just said that we wanted to negotiate on a whole different basis."

The scientists wanted to start a company to develop VEE-based vaccines. University faculty members in California and the Northeast had been spinning off companies for twenty years, including Genentech and Chiron, but in 1997, this remained a revolutionary act for professors at a state institution in North Carolina. "It was just barely okay to do this," Bob said. "Two years earlier, it was absolutely impossible to do. The university wasn't equipped to deal with this. The only precedent I knew was a guy who went to them with the idea of making a company, and they said, 'Sure, but you'll have to resign.' And he did resign to do his company."

Before Bob could approach UNC about a start-up, he had to persuade Nancy, and their collaborator Jon Smith at Fort Detrich, that "if it was gonna happen, we had to do it." Nancy resisted the idea of going into business. She is a modest consumer and an unlikely entrepreneur, the kind of person who doesn't really give a hoot about all the stuff advertised in *Vanity Fair* or *Vogue*. "I'm not a good capitalist. If we were making women's clothes, I would not be in this. Or makeup or sports equipment. It wouldn't be important enough for me," she said. "I think vaccines are about it. They're worth it, and if this is the way, then this is the way."

Negotiations between Bob and the university began in earnest once Wyeth's licensing offer was off the table. "The university offered me a deal where they would retain 80 percent of the company and 20 percent would go to the three founders and we would do all the work—and didn't this sound just wonderful to us. I was stunned at this, because I had originally been told that the university would take between 5 percent and 10 percent. I didn't say anything at all, and then they said, 'Bob, what do you think?' And I said, 'I think you got the names in the wrong boxes.'"

At this point, Bob realized it was time for the scientists to hire suits of their own. This was not hard because Research Triangle Park, only a few miles from the UNC campus, is a regional hub for biomedical and high-tech research companies, an environment that attracts legal and business experts. Bob was able to engage an attorney and a start-up specialist to structure the new company and negotiate with the university. The new company would be called AlphaVax, short for "alphavirus vaccines." In order to pay their consultants and to give the company what Bob called "walking around money," each of the three founding scientists loaned

$10,000 to AlphaVax. Another $10,000 came from Bob's next-door neighbor, a retired investment banker who often hung out on Bob's front porch in the evening, tutoring him about business.

Bob was shocked by UNC's reaction when the new consultants began accompanying him to meetings. "At that point, I became an adversary, as opposed to someone who had worked here for eight years and brought in millions of dollars in grants for them. I was made to feel like some sort of huckster or criminal," Bob recalled. The chairman of his department and other colleagues urged Bob to not give up, to stay calm, and to not tell the university to shove it. His misfortune was to embark on this adventure at a time when UNC wasn't sure how squeamish it was about commercial enterprises launched by professors and partly owned by the university.

"Eventually we worked it all out, and we came to an arrangement that neither party was happy with, so it was probably not an unreasonable compromise," Bob said. UNC would own part of AlphaVax, and the new company would hold the rights to the VEE vaccine technologies and be able to license them to corporate partners.

After the university and the founding scientists had made a deal about ownership of the company, one major hurdle remained: UNC would not hand over the intellectual property rights until AlphaVax raised $1.5 million on its own. "They tied one hand and one foot behind our backs and told us to go out and raise money," Bob said ruefully. Without the licensing rights to VEE vectors in hand, AlphaVax had to convince big pharmaceutical companies they had the technology for making safe and effective vaccines against AIDS and other important diseases.

As they combed the suburbs of New Jersey and New York, beating the manicured bushes for corporate investors, there were times when the scientists wondered whether it was crazy to try to launch a company under these circumstances. "The key was to be absolutely naive, because otherwise you would never do it," Bob said.

●

On May 21, 1997, R. Gordon Douglas went to Capitol Hill to address the Congressional Task Force on International HIV/AIDS. Only a few days earlier, President Clinton had declared the search for an AIDS vaccine to be a top national priority and had challenged scientists to come up with one over the next decade. This announcement followed several months of journalistic fawning over Nobel laureate David Baltimore's new role as federal AIDS vaccine czar.

Gordon Douglas, as president of Merck Vaccines, led a major division at a blue-chip company. And not just any blue-chip company: No matter where Merck ranked in pharmaceutical sales for a given year, it was perennially regarded as one of America's most admired corporations. Anyone who had ever leafed through a business magazine knew that Merck was special. Douglas was the very model of a Merck executive; he was a famous infectious-disease physician at Cornell University Medical College who'd left the Mount Olympus of academic medicine for a position that was just as elevated—and was much better compensated.

Douglas has impeccably trimmed carrot-colored hair, dark horn-rimmed spectacles, and a characteristic facial expression that stops just short of a smirk. More memorable than his appearance is the sandpapery rasp of his deep, distinctive voice. It served him well in the congressional hearing room, where people are inured to promises about all sorts of things. "We are committed to pursue an HIV vaccine with as much vigor and passion that drove [sic] the discovery and development of our HIV protease inhibitor, Crixivan," Douglas intoned. Even politicians with a limited knowledge of medicine read the business pages, and Crixivan was the trade name for indinavir, which had zoomed past competitors to win 52 percent of the protease inhibitor market. They were less familiar with the name of Emilio Emini, who was praised by Douglas as the lead scientist for this achievement.

As wonderful as the new antiviral drugs are, Douglas told the assembly, "Merck believes that to control the HIV epidemic worldwide, a vaccine will be required." This was hardly a revolutionary statement, coming from the president of a vaccine company. Douglas tantalized listeners with the promise of Merck's experiments with naked DNA but cautioned that a DNA vaccine for AIDS remained in the early, laboratory stages of development. When it was closer to the clinic, he assured members of Congress, Merck would be ready for "fast-track development." Margaret Liu was not mentioned.

As befits a top corporate executive, Douglas spent more time talking

about money and policy than about scientific details. Although Merck
and other major companies were striving to create vaccines against AIDS
and other scourges of the developing world, economic difficulties could
keep these lifesaving products from reaching people most in need. The
companies were hampered by inadequate intellectual property protection across international boundaries, national laws that restrict prices or
profits, and the inability of poor countries to pay for costly, high-tech vaccines. He warned that even if Merck or its rivals developed an AIDS vaccine, global use would be impossible without action by governments,
private foundations, and international agencies like WHO and the World
Bank. Still, Douglas said in closing, "I cannot emphasize enough the commitment Merck has made to discover and develop an HIV vaccine."

This noble resolve was not always so obvious at Merck Research Laboratories. Margaret Liu watched as Dave Weiner's HIV vaccine became the
first naked-DNA immunization ever tested in humans. She kept up with
the news coverage as trials got underway, first in Philadelphia with HIV-
infected patients, then with healthy volunteers at Penn and the prestigious NIH Clinical Center.

"I was frustrated because my group had pioneered DNA vaccines and
I didn't want to be left in the dust, and I was really afraid of that. We kept
saying, 'We need to test this, we need to test that.' It costs money to do
these deals or collaborations, and this wasn't something that management wanted to invest in," Margaret recalled in a 1998 interview. As she
saw it, simply getting a DNA vaccine for HIV into clinical trials wasn't the
most important goal. The real challenge would be to modify DNA vaccines so that the immune system would have a stronger, longer-lasting
response to the shots.

Word along the grapevine was that Weiner's vaccine was generating far
lower levels of CTLs than expected. And when Mary Lou Clements-Mann
began testing Merck's flu vaccine in a low-profile Phase I study at Johns
Hopkins, early laboratory results were also disappointing. A letdown was
probably inevitable, given the explosion of hype after Margaret, Dave,
and other naked-DNA pioneers first reported that they had protected
mice against certain diseases.

Four years after that surge of excitement, "I was worried about putting
all our eggs in one basket. Even if naked DNA worked, we wanted to be

testing other formulations or modalities," Margaret said. On one occasion, in early 1997, she and Edward Scolnick, Merck's all-powerful director of research, had a brief but memorable exchange.

"Do you think DNA vaccines are going to work? How much of your salary would you bet on it?" he asked her.

"I'm not betting any part of my salary on it. I'm betting my life on it, Ed, because this is what I'm working on. So it's an understatement to talk about betting my salary. And when I say they'll work, I mean they will work in some embodiment," Margaret replied.

She and other researchers now thought that putting viral genes into plasmids was just a start and that more would be needed to jack up the immune system's response to naked DNA. Figuring out how to accomplish this would take lots of costly experimentation, but support was hard to come by. Margaret was only one of many Merck scientists with the rank of senior director, and they were all scrambling for resources. There was a lot of lobbying, competition, and waiting for the wheels of bureaucracy to turn.

And then, one day in 1997, Margaret had a new boss. Fresh from the Crixivan triumph, Emilio Emini had been given command of Merck's basic-research program for vaccines. It was a homecoming of sorts for him, a circling back to the part of the company that he had joined in 1983, then left for antiviral drug research. Within a few months, Emini was sounding like a man who had never left the vaccine world for even a quick trip to the rest room.

Despite his highly successful adventures in drug development, Emini emphasized that not even the best of current treatments could cure AIDS. For him, the take-home lesson about HIV therapy was that "this isn't penicillin, it's not a matter of one or two shots and the infection is gone. The infection is not gone." Fancy treatment cocktails never work for some people, and for others their effectiveness diminishes over time. "There's no alternative. You need a vaccine," Emini declared after a few months at the helm. And now he was in charge of making one.

●

"The guy in human resources said he'd been telling people that in the vaccine world, having me come is like being a basketball team and having Michael Jordan come to play. I certainly don't view myself like that, but that's the way I've been treated by everybody," said Margaret Liu, newly appointed vice president for vaccine and gene therapy research at Chiron. In September 1997, she traded Pennsylvania farmland for the Left Coast, and her new base of operations was an office with a panoramic view of the San Francisco Bay Bridge. This vice presidency had stood open for ten months, since Kathy Steimer's death.

Like the view, Margaret's professional horizons seemed broader here than in the East. "Merck is a company focused on making drugs, but Chiron is focused more on technologies," she said. "It's a completely different mindset." The one thing that remained constant was Margaret's determination to make an HIV vaccine. Before she agreed to come, she confirmed that Chiron shared this goal.

Chiron's scientific assets matched Margaret's ideas about what it would take to protect against HIV. She thought three elements would be needed: gene delivery to elicit CTLs, proteins to stimulate antibodies, and adjuvant to magnify immune response. Although Chiron's DNA vaccine program was relatively small, a larger group was exploring DNA delivery for gene therapy. Margaret expected to build on the work of both teams. The company also had ample expertise in recombinant proteins, dating back to its hugely successful hepatitis B vaccine, and was a leader in adjuvant research.

Expectations for Margaret were extremely high, as though she was a savior. "After Kathy's death, and before we recruited Margaret, it wasn't clear that we had the horsepower to continue an effective DNA vaccine program," reflected CEO Ed Penhoet. Chairman Bill Rutter saw her as providing "very strong intellectual leadership" that had been sorely missed by the survivors of Kathy's vaccine research program. DNA stalwarts like Susan Barnett were especially glad to have Margaret on board.

Two blocks from Margaret's office with the Bay view, Chiron's clinical department was housed in a renovated warehouse with modish distressed-brick walls, exposed ductwork painted in bright colors, and big windows overlooking a parking lot. The people in this department worked side by side with people from WRAIR, or from NIH, to carry out gp120 clinical trials. When Margaret came on board in late 1997, they were very busy.

The Thai government had just approved a Phase II study of the clade E gp120 vaccine, which was expected to pave the way toward Goal 2000, the U.S. military's long-awaited efficacy trial in that country. Meanwhile, the NIH's Phase II study of the prime-boost approach, which paired gp120 with Pasteur Mérieux Connaught's canarypox vector, had been underway for six months. If results from this trial looked good, then NIH would once again have to decide—for the first time in four years—whether it was ready to sponsor an efficacy trial in the United States.

When NIH first put the brakes on, in 1994, Chiron had been ready to go. But the company faced different realities now. If an efficacy trial was approved and Chiron agreed to participate, large quantities of the gp120 products would have to be made and donated for study. That is what manufacturers are expected to do in exchange for learning, at taxpayer expense, whether their products work. But more than the cost of one trial was at stake.

"The real issue was what do we do with the manufacturing facility in St. Louis, which was costing one heck of a lot of money," Bill Rutter said. The plant had been set up to produce recombinant protein vaccines against HIV and herpes, but by late 1997, the herpes vaccine had been dumped and top executives reportedly had little faith in gp120. Margaret was expected to reinvent vaccinology at Chiron, presumably by emphasizing new approaches such as naked DNA. In this context, Chiron had to decide whether to keep the St. Louis factory running.

One of Margaret's first assignments was to sort out this situation. At the outset, she needed to clarify NIH's real intentions toward a prime-boost efficacy trial. She and other Chiron executives sought to find out from Jack Killen, director of the Division of AIDS, but couldn't seem to get a definitive answer. They came away worried that "Chiron would be left holding the bag if NIH decided not to go ahead."

At this critical juncture, the company decided to call upon David Baltimore and other prominent experts for advice. Baltimore had become the Alan Greenspan of HIV vaccine research. Like the legendary chairman of the Federal Reserve, the chairman of the government's AIDS Vaccine Research Committee was closely observed, and researchers deconstructed his every move for hidden meanings.

Margaret set up a teleconference so that Baltimore and some of the other important players in the AIDS field could weigh in on the future of gp120. Baltimore's advice to Chiron executives was "don't continue to test this garbage," according to Mary Lou Clements-Mann, the famous clinical trialist from Johns Hopkins. She was at the other end of the spectrum, arguing that vaccinologists would learn much from a large-scale study of canarypox and gp120, no matter what level of protection the prime-boost demonstrated. Other participants were reportedly in the middle, less zealous than Mary Lou and less dismissive than Baltimore.

"The outcome of the meeting, though, was that Chiron shouldn't feel it had to commit to a Phase III," Margaret said. If someone else wanted to manufacture enough gp120 for larger trials, that could probably be arranged. Within months, however, the St. Louis manufacturing facility was closed down. As a result, Chiron's clinical trials department would have to dole out the remaining vials of vaccine very carefully, to fulfill the company's obligation to ongoing trials in the U.S. and Thailand. As 1997 drew to a close, however, only Chiron and the participants in the teleconference knew how bleak gp120's future actually was.

On the research front, Chiron's vaccine program was reorganized to work on a smaller number of diseases but a larger number of platform technologies. On the agenda were upgraded versions of DNA vaccines, strategies for packaging DNA so it would be more easily taken up by human cells, a souped-up alphavirus vector, and new adjuvants.

Margaret had a lot on her plate, and the clock was running.

●

In Dave Weiner's fine new laboratory at Penn, the technical complications of refining and testing his HIV vaccine took center stage throughout 1996 and for most of 1997. But at Great Valley Corporate Center in suburban Malvern, his collaborators at Apollon had another preoccupation: money. The company was desperately hungry for cash. There were periodic infusions from Wyeth, and in early 1996, it got $9.7 million more from Centocor, which had spun off Apollon in the first place. This lowered Apollon's anxiety level for a time, but expenses skyrocketed as clinical trials expanded at Penn and began at NIH. It was costly to make GMP batches of vaccine, and the thousands of lab tests generated by clinical trials were expensive and labor-intensive. The burn rate, as they say out in Silicon Valley, was high.

Grasping at straws, Apollon's board decided to try to raise money by going public, announcing plans for an initial public offering of 2.5 million shares of stock with an asking price of $11–13 per share. But when the offer was made in mid-December, investors stayed away in droves. People who could earn 30 percent on blue chips saw no reason to take a flyer on a risky biotech offering. Within a week, the IPO had been withdrawn. In the wake of this fiasco, Apollon's board of directors decided the company was now for sale.

Dave Weiner had no time to worry about any of these business gyrations. In early October, the night before he was scheduled to leave for the army's immunology meeting in Chiang Mai, his wife suddenly coughed up prodigious quantities of blood. The trip was forgotten as Dave was caught up in weeks, then months of nightmarish events in the emergency room and hospital. After a great many tests, the problem turned out to be a vascular malformation that could only be treated by removing the affected part of one lung. Besides attending to his wife's medical crisis, Dave was caring for and comforting his three little girls, who were between the ages of five and ten. Apollon's woes took a back seat to all this.

Eventually, in May 1998, Apollon was sold to American Home Products, parent of Wyeth-Lederle Vaccines. Because clinical trials would grind to a halt without them, scientists and technicians who worked on R&D and manufacturing kept their jobs at the Malvern site. The administrative staff was history.

Apollon's strong suit, and what enabled it to attract NIH support as an academic-business collaboration, was its single-minded focus on Dave's DNA vaccines. Once the little biotech was acquired by Wyeth-Lederle, however, DNA vaccines became only one of many interesting ideas in the bulging portfolio of a giant corporation. The only people Dave really knew at Wyeth-Lederle were two top Apollon scientists, one in R&D and one on the clinical side, who had been retained but shipped off to Pearl River, New York, where Wyeth-Lederle is located.

Dave was now operating in a different world.

●

Since 1993, HIV vaccine trials in Thailand had been the focus of Lieutenant Colonel John McNeil's life. By early 1998, he had traveled there more than three dozen times, laying the groundwork for the Goal 2000 study. If he could keep it on track, this would be the first trial to evaluate three vaccine concepts at once. One arm of the study would measure antibody responses to gp120 alone; the second would look for CTLs and antibodies elicited by a canarypox prime and a gp120 boost; and the third would look for CTLs and antibodies following naked-DNA immunization.

As the officer responsible for coordinating all this, John had to operate with confidence in two very different worlds. In Thailand, he had to meet the logistic and diplomatic demands associated with an international clinical trial; in the United States and France, he had to negotiate with the corporations whose products the military wanted to test.

The Thai component was going well. In late 1997, Chiron's clade E gp120 had sailed through its initial safety study, and the Data and Safety Monitoring Board for the trial had approved expansion to nearly 400 volunteers. This Phase I/II study would determine whether the clade E gp120 alone, or a bivalent gp120 B/E, stimulated a more powerful antibody response against HIV. The winner would be an integral part of the Goal 2000 study, where it would be tested by itself and as a boost in volunteers who had been given Pasteur Mérieux Connaught's canarypox.

There was considerable pageantry when the Phase I/II trial was launched in mid-January 1998. John McNeil and Debbi Birx flew to Bangkok for an opening ceremony arranged by the Royal Thai Army and the Ministry of Public Health. Speeches praising the experiment were made by the U.S. ambassador's first deputy, the RTA's chief of staff, top MOPH officials, and the presidents of Mahidol and Chiang Mai Universities. In U.S. terms, this was like having a clinical trial kicked off by the presidents of Harvard and Yale, the director of NIH and his deputies, and the chairman of the Joint Chiefs of Staff.

It was a great day all around, the launch of the largest HIV vaccine trial ever carried out in Asia. On the long flight back to the States, John felt optimistic about Thailand's role in the undertaking. Clinic staffs were well trained, and they were fired up to recruit people and get the trial off to a fast start. The crucial immunology studies would be split between labs in Thailand and at WRAIR, and by early 1999, the investigators should be able to tell which of Chiron's two gp120 products would be more likely to protect people in the efficacy trial.

The manufacturing companies were more worrisome. Everyone in the vaccine world had heard that Pasteur Mérieux Connaught was having trouble making canarypox vaccines in large quantities, but there was no point in agonizing over that. PMC had promised to supply vaccine for the trial, and it was up to the company to solve its technical difficulties. As for Apollon, the failed public offering had made news in December, and now the company was reportedly for sale. Given all this, it did not appear that the naked-DNA vaccine would be ready in time for Goal 2000.

The biggest source of uncertainty and disappointment was Chiron. This company had been one of the military's strongest corporate partners since 1993, when Kathy Steimer first pledged to create a clade E gp120 for Thailand. Now the Chiron vaccine that looked better in the Phase I/II study would play a pivotal role in Goal 2000. But would Chiron come through?

Rumors swirled about what was going on in Emeryville. Margaret Liu's hiring seemed to signal that Chiron was serious about making an AIDS vaccine, but no one expected her to be enthusiastic about gp120. Word had also spread about the conference call when David Baltimore and the other heavy hitters blessed Chiron's decision to cease making gp120. This was clear enough. Less certain was Chiron's commitment to its partners, such as PMC, the U.S. military, and the Thai government, and to ongoing clinical trials.

"Everybody hears a thousand different things about Chiron," John said, and the other players needed to know what was happening. If Chiron was going to walk away from the Goal 2000 trial, delay would be inevitable and major retrenchment essential. The Thai Food and Drug Administration, like its American counterpart, did not approve of switching horses in midstream. The product that plods through Phase I and II studies is the only one that can advance into a Phase III. If products are paired for testing, such as PMC's canarypox and Chiron's gp120, then only that duo can move forward. No substitutions are allowed. If one product becomes unavailable and another takes its place, then it's back to Phase I.

The reckoning began on February 10, in Bangkok. Representatives from Chiron and PMC, along with John McNeil, did a triathlon of meetings. They started with the principal investigators from the four sites where Chiron's vaccine was being tested and moved in the afternoon to Dr. Natth Bhamarapravati's scientific subcommittee on HIV vaccines. The next morning, they joined a three-day public forum on HIV vaccine research, which drew hundreds of scientists, doctors, nurses, and public-health workers to the Siam City hotel.

The real business was transacted in the small meetings, where Thai scientific leaders were not pleased with what they heard from Chiron. For starters, the company had sent Lori Hansen, the project manager for gp120, a young administrator who was a stranger to them. Rank and formality matter in the Thai scientific establishment, and they preferred to deal with corporate officers or with physicians like Chiron's Anne-Marie Duliege, who had come often to Thailand and had an established track record. Never mind that Hansen had a Ph.D. in microbiology, adequate corporate experience, and the authority to speak for the company. As far as the Thai scientists could see, Chiron had not done them the honor of sending an important person.

"Chiron was interested to the point that they send a vice president here once, but that was a long time ago," Dr. Natth said. "We are only small people here," he added with an eloquent shrug. "We cannot influence a big company like that."

Chiron's official position was that it wasn't "bailing out" of current and future trials, it was "regrouping." The company was committed to finishing the Phase I/II study now underway, and what happened next depended on results from that trial. If lab tests showed that immunized volunteers made neutralizing antibodies against primary isolate viruses, then the company would think about further development. By this Chiron meant participating in prime-boost studies, not testing gp120 as a solo agent. The company was also unwilling to pick up the cost of making more gp120 when the current supply was exhausted.

This was a long-winded way of saying that Chiron was finished with gp120. If the U.S. and Thai collaborators were determined to keep the prime-boost effort on track and were certain that Chiron's gp120 was the best boost, John's current budget couldn't handle the $1.5 million to $3 million needed to make another batch. The company's decision meant that the Goal 2000 trial was receding into the distance, turning into a Goal 2001 or 2002 study.

Back at WRAIR, one month after the round of meetings in Bangkok, John looked tired. He was still coming to grips with the delay of the Thai trial. The worst thing about this was its impact on the military's partnership with the Thai government. Years earlier, John had given his word that government officials would always be in the loop, that they would have time to review and make thoughtful decisions, and that their people and laboratories would be strengthened by collaborating with WRAIR. John had spent years making good on these promises, and he felt confident that when the time came, Thailand would host an efficacy trial.

But for now, he was in limbo. "I worried about the country, and I should have been worrying about the companies," he said ruefully. John had not given up on a Thai trial, not by a long shot. But this summer he was going to coach his eleven-year-old daughter's softball team, instead of spending quite so much time in Thailand.

●

Back in North Carolina, it took nine months for AlphaVax to raise the $1.5 million that UNC demanded. Ironically, the source was Wyeth-Lederle, the very company that originally offered $60,000 for the rights to VEE vaccines. For $1.5 million, Bob Johnston and his cofounders agreed to sell Wyeth a "tri-exclusive" license to vaccines for five viral diseases: parainfluenza, respiratory syncitial virus, herpes 1 and 2, and human papilloma virus. For each vaccine, this meant that Wyeth "could have a license to it, AlphaVax would retain a license to it, and we would have the right to license it to a third party if we chose," Bob said. The difference between an arrangement like this and an exclusive license, he added, "is how much money the licenser is willing to pay."

Carefully excluded from this deal were vaccines against HIV and influenza. Unless AlphaVax mushroomed into a giant company, with sales representatives visiting doctors' offices to push products, these vaccines would eventually be licensed to a big corporation. But not just yet. There was a lot of public funding available for AIDS research, and although the army was their only government backer so far, Bob was willing to roll the dice and see what happened. He believed that he could raise enough money to develop HIV and flu vaccines in-house, then license them at a higher price when they were further along.

Finally, the seemingly endless negotiations culminated in a meeting between the AlphaVax team, the UNC intellectual property staff, and Wyeth-Lederle. It was January 12, 1998, when they gathered in a conference room near the tech transfer office. After "a little more discussion, and whining and carrying on," as Nancy described it, the agreements were signed.

Afterward, Nancy, Bob, and four of the consultants who had pulled together the deal strolled across campus to the faculty club. It was all dark wood and plaid upholstery, with lots of UNC insignia and heraldry on display. They drank a toast to AlphaVax, saying, "We're off!"

As soon as Wyeth's check cleared, they rented space for AlphaVax at 710 West Main Street in Durham, less than ten miles from the UNC Medical Center. The white marble cornerstone on this red-brick building reads: "Research Laboratory, Liggett & Myers Tobacco Company, 1949." It is part of a complex of tobacco warehouses and cigarette factories that sprawl over several blocks of downtown Durham. An elevated, enclosed walkway soars over Main Street, so that employees cross several stories above traffic.

The old L&M building is no longer used by tobacco researchers, and there are no laboratory rats puffing away on smoking machines. Instead, it is now an incubator for biotech start-ups like AlphaVax, which rent space until they can afford something more suitable. Footsteps clatter noisily in the hallways, where sounds bounce off ceramic-tile walls the color of a wet cigarette.

AlphaVax rented offices and lab space on the second floor, and no sooner was this done than the company's research director "lost heart and left" according to Nancy. He was an alphavirus expert who had previously worked for a company acquired by Chiron, and he returned there to join Margaret Liu's new vaccine and gene-therapy team.

Because there was no time to waste and somebody needed to get vaccine research moving, Nancy considered taking the position herself.

But she had spent her life in academia, and she loved working at UNC. "I didn't want to work in a company," she said. But for the vaccine, and for AlphaVax, she was willing to consider it.

Fortunately, Bob came up with an alternative He contacted Bob Olmsted, who in the early 1980s was the third Ph.D. candidate he mentored at North Carolina State. Olmsted was a small-town boy from upstate New York, who after his undergraduate years ran off to South Florida to tend bar and live a Jimmy Buffett kind of life. "I had a nine to five job," Olmsted says with a twinkle in his eye. "It just wasn't during the daytime." Bob held none of this against the young man, who thrived in grad school and proved to be an excellent microbiologist. His next stop was NIH, where he spent his postdoc years working with numerous "hot viruses" and learning about using SIV in monkeys as a model for AIDS.

Olmsted then joined Pharmacia & Upjohn, in Kalamazoo, Michigan, where he searched for antiviral drugs for hepatitis C. And that's where he was when Bob Johnston called and invited him down for the weekend. At the L&M building, he met with Bob, Nancy, and Jon Smith, who had come down to Durham from Fort Detrick. AlphaVax had no furniture yet, so its founders had borrowed a conference room that did. They spent hours going over data from animal studies and talking about their dreams for the new company.

Olmsted had always wanted to return to North Carolina, where he enjoyed living as a graduate student, but now he was older and had a steady job with a major company. The former bartender had more to lose, and AlphaVax was a high-risk venture. A few months later, he was swayed by news about a primate experiment using Marburg virus, a close relative of Ebola.

Monkeys were immunized with VEE replicon particles carrying genes for Marburg proteins, then challenged with a lethal dose of the virus. Three monkeys given a placebo vaccine were dead within ten days. But the immunized animals had no detectable infection. "It's a very nasty virus. This was the first demonstration of any vaccine strategy against this class of viruses that was shown to be completely efficacious in nonhuman primates. I signed up after that," Olmsted recalled.

"The science was solid, the opportunity of working with these people, and the challenge of starting a new company—these sorts of opportunities don't come along very often. At the time I made the jump I was forty-five, and if I was going to do it, it was going to be now."

"It was a miracle that he would do this," Nancy said. "He had a great job at Pharmacia & Upjohn, and they tried hard to keep him. And he came anyway." Of course, she adds with a knowing smile, there might have been other reasons. Olmsted is a great golfer, and in North Carolina you can play year-round. Kalamazoo, Michigan, couldn't compete with that.

13

THE CATBIRD SEAT

WHEN BOB NOWINSKI thought about the gp120 vaccine, he imagined a train that had been halted, time and time again, by flashing red stop signals. And VaxGen was the crane he and Don Francis had constructed to "lift the train up and put it on a new track"—a company capable of staging the world's first efficacy trials of an AIDS vaccine, without asking for government help. In order to do this, Bob told Don and Phil Berman, whose egos were understandably tied up with the vaccine, that they were going to behave differently from now on. They would stop trying to convince the David Baltimores and Tony Faucis of the world that gp120 could prevent AIDS. They would no longer engage in floor fights at scientific meetings, where Phil Berman had to fend off academic critics. Instead, Bob said, "We are going to open the way to free-flowing development."

The spin-off agreement between Genentech and VaxGen required that the new company raise $18 million before Genentech would give them the gp120 patents. The efficacy trials that Don was planning for the United States and Thailand would cost more than that, but VaxGen would deal with that later. The immediate challenge was to pull together $18 million in less than twelve months. Genentech also specified that fund-raising begin in December 1996, a schedule Bob hated because the holidays would sap whatever momentum they'd gained. There was no point in arguing, however.

Bob first turned his attention to Seattle, a city that had been very, very good to him already. Unlike California and the Northeast, where venture capitalists and institutional investors rule, Seattle abounds with individuals who are willing to put their own money into bootstrap operations. He had started four companies in this city, and he knew several hundred people who had profited from those ventures and would consider putting $30,000 to $50,000 into VaxGen. He moved quickly to give them that opportunity.

Don and Bob set up shop in an intimate meeting room at the Four Seasons Olympic, a grand hotel of the 1920s, and began making their pitch to ten or so people at a time. "We were two guys with thirty overheads and a licensing agreement from Genentech," said Don. The business they described to potential backers was far from a sure thing. Could VaxGen hire the experts needed to carry out an efficacy trial? Would the FDA approve it? Could the company recruit enough volunteers? Could they actually complete the study? "There were an immense number of risks if you looked at the overall company," Don said.

Don's part of the presentation focused on the scientific and public-health aspects of the vaccine, now trade-named AIDSVAX™. He emphasized the global need for such a product, its history so far, and what efficacy testing would entail. Then Bob described how the company would be set up and run, explaining why he thought investors could expect a return on their money. Sitting at the back of the room was a broker with a stack of subscription agreements.

Although the formal presentation took about one hour, people asked so many questions that most sessions took twice that long. Those who had done their homework often asked why Genentech was giving the vaccine away if it was worth anything and why NIH hadn't paid for efficacy testing two years earlier. People who hadn't studied gp120's history, but did follow the news, were interested in David Baltimore's recent appointment as the savior of the federal AIDS vaccine program. Baltimore had been quoted as saying that none of the products in the pipeline were likely to work. Was the great Nobelist wrong?

Don told his own version of the gp120 story. He said NIH had abandoned the vaccine on the advice of a large group of people, many of them not vaccine experts, and attributed this to the complicated politics of the AIDS epidemic. He handed out copies of Jesse Green's "Who Put the Lid on gp120?" a major *New York Times Magazine* piece sympathetic to Genentech and Chiron. This article covered Don's role in developing a vaccine against hepatitis B and made much of his long experience battling dangerous bugs of all kinds. Baltimore, in contrast, was a distinguished basic scientist with no track record in vaccines.

Bob saw the government's stand on gp120 as a head wind that VaxGen would have to overcome. Bob's strategy was to spend lots of face-time with potential investors, answering their questions and establishing rapport. Unlike portfolio managers, who have limits on how much risk they can take with clients' money, "individuals are able to make decisions based on what they feel. There were a significant number who invested for financial reasons and a significant number who invested for altruistic reasons, but everyone basically invested because they met Don and myself," Bob said.

After two and a half weeks of meetings in Seattle, Don and Bob had been promised close to $10 million. Don was stunned: "I had no idea, looking at these people's faces, whether they really were interested in investing or not." When the two reluctantly took time off during the holidays, Don was beginning to feel that VaxGen just might succeed.

January 1997 was bleak, however, with a series of dispiriting meetings in the San Francisco area. Socially committed rich people whom Don knew from his public-health days balked at investing in a preventive vaccine, though many of them gave generously to organizations for AIDS patients. But there was little time to brood about this. By midmonth, the VaxGen team took the show on the road for real, trooping from city to city, hotel to hotel, showing the same overheads to new faces.

A typical meeting drew eight or ten people, but sometimes only one actually showed up. In one city, they scheduled a 5:30 meeting on the top floor of a very tall building, only to find that the elevator automatically shut down at 5:00. Adversity strengthened the bond between the two men and gave them something to laugh about. Repetition made their presentations slicker as they learned to pass questions back and forth and enlarge on each other's answers. At the same time, there was no getting around it: Raising millions of dollars was hard work. "I got awfully tired of doing it, over and over and over, so that sometimes I didn't even know what town we were in," Don recalled.

In February, they spent some especially grueling days in New York, ricocheting between meetings with friendly private investors and dismissive institutional managers. When they finally left New York, their destination was West Palm Beach, Florida. "It was the most dreadful trip imaginable. Every plane was late, we arrived and couldn't get a rental car at first, the broker we were traveling with was too big to get into the rental car that we did find, and we finally had to get a van," Bob remembered. It was 1:00 A.M. when they located the Holiday Inn where they'd been booked for the night, which turned out to be a dumpier-than-usual version of the archetypal Florida motel. Bob's assistant surveyed the asphalt parking lot, the two floors of rooms, and the open breezeways and said it looked like a place where "guys who bump off liquor stores stay."

As they fell into bed, none of the VaxGen team had high hopes for the presentation they would deliver the next morning. They had come to West Palm at the invitation of one of Don's distant relatives, a physician who lived in the area. He asked Don to come and pitch his new company to a group of local doctors who might want to invest. "It was as a favor to him that we went," Don said. Bob might have nixed the idea, except that his elderly parents were spending their traditional Florida vacation at a condominium nearby. It was a chance for him to see them, and for them to see their son in entrepreneurial action.

When Don and Bob walked into the motel's meeting room, it was packed with about seventy doctors affiliated with the same hospital as Don's relative. The only nonphysicians in the audience were Bob's beaming, eighty-year-old parents from Brooklyn. Nothing prepared the VaxGen team for what happened next. "It was the most electric audience I've ever witnessed," Bob marveled. "We gave our talk and then there was an extensive question-and-answer period, and when we finished, literally the whole crowd stood up and grabbed copies of the subscription agreement." The big broker who had come along to handle the paperwork was mobbed.

Don and Bob were still reeling from the West Palm Beach experience when they boarded their flight back to San Francisco. On the plane, they started adding up what they had been promised during their multi-city tour, and the result was close to $27 million—well over the amount that Genentech wanted to see before handing over the patents. Don had trouble believing that it was real, but it was. By March, they were not only ahead of schedule by nine months, but they had also exceeded their financial goal for starting the company.

During the tour, it was obvious that many potential investors chatted up Don because they had read *And the Band Played On* or had seen the HBO movie. And this was probably the deciding factor for some people. "They knew that here was some guy who knew about AIDS, even if they never read more than the preface to the book or the poster for the movie. But that was enough to give them confidence that someone standing up there was a notable person. If it weren't for the book and the movie, I don't know whether we'd have been able to fund this."

It was bizarre and troubling to Don to realize that HIV vaccine development could be driven by his own celebrity. Although he wasn't about to turn down money from starstruck investors, he worried that "something as important as an AIDS vaccine shouldn't be so haphazard."

But no matter. The road to an efficacy trial was paved with the cash they had just raised.

●

In 1996, when Don and Bob were negotiating the spin-off agreement, part of Genentech's contribution to VaxGen was to let Phil Berman resume work on gp120. The big company would give him what he needed to make new, improved versions of the original MN-based vaccine. These would be bivalent products, containing antigens from not one but two types of gp120. AIDSVAX B/B™ would incorporate gp120 proteins from two clade B viruses: the original MN strain, plus a primary isolate like the ones that had caused breakthrough infections in earlier clinical trials. Phil had been eager to make a B/B combination since 1993, when scientists first realized that some strains were harder to protect against than others. His idea was that two gp120 antigens would induce a broader, more protective antibody response than one.

Only after VaxGen was launched, however, did it become clear that Phil would need to develop a different bivalent construct for Thailand. AIDSVAX B/E™ would pair the original gp120 with gp120 derived from a clade E virus isolated from a Thai AIDS patient. For scientific reasons, a B/E combination was essential. And it was also essential for political reasons.

The overseas testing of American-made pharmaceuticals had been a hot-button issue for decades, and by this time, developing nations were on guard against exploitation. People in poorer countries might serve as guinea pigs for experimental products, risking exposure to unknown harms, only to find that these products were too expensive or otherwise inaccessible once they were on the market. This happened with oral contraceptives, which were tested among poor women in Puerto Rico and then not sold there.

On the other hand, developing countries did not want to turn away ethically conducted clinical trials that could benefit the health of their citizens and maybe even their economy. AIDS had hit Thailand hard, and the country embraced its role as one of the World Health Organization's preferred sites for vaccine testing. A Phase I trial of Genentech's original clade B vaccine began in February 1995, recruiting volunteers from a population of recovering heroin addicts in Bangkok. The company and Thai officials saw this as a perfect fit for this product: Studies showed that the viruses being spread by dirty needles were clade B, the type the vaccine was meant to block.

This picture of AIDS among IV drug users had emerged from a special laboratory operated by the U.S. Centers for Disease Control and the Thai Ministry of Public Health. Every four months, this lab analyzed blood samples from a research cohort of 3,000 participants in a municipal treatment program. In 1996, one of these periodic surveys generated an extraordinary result: among those who had just tested positive for the first time, there were three times as many clade E as clade B infections.

Epidemiologist Timothy Mastro, who was in charge of the CDC field station outside Bangkok, was astonished by what he described as "a remarkable switch from a clade B epidemic to 80 percent E." The implications for vaccine research were unmistakable. "A B-only vaccine trial would have been inappropriate on all counts. It was now an E epidemic, and clearly you needed to develop an E vaccine."

Phil had gotten samples of Thai E viruses from the army in 1993, when John McNeil first urged Genentech and Chiron to design vaccines for Thailand. Kathy Steimer had immediately begun developing a gp120 E at Chiron, but Genentech was more interested in the clade B epidemic among Bangkok drug users. If their original gp120 could be tested in Bangkok, it didn't make sense to spend several million dollars making a new version. Once clade E became rampant among IV drug users, however, there were sound scientific reasons for making a construct that incorporated E as well as B antigens.

Hardly anything gets done for scientific reasons alone, however, and observers say that Dr. Natth Bhamarapravati, chairman of Thailand's most powerful AIDS vaccine committee, applied considerable political muscle to VaxGen. Dr. Natth's message was "if you want to go further with a vaccine trial in this country, you need to produce a vaccine for the strains circulating here."

As a result, Phil developed a new clade E antigen that could be combined with B in a bivalent vaccine for Thailand. In March 1997, just as Don and Bob wrapped up their financing tour of the United States, Genentech began manufacturing AIDSVAX B/E™. This sent a clear message to Thai officials that VaxGen, which would soon own the new vaccine, was serious about doing clinical trials in their country. Although Thai officials could not guarantee this product an effortless climb up the salmon ladder of bureaucracy, at least the B/E vaccine had a fighting chance. A vaccine based on B alone would never survive the trip.

●

In early 1997, the vaccine world buzzed with the news that VaxGen had raised enough money to launch an efficacy trial on its own. This toppled the assumption that only the National Institutes of Health or a pharmaceutical superpower like Merck could propel an HIV vaccine all the way to a Phase III study. The realization that an upstart biotech might get an efficacy trial underway, while NIH regrouped and focused on basic science, stunned those who wrote off gp120 as a failure and Don Francis as a wacky, West Coast zealot. The conventional wisdom was that the prime-boost strategy, just about to enter Phase II testing at NIH expense, would be the first product to win approval for efficacy testing in the United States. Now all bets were off: VaxGen was marching toward large-scale tests not only in the United States but in Thailand as well.

Being in the lead made both VaxGen and the Thai government, which was evaluating the company's request for clinical trials, vulnerable to attack by people who saw gp120 as worthless. One such attack was instigated by a maverick member of Dr. Natth's Subcommittee on AIDS Vaccines, who invited some of gp120's most outspoken American critics to weigh in on the Thai trial. He solicited a letter from David Ho, director of the Aaron Diamond AIDS Research Center in New York, and his collaborator Steven Wolinsky, an infectious-disease expert at Northwestern University in Chicago. Along with John Moore, also of ADARC, they had been involved in analyzing infections among volunteers in the Phase II study of gp120 vaccines made by Genentech and Chiron. These three researchers concluded the vaccines had no protective effect. They also believed the viruses that "broke through" to infect immunized volunteers were not unusual, as Phil Berman contended they were, but perfectly ordinary. These were the same issues that Phil and John Moore had disputed during the 1996 AIDS conference in Vancouver.

Ho and Wolinsky reiterated these negative findings in a letter to the Thai scientist who solicited their opinion. Once that letter hit Bangkok, it sped through Thailand's public-health establishment and the U.S. vaccine community faster than an e-mail joke. The more widely distributed the letter was, the more imperative it became for Thai decisionmakers to come up with a wise and dignified response.

The pressure on them increased in May, when Ho came to Bangkok in person. In a speech during a medical conference, Ho summarized gp120's history in the United States and said, "For me, as part of the Asian minority in the U.S., I feel it's important for the Thai people to be aware of the possibility of exploitation. If a product is rejected elsewhere, why should you take it?"

Although Dr. Natth and other prominent Thais knew about the ill will that had festered between Ho's group and the VaxGen scientists for some years, they could not simply write off either viewpoint. The National AIDS Committee, and especially Dr. Natth's subcommittee on vaccines, had to sort out tough scientific and ethical issues while the world watched.

In a flash of brilliance, Dr. Natth asked UNAIDS to consider the merits of gp120 and the wisdom of proceeding with what would be not only the world's first international efficacy trial but also the first ever funded by a private company. UNAIDS called on five members of its Vaccine Advisory Committee and eight outside scientists who were knowledgeable in the field. This panel was given letters from Ho and Wolinsky, and from Phil Berman and Don Francis, explaining their conflicting interpretations of the Phase I/II results in the United States. They were also supplied with unpublished articles by John Moore and Phil Berman about the breakthrough infections, as well as additional data from the trials.

In July 1997, the panel sent a report to Dr. Natth that included detailed criticisms and sweeping recommendations. Many reviewers faulted the Ho and Wolinsky letter for perpetuating errors that had originated in Moore's article. Panelists said he had categorized some infected placebo recipients as vaccinees and in one case counted a healthy person as being infected. Both made the vaccine look worse. The UNAIDS group did not think Berman's analysis was perfect, but saw it as less flawed than Moore's report.

When the panelists stepped back and looked at the big picture, they agreed on three points. First, gp120 was safe. Second, it definitely stimulated an antibody response, although the protectiveness of that response was unknown. Finally, they did not expect this antibody response to protect more than one person in three, a moderate efficacy level that would be detectable only in a very large clinical trial.

Asked to vote on the value of going ahead with a Phase III trial in Thailand, ten panelists said the trial should be done, two said it should not be, and one said no decision should be made until Phase II data were analyzed. UNAIDS's policy was that each country should choose what clinical trials it would accept, and Thailand had decided to consider only products with a chance of protecting against clade E viruses. The UNAIDS reviewers agreed that VaxGen's new bivalent B/E was a more appropriate candidate than a B-only vaccine.

The U.S. military, of course, also had E-based products in the works: a gp120 B/E made by Chiron, an E-carrying canarypox vector from Pasteur Mérieux Connaught, and an early-stage DNA vaccine with clade E genes made by Dave Weiner at Penn. Even with UNAIDS's advice in hand, members of Dr. Natth's subcommittee still faced tough choices of their own. A large-scale trial in Thai clinics staffed by Thai professionals was going to burn up Thai baht as well as U.S. dollars, regardless of support from international sponsors. The challenge was to get the best return on Thailand's investment, in terms of acquiring new knowledge and technology.

Would Thailand end up giving the green light to VaxGen, the army, or both? In late 1997, no one knew.

●

At 8:10 on the morning of June 6, 1997, the Food and Drug Administration's Vaccines and Related Biological Products Advisory Committee convened at the Holiday Inn in Bethesda. Crowded around the table were more than two dozen top FDA officials and advisory committee members. Don Francis, Phil Berman, and other colleagues from Genentech and VaxGen, along with lower-level FDA staff, were seated around the perimeter of the Versailles Ballroom. Although this meeting room was less grand than its name implied, at least this Holiday Inn was better suited to bureaucrats than guys on the lam.

FDA officials often make their own judgments about clinical trials and drug licensure without seeking advice from outsiders. On this landmark occasion, however, the agency wanted counsel. AIDS had been killing people for sixteen years, and for the first time the FDA was being formally asked to approve Phase III testing for a vaccine that might, just might, prevent enough infections to slow the epidemic. The FDA had summoned members of its standing committee on vaccines, augmented with eight "temporary voting members," appointed because they had specific types of AIDS expertise.

Three years earlier, in a fancier hotel several blocks further south, an NIH committee had scuttled efficacy testing of Genentech's original gp120 before the proposal got as far as the FDA. Now the future of VaxGen's two bivalent gp120 vaccines hinged on this meeting. To prepare for this day, Don and Phil had made themselves focus on Bob Nowinski's Rules for Living: Keep your head down, ignore your critics, and work like hell to get the trials underway. They had to shut out the mischief that

David Ho had stirred up in Thailand, as well as all other distractions, and focus on the unusual strategy they would lay before the advisory committee.

Instead of seeking approval only for Phase I and II studies, then coming back later to petition for Phase III approval, VaxGen had decided to roll the dice on all three phases at once. Although this wasn't standard practice, the FDA was open to the idea because the safety of gp120 vaccines was not an issue: These products had not caused any problems for the more than 1,000 volunteers who had already received them. VaxGen's bold plan was to do Phase I/II studies quickly and to make the decision about proceeding with the efficacy trial before—not after—they were completed.

Phil, VaxGen's first presenter, later recalled feeling a surge of adrenaline and anxiety as he rose to speak. He described making new antigens, one from a U.S primary isolate and the other from a Thai virus, and combining these with the original MN antigen to make AIDSVAX B/B™ and B/E™. Although some committee members questioned how immunogenic these new candidates might be, no one wrote them off as worthless or poorly designed.

Don's presentation used findings from human and chimp studies to argue that early in a vaccine trial, it's possible to make a "pass-fail judgment" about whether the bivalent vaccines merit efficacy testing. In previous experiments, the level of anti-HIV antibodies measured after the second injection reliably predicted how high an individual's antibody level would be when the seven-shot regimen was complete. In these earlier trials, at least 75 percent of volunteers made antibodies against HIV after two shots. And although these studies were not large enough to reveal how well these antibodies might protect someone exposed to HIV, Don believed they would work. Although the prevailing opinion was that chimp models were flawed, Don still put considerable stock in Phil's experiments at Genentech. And those showed that chimpanzees with high antibody levels, after two immunizations, were later protected when challenged with HIV.

For Phase I/II studies of the new bivalent vaccines, VaxGen planned to measure antibodies two weeks after the second immunization, which would be only six weeks after each volunteer entered the study. Test results would be handed over to the FDA, and if 50 percent or more of vaccinees had made antibodies, the Phase III would be authorized and planning could begin. The Phase I/II study, meanwhile, would continue. This way, no additional paperwork, meetings, or formal approvals would be required: If enough vaccinated volunteers responded, the efficacy trial would go forward. That's what the FDA advisory committee was asked to approve.

Don described a Phase III protocol consisting of two double-blind, randomized placebo-controlled trials: a U.S. study enrolling 5,000 gay men and a few hundred women with HIV-positive partners, and a Thai study with 2,500 IV drug users in Bangkok. These parallel experiments would tell researchers how well the vaccines protected against sexually transmitted HIV as well as virus introduced directly into the bloodstream by a dirty needle. These high-risk volunteers would receive seven immunizations, spread over thirty months, and would be observed for an additional six months. Blood samples would be tested regularly for signs of HIV infection, and researchers would measure HIV levels, or viral load, in blood from the several hundred people who would probably become infected—either sexually or by injecting drugs—over the course of three years.

In addition to getting off to a fast start on the Phase III trial, VaxGen also wanted to give itself the shortest possible route to marketing approval. In earlier negotiations, the FDA had agreed that interim analyses be done after participants had been in the trial for eighteen months, and again after twenty-four months. The agency had also agreed that if the vaccine showed efficacy greater than 30 percent at either of these times, the trial could be halted early and the company could seek final FDA approval. If interim analysis didn't establish that the vaccine protected more than one person in three, the company would see the trial through to the end. After a moderate amount of wrangling about statistical aspects of this proposal, the FDA committee endorsed it.

By the end of the day, all VaxGen's ambitious plans for testing its new vaccines had been approved. "We went out of there pumped," Don said. All things seemed possible: By September 1997 they would get the go-ahead from Thai authorities, then Phase I/II trials could begin immediately in the United States and Thailand. By early 1998, he expected efficacy trials to be approved for both countries, and he anticipated that the smaller study, in Bangkok, could get underway as soon as early as February 1998. In reality, of course, everything takes longer than you think.

●

Don wasn't far wrong about the timetable for domestic Phase I/II trials of the two bivalent vaccines; these got off the ground in several cities in November 1997. AIDSVAX B/B™ and B/E™ were each tested in sixty volunteers recruited because they were at very low risk for HIV infection. At a public-health clinic in Denver, Don himself was among those who rolled up their sleeves.

Thailand's FDA soon followed in the footsteps of its U.S. counterpart, authorizing Phase I/II testing with built-in provision for speedy approval of a Phase III trial. This looked fine on paper, but in fact the path to efficacy testing was still under construction in Thailand. Various offices and committees within the Ministry of Public Health would have to sign off on the plan, and government officials were using VaxGen as a test case for deciding how future trial requests would be processed. The National AIDS Commission, especially the technical and ethics subcommittees, were determined that the study would be bullet proof. "They were inventing it as they went along, and they put in layer after layer of review. They wanted Thailand to be respected, and certainly not to be criticized as carrying out an unethical, technically unwise, or half-assed research effort," Don said.

Dr. Natth and other leaders had also resolved that Thailand's scientific community would understand the trial, support it, and be involved at every step along the way. VaxGen had already formed partnerships with researchers at Mahidol University, the Bangkok Metropolitan Administration (BMA), and elsewhere. Researchers and physicians who weren't directly involved had a chance to review VaxGen's plans during the February 1998 meeting at the Siam City hotel, the event where Chiron ditched its Thai vaccine.

Although it was important to hold this public discussion, what was said there broke no new ground. The loyal opposition to gp120 reiterated its doubts about the vaccine's ability to rouse protective antibodies, an uncertainty that would not be resolved until an efficacy trial was carried out. Others raised the doomsday scenario that comes up whenever American companies do clinical trials in other countries. The fear is that a rich corporation will sweep in, shamelessly exploit local volunteers, prove that the product works, and disappear without a trace. The host population won't benefit from the results, because people won't be able to afford what was tested on them. Everyone wanted to make sure that wouldn't happen.

Because AIDS has been the most politicized of all diseases, international trials having anything to do with HIV were especially highly charged. A battle was raging over placebo-controlled trials of a low-cost antiviral regimen that reduced the transmission of HIV from infected mothers to their babies. These trials had been conducted in Africa and Thailand; they would not have been approved in the United States, where instead of placebo the low-cost preventive drugs would have been compared with a lengthier, more expensive approach already being used to protect infants.

Placebo control was not an issue for international vaccine trials, because this was the only choice. The only way to test an HIV vaccine was to randomly assign volunteers to receive either the vaccine or an inert substance and to judge the vaccine's effectiveness by comparing the number of infected people in each group.

When Don Francis talked about the ethics of vaccine testing, he emphasized that HIV was spreading at the rate of 16,000 new infections every day and that the main imperative was to seek a vaccine that could slow this catastrophe. He believed this could be accomplished while meeting all the usual ethical standards. Informed-consent procedures for volunteers should be clear and understandable, their efforts should not be wasted on a worthless study, and their safety should be closely monitored and guarded. These were Mom-and-apple-pie values that everyone could endorse.

A more controversial provision of Don's plan for the VaxGen study was that participants who became infected "would receive care consistent with the current standards of practice." In the United States, this would mean treatment with highly effective antiviral cocktails that cost upward of $10,000 per year, paid for not by VaxGen but by private insurance or government drug programs. In Thailand, where state-of-the-art care was available only to a handful of wealthy people, VaxGen proposed that infected volunteers be treated however Thai health authorities thought best. This would almost certainly mean that Thai volunteers would get less sophisticated care than their American counterparts.

Was this acceptable? Medical ethicists in the industrial world were sharply divided on this question. At one extreme were the hard-liners who said that all infected volunteers should receive the best medical care in the world, until they died, at the expense of the trial's sponsor. Others said that people in clinical trials should get exactly the same care as anyone else in their country. Some claimed that offering a higher level of care would be coercive, unfairly enticing people into vaccine trials so that if the worst happened, they would be assured better treatment than their neighbors. Cynics said corporations withheld treatment just to save money, and they suspected that scientists wanted to see whether immunization altered the severity or course of disease in untreated people. There were dozens of vociferously expressed opinions.

Lost in the rhetoric was the small number of people who would be affected. Statisticians familiar with infection rates among Bangkok drug users estimated that about 110 people in the 1,250-member control group would become HIV-positive during the three-year study, plus an unknown number of people in the vaccine group. If the efficacy level of the vaccine was 50 percent, about 55 vaccine recipients would be infected.

After much discussion, VaxGen and Thai officials came up with a plan for handling infected volunteers. The Bangkok Metropolitan Administration, which ran the drug treatment clinics where the trial would take place, selected the treatment regimen. Newly infected participants would be treated with two antiviral drugs, neither of them an expensive protease inhibitor, and supplied with medicine to help ward off tuberculosis, pneumonia, and other opportunistic infections that take advantage of immune systems weakened by HIV. As part of the vaccine study, their immune responses and HIV viral load would be monitored regularly. In addition to covering the lab work, VaxGen donated money to the BMA to help cover the costs of medical care.

●

By February 1998, it was clear that the VaxGen efficacy trial was going to be approved by the Thai government. Yet Don still flew from San Francisco to Bangkok every month, negotiating aspects of the study that would affect not only Thais at risk for AIDS but the country as a whole. Many of these discussions were between Don and Dr. Natth, two men with radically different styles.

"He is not an easy person to deal with," Don said of Dr. Natth. "The first time I met with him, he told me, 'Don, don't come in here and do parachute research. If you want to come in, there are things I want left here. It has to be good for Thailand.'" When Don looked at Dr. Natth, he saw a man in a starched white shirt and silk tie, in his sixties but so solid that he appeared to be built of stacked cannonballs. Using access to high-risk volunteers as leverage, Dr. Natth was determined to create a vaccine industry in Thailand. He was a savvy negotiator who would not rest until VaxGen met his conditions for training clinic and laboratory staff so that they would be prepared to team up with other companies in the future.

Dr. Natth had expected the U.S. military to win approval for Thailand's first HIV vaccine efficacy trial. Clearly that was not the case now, and he saw two reasons for that turnabout. The first was Kathy Steimer's death, which Dr. Natth believed cut short Chiron's commitment to an HIV vaccine for Thailand. And the second was Don Francis's tenacity. Despite his casual clothes and loose-limbed tendency to rock back in his chair while talking, Don had proved very, very persistent. "Don Francis is a crusader. He is a missionary kind of person, that keeps pushing on this unbelievably. And he has an absolute confidence in his vaccine," Dr. Natth said.

Don agreed that VaxGen would meet nearly all the technology transfer requirements that Dr. Natth set forth. The two also reached what Dr. Natth called "a gentleman's agreement" about the future accessibility of the Thai gp120 vaccine, should it prove successful in clinical trials. VaxGen would be willing to send bulk shipments of the product to Thailand, where a government-run pharmaceutical plant could package it in doses more cheaply than a U.S. facility. This would be the first step toward a joint manufacturing agreement, which would further reduce the price of the vaccine in Thailand and other developing countries. Although there was definitely wiggle room in the letter of agreement they signed, this was the most significant business commitment that a vaccine company had ever made to Thailand.

In addition to planting the seeds for a future vaccine industry, Dr. Natth and his technical subcommittee weighed in on some ethics issues as well. For example, the committee suggested that both the U.S. and Thai trials be overseen by a single Data and Safety Monitoring Board, made up of Thai and American members. The DSMB is a watchdog group of clinical research experts, who meet periodically to scrutinize data from the study while it's underway. Their role is to protect volunteers against exposure to undue risk, and they could stop the trial if the vaccine appeared harmful or if it was so obviously effective that no additional data were needed.

The technical subcommittee also proposed that one of its own members, a highly respected, politically connected social activist named Jon Ungpakorn, lead an independent monitoring effort that would keep an eye on the BMA clinics where the trial was being conducted. A perennial concern about vaccine trials is that busy clinic staff might give short shrift to risk-reduction counseling, and the role of the independent monitors was to make sure that didn't happen. "This is an experiment," Dr. Natth said. "No one has done it before, and in a developing country. We are ready to try it."

●

Back in the United States, the pieces were falling into place for the Bangkok trial, and they were being nailed down by Marlene Chernow, the ace clinical-trials coordinator whom VaxGen had lured away from Genentech. She was the one who had to deliver whatever goods Don had promised. A red-haired, green-eyed Smith College graduate who began her working life in a biochemistry laboratory, she had spent seven years running clinical trials for Genentech and a few years before that at a different company. In early 1997, she was hired as VaxGen's third employee. She hit the ground running, immediately drafting the clinical-trial protocols that the FDA approved in June 1997.

Friends told Marlene that she was crazy to take a risk on a little start-up like VaxGen. But she had known Don since the late 1970s, when they had met on the East Coast, and she was passionately interested in working toward an AIDS vaccine. If she could have a hand in defeating AIDS, it would mean far more to Marlene than the other drugs she had helped bring to market. As for setting up clinical trials in Asia, that was part of the adventure. Although she had never been to Thailand, "I had done this work for a long, long time, and part of the intrigue is variation on a theme, putting it in a new setting."

On her first couple of trips to Bangkok, Marlene sat back and watched Don, hoping to figure out "what went well and what didn't in terms of communication, how people wanted to be treated, what was respectful and what wasn't." By mid-1998, she was practically living there. At times, Marlene worried because so few of her new colleagues had any experience with clinical trials. But she soon discovered that "the Thais are really anxious, and really good learners, and eager for the technology transfer." Marlene came to like the East-meets-West feel of Bangkok, where ancient Buddhist temples stand side by side with glitzy, high-rise shopping malls. And she found that the Thai nurses and counselors in the BMA clinics, and in the labs and data center at Mahidol University, were not so reserved as they first appeared. They worked hard, but they knew how to kid around over a beer.

●

The individuals who joined VaxGen's team were often crusaders, people inflamed by Don Francis's passionate conviction that gp120—if only they could do an efficacy trial—would prove to be a successful AIDS vaccine. And although they knew that much of the scientific community was extremely skeptical about what they were doing, they were too busy to care.

VaxGen's underdog status was apparent to visitors who came to the offices Genentech provided as part of the spin-off deal. The new company had a small suite of rooms in one corner of Building 54, a low-rise loaf of a structure across the street from Genentech's shipping and receiving operation. A company shuttle connected this satellite area with the main campus of Genentech, where Phil Berman's people occupied the corners of laboratories in three different buildings. Although the new administrative offices were small and overlooked a parking lot, at least they were stationary. This was an improvement over their early days as the nomads of Building 7, when Bob Nowinski wheeled his belongings from place to place on a swivel chair.

When the May 8, 1998 issue of *Science* hit their desks, Don and Phil were vividly reminded that many scientists expected—even hoped—that gp120 would fail. Inside this issue of the journal was a letter, signed by some seventy-five people in support of NIH's stand on AIDS vaccine research, most notably the decision to hold off on efficacy testing and invest heavily in basic science. Most of the signers were themselves engaged in basic research, funded by NIH grants at universities or working for NIH's intramural programs in Bethesda. The remaining signers were AIDS advocates, the men that Tony Fauci had wisely invited to sit among the greats on advisory committees and councils.

The letter also leapt to the defense of David Baltimore and Harold Varmus, whose role in derailing Phase III vaccine trials had recently been branded a "human rights violation" by Jonathan Mann, a pioneering AIDS epidemiologist who was now dean of a struggling public health school in Philadelphia. Like Don, Mann had worked for CDC during the early days of the epidemic; later, he became the first director of the World Health Organization's Global Programme on AIDS, the forerunner of what is now called UNAIDS. Mann was famous for overheated rhetoric and had excoriated the NIH leadership at a meeting of the President's Council on HIV and AIDS back in March. News of this speech spread fast, sparking the letter to *Science*.

Angry mainstream AIDS researchers defended NIH as "the federal agency most suited to supporting the development of this vaccine." Their letter left no doubt that VaxGen, although the company was not named in the letter, had gone tooting off on a fool's errand. This impression was reinforced by a second letter in the same issue of *Science*, in which the head of the French government's AIDS program trashed the idea of efficacy testing for gp120.

Several years later, Phil Berman acted as though he wasn't bothered by people who attacked his life's work. "I was used to cheap shots," he said of the letters to *Science*, David Ho's advice to Thai authorities, and similar events. But Bob Nowinski's recollection is different. Phil and Don "found these attacks unbelievably insulting, and I would have to say, 'Guys, you gotta let it go. This is talk about old stuff, it has nothing to do with us, and you have to let it go.'"

Meanwhile, Phil's top priority was analyzing blood samples from the Phase I/II studies that had begun recruiting volunteers in November 1997. The FDA had agreed that if at least 50 percent of vaccinees made antibodies against HIV after receiving two shots, the agency would automatically approve an efficacy trial in the United States. It had taken time to fill all the slots in the trial, immunize everybody twice, and collect blood two weeks after the second shot, but by May the samples were flooding in.

Volunteers were immunized with either AIDSVAX B/B™ or B/E™. Whichever vaccine they received, it was possible that the two gp120 antigens would interfere with each other. "This was the first time that anyone had ever mixed two antigens together, and there was a lot of stuff in the literature about original antigenic sin. [The idea is] that if you make a response to one thing it's going to be hard to respond to the second," Phil said. His laboratory had tools that could distinguish antibodies against the two types of clade B virus and against Thai E, but there was no way to predict what would turn up in the blood samples.

Phil had two lab technicians on the VaxGen payroll, along with one borrowed from Genentech, crammed into a tiny room in Building 20. "Everyone involved thinks of this as the most stressful thing they've ever been through," Phil recalled. The techs bumped elbows at two lab benches crowded with computers and equipment, logging in samples and testing them, over and over, as fast as possible. VaxGen's whole future hung in the balance, because if the FDA didn't see what it was looking for, the Phase III trial would be history.

Early results indicated that about 70 percent of immunized volunteers were cranking out antibodies against both antigens in whichever bivalent vaccine they'd been given. This was well over the threshold that the FDA had set for approving the Phase III trial, and Phil was thrilled and relieved. He rushed to share the results with Don. "We were dancing in the street," Don recalled. Because FDA officials had spelled out exactly what results would trigger approval, Phil and Don felt certain the Phase III study would be okayed by the FDA. And they were right.

News of the approval hit the papers on June 3, 1998. Prominent stories in the *New York Times, Wall Street Journal,* and other major media outlets hailed this as a milestone in the lengthy battle against AIDS, the first time that a candidate vaccine had gotten so far in human testing. Reporters also gave prominent play to the low expectations of David Baltimore, Tony Fauci, John Moore, and other scientists. Baltimore and Moore, in particular, seemed to have talked to every reporter who covered the story. Their message was that gp120 would probably fail to protect people and might damage the overall quest by using up volunteers before other, more deserving candidates were ready for testing. Fauci, interestingly enough, took a slightly softer line. Although he doubted that the vaccine would prove very effective, he thought that if it protected even a few people, then results of the trial might help scientists design better vaccines in the future.

●

On the morning of June 23, 1998, television crews from four network affiliates crowded into a nondescript examining room at Philadelphia FIGHT, a nonprofit AIDS clinic in City Center. The cameras were pointed at a burly, barrel-chested man with close-cropped, graying hair and a dark goatee. The left sleeve of his plaid shirt was rolled up, revealing a tattooed Celtic braid encircling his upper arm. While the videotape rolled, a doctor resembling the young Sonny Bono, with longish hair and a droopy mustache, pushed in a syringe just above the tattoo.

"It hurt," said the man in the plaid shirt, smiling a bit ruefully after the syringe was withdrawn. He was Mark Watkins, a thirty-eight-year-old physician more accustomed to giving injections than receiving them. He was also a sexually active gay man, who had lived his adult life in the shadow of AIDS. As a doctor, he had been treating AIDS patients for more than a decade and had lost many of them, not to mention many friends, to the disease. Watkins had ample reasons, both personal and professional, for going public as the first volunteer in the VaxGen Phase III efficacy trial.

Watkins told reporters that he was confident the vaccine wouldn't do him any harm and hopeful that the trial would show it could protect people. "If this vaccine works, it will be a milestone in medical history," he said, and even if it didn't work, "this is an important study that needs to be done." Watkins knew that many experts expected gp120 to fail completely and said he didn't expect it to be 100-percent effective. "I'll be happy if it protects just 10 to 25 percent of the people," he told the *Philadelphia Inquirer*. "But we're not going to know how effective it is unless we test it."

Before the efficacy trial was complete, sixty more individuals would have the distinction of being the first person immunized in their cities. And most, if not all, of them would make the papers and the evening news. This type of exposure can be a big step for some people. Don Francis mused, "Do they want their grandmother to see them on national TV? That really brings you out of the closet. We have high-risk gay men and heterosexual women, and it's pretty clear which group you're in just by looking. One of the things we assess in this study is social harms, and we do not want social harms to come from us putting somebody in front of a TV camera."

Pioneering volunteers understood that media coverage was an important tool for recruiting enough people to fill the study. Although there was nothing wrong with advertising in alternative newspapers or posting notices in gay bars and bookstores, the impact was far greater with a couple of minutes on the evening news. As each site opened, local investigators emphasized that this was an unprecedented study, offering a chance to be part of an experiment that might ultimately save millions of lives around the world. The pitch appealed mainly to altruism; the only personal benefits were free blood tests for HIV, sessions with counselors, and limited reimbursement for travel expenses.

Most experienced AIDS journalists left no doubt that the trial was a marginal venture. Their stories emphasized that the trial was sponsored by "a small biotech company in South San Francisco, California" and reminded readers that the NIH had refused to pay for such a study back in 1994. Every reporter's Rolodex seemed to hold John Moore's phone number, and his colorful denunciations of the trial were even more widely reported than the doubts of the far more prominent David Baltimore.

•

Behind the scenes at VaxGen, a heroic effort had been needed to get the study off the ground. As soon as FDA approval was granted, VaxGen hired two clinical trials experts who had previously worked for the Division of AIDS at NIH. The medical director for the launch was Nzeera Virani-Ketter, a physician who worked out systems for collecting, processing, and analyzing clinical information. Her role was to begin laying the groundwork that would be needed and, if all went well, to apply for marketing approval after the trial ended.

John Jermano was the person who shouldered day-to-day responsibility for making the trial work. He was from the East Coast, a gay man in his late thirties who was trained first as a nurse, then as a public-health epidemiologist and biostatistician. Another San Francisco biotech had moved him to the area only one year earlier. Until John got a surprise call from VaxGen, he had assumed gp120 was moribund following NIH's 1994 decision. He was astonished to learn it was still alive and "THE Don Francis" wanted to talk with him.

He hung back when VaxGen made him an offer, thinking it would be wrong to change jobs so soon. But the second round of interviews convinced John it was the right thing for him to do. Unlike companies where people seemed motivated mainly by their mortgages, the atmosphere at VaxGen was alive with a sense of mission. He was impressed. "Cynicism is very vogue, but if you didn't have people believing in things, not a heck of a lot would get done," John said.

When John came on board in April 1998, his mandate as clinical program manager was simple: Launch the study. By June the protocol had been finalized, the first sites selected and their staffs trained, and the data-management system put in place. Four people had been hired for John's team, but in fact "everybody in the company worked on launching the trial," including Nicole Lynch, the company's one-woman public-relations department. A journalism graduate of the University of California-Berkeley, on the job Nicole had proved to have an aptitude for science and a prodigious capacity for work.

Every clinic that signed up was embedded in a bureaucracy of some sort. Although many sites were located at academic medical centers or major hospitals, others were part of nonprofit AIDS organizations or community clinics. Each required an individually negotiated contract covering payment for the clinic's services, approval for the trial by the local Institutional Review Board, training for staff, and shipment of vaccine from Genentech to the site. The national trial began at Philadelphia FIGHT because that group had completed this obstacle course faster than anyone else. Runners-up were in St. Louis, Denver, Chicago, and Rochester, followed by a long list of other cities.

But sometimes Murphy's Law is inescapable. Washington, D.C., has more than its share of reporters, and a good number of them were expected to attend VaxGen's press conference for the kickoff at D.C. General Hospital. Don was flying in, and the first volunteers were ready to be videotaped as they were inoculated. All was well until John Jermano discovered, twenty-four hours before the July 30 event, that Genentech had never shipped any vaccine to D.C. General. He had to move heaven and earth to convince Genentech that it was permissible to release a Styrofoam cooler of vaccine to him, as opposed to a commercial shipper.

John put the cooler on a nonstop flight to Washington, nestled in the arms of a woman who had been hired only a few days earlier as a clinical research associate, or CRA, one of the people who would monitor the performance of the trial sites. She landed in Washington at night and drove to D.C. General, a grim, red-brick institution on the same grounds as the city jail. On this occasion, the hospital was lit up with flashing red and blue lights and ringed with heavily armed men, including SWAT teams, military police, and Secret Service agents. Earlier in the day, a disturbed gunman had opened fire in the Capitol Rotunda, killing two security men before being brought down. The wounded shooter was hospitalized at D.C. General, and hundreds of reporters were camped out in the sweltering summer night, waiting for news.

The woman with the cooler eventually threaded her way through the checkpoints and delivered the vaccine. The next morning, reporters had to be patted down and escorted into the hospital for the first immunizations and the press conference. Despite its precarious beginning, this site enrolled more participants than any other by the end of the study.

The Phase III protocol specified that more than 90 percent of volunteers should be high-risk homosexual men. Don's relationship with the gay community had been bumpy over the years: He was perceived first as a hero, then as an enemy when he advocated closing gay bathhouses and sex clubs. When the efficacy trial was getting started, the idea of courting the gay community still didn't sit well with him.

"I did not need the gay community; I needed 5,000 volunteers," Don said. "I wasn't looking for every gay man. I was looking for a small number of gay men that I know are out there. It was a matter of letting them know that we're here." Gay men had flocked to the hepatitis B vaccine trials that Don had led in the early 1980s, and he was confident this would happen again.

It was good to have faith, but John Jermano knew that finding those 5,000 individuals could easily consume more time and money than Vax-Gen had. The company needed to reach thousands of high-risk gay men and about 400 women with HIV-positive partners. The people they found also needed to remain in the trial for the full three years, or else the results could be inconclusive. The key to retention was attracting people who understood that keeping appointments for seven injections and numerous blood draws was time-consuming and inconvenient, but nevertheless worth doing.

Logical places to find potential volunteers were AVEG and HIVNET, the two vaccine-trial networks that NIAID had created, maintained, and never used to the fullest. Although the six AVEG sites recruited low-risk volunteers for safety studies, people who weren't good candidates for this trial, the seventeen HIVNET sites had extensive experience with gay communities and IV drug user populations. Both networks had highly trained clinic staffs who knew how to do research. Although thousands of people had participated in HIVNET's vaccine-readiness studies, NIH had never given them an efficacy trial. Instead, they had mostly tested non-vaccine prevention strategies, such as antimicrobial gels and contraceptives.

VaxGen assumed it would be shunned by NIH-funded researchers who had been on hand when gp120 was dumped by NIH in 1994. John didn't think this was the case. He suspected that the doctors and nurses on the front lines, burned out from seeing patients fall prey to HIV, might jump at the chance to participate in world's first HIV vaccine efficacy trial. They might be especially willing now that HIVNET and AVEG were being dismantled while NIH set up the new HIV Vaccine Trials Network. If researchers in the original networks wanted to do an efficacy trial during the next several years, then VaxGen was the only game in town.

"So we set out on a quiet little campaign to accrue the HIVNET sites and recruit the AVEG sites. There was a certain amount of resistance at first—disbelief, a little surprise," John said. Soon the reluctance of these investigators, who relied heavily on NIH for support, melted away. This was partly because John and Nzeera Virani-Ketter had both done AIDS research in Bethesda. John's first job at NIH had been caring for AIDS patients on the ward where Tony Fauci practiced medicine and met his future wife. Later, John moved to the Division of AIDS, where Virani-Ketter also worked. "We had been part of the family. Like the Cosa Nostra, once you're in the family, you're always in the family. I think that increased the trust level." It took less than six months for the majority of AVEG and HIVNET sites to sign on with VaxGen.

●

While John Jermano's group was establishing rapport with NIH-funded investigators out in the field, relations at the top of the pecking order were tense between VaxGen and NIH. Since early 1998, when Chiron had decided not to supply gp120 for future prime-boost trials, NIAID had been trying to arrange a marriage of convenience between Pasteur Mérieux Connaught and VaxGen. NIH had thrown its weight behind the prime-boost strategy and repeatedly touted it as the leading candidate for efficacy testing. In NIH-sponsored studies, more volunteers had been inoculated with canarypox than any other experimental vaccine. But canarypox would be deader than a caged bird in a coal mine if there was no boost available to test with it. VaxGen was the logical place for NIAID to turn.

But PMC and VaxGen were having a hard time working out a deal, in part because AIDSVAX B/B™ was in short supply. The vaccines were still manufactured at Genentech, which had made an amount thought to be ample for the domestic Phase III study. But when statisticians recalculated the trial size, it was obvious that there was barely enough. VaxGen had to husband every vial for its own efficacy trial, and no more was going to be made until VaxGen and Genentech worked out a manufacturing agreement.

A second barrier to VaxGen's participation in prime-boost studies was that NIH officials and investigators couldn't seem to stop bad-mouthing the product. Although the NIH vaccine program desperately needed gp120 as a boost for canarypox, the top brass freely criticized Vax-Gen's efficacy trial. When the newspapers quoted David Baltimore as saying the vaccine would never work or Tony Fauci as saying that it probably wouldn't work, Bob Nowinski was not happy. It seemed to him that NIH leaders were talking out of both sides of their mouths.

Bob had a reputation for playing hardball, and the message he sent to NIH was simple. "I literally said we may not be able to help you with your work if you continue doing this. We want to work with you, but we can't provide material if you're going to talk negatively about it." He put this threat in writing, and after a series of meetings and phone calls, NIH and VaxGen agreed that it was time to bury the hatchet.

On August 18, NIAID distributed a press release announcing plans to collaborate on VaxGen's trial by funding additional studies of "immune responses induced by AIDSVAX™, as well as use of AIDSVAX™ in combination with other vaccines currently studied by NIAID. Additional joint research aimed toward creating formulations of AIDSVAX™ for viruses prevalent in developing nations is also under discussion." The tone of NIAID's comments on gp120 shifted after this. "Now it was 'I'm not sure if this is going to work,' instead of 'This is baloney,'" Bob said.

Some observers guessed that Fauci, a man known for covering all the bases, did not want to be out in the cold if VaxGen's trial proved successful. "At this point, in a political sense, you want to get in the tent. You don't want to be an outspoken critic in case it really works," Don said. NIH's top brass were the last to climb on board. Lower-ranking Division of AIDS staff were already saying privately that the government owed Don and his company a huge debt of gratitude. VaxGen had proved that you can dive off the ten-meter board and survive, a demonstration that might help the NIH find the courage to climb the tower.

●

By September, more than thirty clinics had decided to participate in the VaxGen trial, although only six had completed all their paperwork so they could actually inject volunteers. Nearly half of the clinics had been part of HIVNET or AVEG. This was a time of rapprochement for NIAID and VaxGen, and John Jermano had what he called "a crazy idea" about how to seal the deal. Like most sponsors of large clinical trials, VaxGen would periodically bring scattered investigators together to talk about how things were going. These events are mostly business, but it's also traditional to stage a banquet for all the participants.

John's brainstorm was to invite Jack Killen, head of the Division of AIDS, as the banquet speaker at the trial's inaugural dinner. Killen was not a favorite of the VaxGen leadership, who associated him with gp120's defeat in 1994. John was not burdened with this history. "I've known Jack for a long time. I knew he would say yes, and I thought that symbolically, this shows NIH investigators that it is okay to participate in the VaxGen study, that it's a good thing. It shows that VaxGen was first, and that we're inviting NIH to our dinner, not the other way around." As John predicted, Killen did speak at the banquet, which was held at a freshly opened Hyatt Hotel near McCormick Place in Chicago.

Being wined and dined by VaxGen probably inspired some of the clinic staff to go home and work even harder to round up healthy men for the trial. Others had more bureaucratic hurdles to surmount before getting to that stage. Back in California, John Jermano and his colleagues began to worry that it might not be possible to fill all the slots in a single year, which the FDA expected. The protocol specified that 5,000 gay men and several hundred high-risk women would be enrolled and receiving shots by June 1999.

If they'd been able to step back and gain more perspective, John's clinical team would have marveled at how far they had come. After all, they had been building a rocket and blasting off at the same time. But they didn't pause to reflect, because all they could think about was the deadline for enrollment, which was hurtling toward them like an asteroid in a sci-fi movie.

On December 1, World AIDS Day, John had the first of many strategy sessions with Nicole Lynch from PR and a few core members of his team. They could see that some clinics were enrolling at a rapid pace, while others were getting nowhere fast. They had left recruitment up to the locals, but clearly more was needed. The SWAT team, as this core group soon called itself, came up with two advertising campaigns for the sites to choose from: "Let's talk about SEX and a vaccine for AIDS" and "Make it safer for future generations." Nicole used her media skills to generate display ads, T-shirts, posters, and other materials for clinics to use.

These efforts were just getting off the ground in mid-December, when the latest count showed that only 700 volunteers had signed up at twenty-four clinics. Several newspaper articles described the efficacy trial as "falling short of volunteers." At scientific meetings, the hallway gossip was that the VaxGen trial was doomed, because gay men were too savvy to sign up for a low-tech vaccine like gp120.

●

Like Don Francis in the early days of AIDS in the United States, Dr. Supak Vanichseni stuck her neck out when the epidemic first hit Thailand. In 1979, she had helped launch the first of Bangkok's free public clinics for IV drug users, a system that had since expanded to seventeen locations in some of the city's dirtiest, most frightening slums. "In 1988, we had a seminar about HIV infection, and I attended that seminar and heard about transmission by IV drug use," she recalled. "At that time, I was in charge of the Drug Division for Bangkok Metropolitan Administration, so I asked for reagents to use the ELISA test for HIV."

Using blood samples obtained from 1,600 drug users in early 1988, Dr. Supak's lab determined that 15 percent were already infected with HIV. But no one wanted to hear about her discovery. "I was told to keep this down. Because like every country that has these epidemics, politically and nationally they have denial of the problem. And then we had the second seroprevalence survey, six months later, and it was 42.7 percent." At this point, government officials could no longer close their eyes.

Although heroin use is as reviled in Thailand as in the United States, the philosophy of the BMA clinics is that drug users are medical patients, not criminals. Faced with an astronomical rise in HIV infection, Dr. Supak's public-health training told her that immediate steps should be taken to slow transmission of the virus. She called international experts for help putting together educational videos, posters, and brochures. These emphasized the importance of not sharing syringes and of using bleach to clean needles between uses. The BMA clinics began by handing out bleach, then launched their first-ever methadone maintenance program.

Addicts in the BMA treatment program were bombarded with preventive tips on safe drug use, and they were not exempt from massive public campaigns aimed at promoting condoms. All this had an impact, and after 1989, the prevalence of HIV infection among BMA clients stabilized between 38 percent and 44 percent. People continuously come and go from the clinic population, however, with some recovering or dropping out as new ones enter the system. So even though the overall percentage of infected people has been stable, the incidence rate for new infections among IV drug users remained at 6 percent to 10 percent each year.

Dr. Supak looked at this stubborn incidence rate, which persisted despite counseling, clean needle campaigns, and methadone, and knew that more was needed. The next step presented itself in 1993, when she was invited to a World Health Organization workshop for countries that might be willing to be considered as sites for HIV vaccine trials. "It would be good for Thai people to have vaccines, so I made the decision to tell the Deputy Governor that I wanted to do this." This is how Thailand became one of WHO's four preferred locations for international trials.

As a result of Dr. Supak's interest in testing vaccines, the BMA clinics forged new ties with WHO, the Vaccine Trial Center at Mahidol University, and the HIV/AIDS Collaboration, or HAC, itself a partnership between the U.S. Centers for Disease Control and the Thai Ministry of Public Health. It was HAC's sophisticated virology lab that detected the shift from clade B to E infections among Bangkok addicts, which in turn led Phil Berman to design AIDSVAX B/E™ for Thailand.

This consortium had tested Genentech's original monovalent, clade B gp120 vaccine in early 1995, when Don could think of no other way to keep the vaccine project alive after the 1994 NIH decision. This was a small study, but it gave the BMA and its partners an opportunity to begin figuring out how to run vaccine trials. The only staff with actual clinical trial experience were at the Vaccine Trial Center, a specialized research operation on Mahidol's medical school campus. Rather than trying to entice drug addicts to this unfamiliar place, VTC staff fanned out to the bad neighborhoods where BMA clinics were housed.

Heroin use is as illegal in Bangkok as it is in New York. But over the years, addicts have learned that the BMA nurses and counselors won't turn them over to the police. So when familiar staff members brought new faces from the VTC into the drug clinics, the newcomers were accepted. The result was a win-win situation: VTC researchers gained access to a large number of high-risk people, and BMA staffers began learning how to carry out research and manage data according to rigorous FDA standards.

Marlene Chernow's training programs for the Phase III trial built on this earlier foundation. In the seventeen clinics of the BMA, she confronted a world that in San Francisco, where she lives, has been driven mostly out of sight by wealth and gentrification. Every day, several hundred men and a few women line up at each of the clinics. At Taksin Hospital, the line forms in a *soi,* or alley, crowded with food vendors and scrawny stray dogs. Inside, clients fill rows of plastic chairs, waiting their turn at the dispensary window. One by one, they step up to the counter, show a picture ID to the nurse on the other side of the glass, and receive a small stainless steel cup containing the yellow, slightly viscous methadone. They drink it down and leave, about half of them going to jobs they hold despite their illness.

More than 95 percent of narcotics users in Thailand are men, and the mean age of those who seek help from the BMA is thirty-two. The oldest clients in the program are in their fifties, the youngest in their teens. Dr. Supak's view is that they became addicted by accident, often through a process that began as a dare or a night on the town. This may explain why so few of the addicts are women. "Our Thai women do not like to take adventure, and the prime cause of taking the drug the first time is experimental. Men like to experiment," she said.

On March 24, 1999, six of the Bangkok drug addicts embarked on a different kind of experiment: They rolled up their sleeves and were injected with a syringe containing not heroin but either AIDSVAX B/E™ or a placebo. The setting was the BMA clinic in Klongtoey, an area described by Dr. Supak as one of the city's most famous slums. It was not the sort of place that visiting Americans, including famous scientists, would see on a tour of Bangkok.

These men were the first of 2,500 who would ultimately volunteer for the Thai trial. In order to qualify, each had tested negative for HIV infection and been examined by a doctor, had taken part in group and one-on-one education sessions, had passed two comprehension tests covering risks and benefits of participation, had undergone HIV prevention counseling, and had signed an informed consent document. They were also promised confidentiality. These safeguards not only met, but exceeded, international standards for clinical trials.

Potential volunteers were questioned about why they wanted to join the trial, and Marlene could not help comparing their responses with those from U.S. participants. "In the U.S., a lot of people are doing this for purely altruistic reasons directed toward the gay community. They are from an era where they were affected, their friends died of AIDS, and they want to do something for the community. In Thailand, there's more of a nationalistic altruism: We're doing this for the people of Thailand."

One newspaper story quoted a vegetable vendor as saying he volunteered "for the millions of AIDS victims all over the world." Another volunteer told the same reporter, "It is good for a drug user normally looked down upon by others to do something for society."

There were practical, as well as theoretical, benefits to participants. They got increased personal attention from counselors, and nurses monitored their overall health more closely than in the past.

Before the trial began, VaxGen and the BMA agreed that people who became HIV-positive during the trial would get limited antiviral treatment, as well as drugs to prevent some common opportunistic infections. This was better care than the BMA clientele could ever expect to obtain on their own. If people who couldn't stop shooting heroin realized that superior care was part of the deal, they might sign up for this reason alone. They might forget all about clean needles and condoms, figuring that if they did get infected, their medical care was assured.

This was precisely the sort of lure that some ethicists viewed as coercion and warned against whenever an American drug company launched an international trial. In an effort to skirt this quagmire, the Thai researchers who drafted the consent form opted for deliberate vagueness about treatments for the infected few. "You will receive counseling and care according to the policy and standard of the BMA," the consent form stated, leaving it at that. The Thais had come up with an elegant solution that might never have occurred to American investigators: Although they were going to provide superior medical care, which most people would view as a good thing, they kept quiet about it.

●

When Don Francis and Bob Nowinski hit the road to promote Vax-Gen's initial public offering, their tour was like a Bonzai presidential campaign. For three intense weeks in June 1999, they traveled to a dozen places, including Seattle, Chicago, Boston, New York, Philadelphia, West Palm Beach, Houston, Los Angeles, Orange County, San Francisco, and Denver. In some locales they did two or three presentations each day; in others, as many as six or eight.

"It's not the most fun," Don said, grimacing at the memory.

"It's a real recipe for exhaustion," Bob concurred. "But it was interesting to see the difference between Don and myself. When we finished a presentation, Don would take a walk and I would take a nap." He gave a slightly crazed laugh.

Investors who had gotten in on the ground floor, subscribing to earlier private offerings, were invited to attend one of these IPO sessions and bring their friends. Like political candidates, Don and Bob stuck to their stump speech. "You make the identical presentation over and over again, in groups from two to 100 people. We still had about thirty slides, but we had a little more to say this time." In fact, they had a lot more to say now than two years earlier. VaxGen had launched the first domestic and international clinical trials large enough to demonstrate whether a vaccine could interfere with the spread of AIDS, a feat no other government agency or company had duplicated. Private investors had made this possible.

VaxGen's research had also been validated by the NIH, which disdained their efforts in the beginning, and by the supportive but chronically underfunded Centers for Disease Control. Bob didn't tell future stockholders that some strategic arm-twisting on his part motivated NIH to get involved. And Don didn't emphasize that his old CDC chums had goaded the Atlanta-based agency to resume AIDS vaccine research, fifteen years after it ceded the field to NIH. All stockholders needed to know was that VaxGen's trials were stamped with the imprimaturs of the NIH and the CDC.

In general, the field of AIDS vaccine research had a higher profile now. Microsoft founder Bill Gates added celebrity glitter in May 1999, when the William H. Gates Foundation donated $25 million to the International AIDS Vaccine Initiative. IAVI's ambitious goal was to develop vaccines for the hardest-hit countries in Africa and Asia, but so far its budget had permitted investment in only two potential vaccines. One was the VEE vaccine invented in North Carolina by Bob Johnston and Nancy Davis; the other was an updated vaccinia vector made at England's Oxford University. The Gates Foundation windfall, hailed as the largest private donation ever made to AIDS research, would enable IAVI to expand its good works.

Vaccines made headlines again while Don and Bob were on their IPO tour in June 1999. Potential investors saw TV and newspaper coverage of President Clinton, dedicating the $26-million building that would house the Dale and Betty Bumpers Vaccine Research Center at NIH. This state-of-the-art facility, due for completion by early 2001, was part of the AIDS vaccine effort the president unveiled in May 1997, when he challenged scientists to develop an AIDS vaccine within a decade. The new center wasn't up and running yet, and the director's job had taken nearly two years to fill, but eventually it was expected to do great things.

It was impossible to say whether such news events made potential shareholders more receptive to the VaxGen pitch. Bob had done IPOs before, and he napped rather than worried. But the tour was a new experience for Don, and he found it an exercise in uncertainty. For the private placement, they had established a share price and a minimum number of shares that could be purchased. Investors could accept the deal or not. This time, the Bob-and-Don road show was different: Their goal was to sell 3.1 million shares at $13 to $15, but they had no control over what people would pay.

When the IPO was launched on Wednesday, June 30, 1999, the shares sold out at $13; by Friday, the price had climbed to $17.31. Don breathed a sigh of relief: "We raised all $42 million and that's it." They estimated that about $30 million would be needed to complete the clinical trials in Thailand and the United States, which were scheduled to run into the year 2003; the company was also investing heavily in laboratory facilities, new product development, and setting up a regulatory office to manage licensing.

Bob was pleased with the IPO. Not only had they met their financial goal but also the majority of stock buyers were people who had backed the start-up. The conventional wisdom was that a company couldn't go public by relying on its private investors, and Bob was always happy when he did what others said was impossible.

Back at VaxGen, the IPO created far less hysteria than these events bring at dot-coms, where the top executives are in their twenties. "A lot of us have had experience with this," Phil Berman said in a blasé manner. He, Don, and Bob were all past fifty, and many of their employees were over thirty. Nor was the financing structured in a way that sent employee stock options into the stratosphere. "It wasn't like everyone was getting rich, as it is with some IPOs," Phil said. Unlike the early days at Genentech, where stock prices were reflected in the shiny Porsches parked outside, there were no new luxury cars at VaxGen.

●

Bob Nowinski had promised, at every stop on the IPO tour, that Vax-Gen's domestic efficacy trial would be fully enrolled by the end of the summer. According to the protocol filed with the FDA, the last of the 5,000 slots should be filling while he and Don were on the road. In reality, total enrollment was nowhere near complete. Drug development is a chain reaction where front-end delays have consequences all down the line. The slower the slots were filled, the longer it would be before VaxGen could file for FDA approval. In the meantime, every additional day cost money.

Bob saw no point in worrying about the smaller trial in Thailand, because timing was controlled by the company's Thai collaborators and the whole enterprise had, as he said, a very different momentum from the U.S. experiment. So Bob focused exclusively on the stateside operation.

The man responsible for getting the trial done was the most significant new hire VaxGen had made so far. John Curd had been vice president for clinical development at Genentech, where he had proved, three times in nine years, that he could go the distance: taking drugs all the way from early clinical trials through FDA licensure and marketing. His best-known project was Herceptin, Genentech's genetically engineered miracle drug for metastatic breast cancer.

Curd had a great run at Genentech but felt that his career was capped there. When he began looking around, other major pharmaceutical companies wanted to hire him. "But it just didn't appeal to me, moving to New Jersey and working in the bowels of a 10,000 person company, even if I was the vice president." He was fifty-four years old, a Harvard-educated physician, a funny, articulate man who looks like a more genial, better-groomed cousin of Salman Rushdie. Three years earlier, he had survived major neurosurgery to remove a benign brain tumor, his kids were mostly through college, "and for the first time in quite a while, I could take more risks."

So he cast his lot with VaxGen. John Curd had known Don Francis for years; in fact, he was the one who hired Don at Genentech. He saw the pursuit of an AIDS vaccine as one of biomedicine's most important challenges and believed he could help make it happen. At Genentech, hundreds of people contributed to the success of a product like Herceptin. Even though John was in charge of the project, there were aspects that he knew little or nothing about. At tiny VaxGen, it would be different. "Here, if you make a big contribution, you can see it and feel it," John said.

When John came to VaxGen in May 1999, he immediately saw that John Jermano and the SWAT team were running on fumes. "It was a small team that pushed themselves at a frenetic pace, facing a huge challenge, and they were exhausted." Bob Nowinski was pushing them hard to finish enrolling the study by the end of summer, which they didn't believe could be done. At this point, fifty-six clinics in the United States, one in Puerto Rico, and one in Amsterdam had signed on for the efficacy trial, though not all of them had begun vaccinating. Three more sites in Canada were going to join over the summer, their entry having been slowed by regulatory paperwork.

So far, about 2,500 volunteers had signed up. When John Curd ran the numbers, he saw that seventy-five to ninety new participants were enrolling each week. Seven months remained in 1999, and he projected that the trial would be fully enrolled—with 5,000 gay men and about 300 women—"before the end of the year." When he presented his estimate at an executive committee meeting, "nobody reacted particularly strongly."

The following weekend, Bob Nowinski phoned him at home. Bob told John that finishing by the end of the year "was not acceptable." He was preparing the IPO, and it was going to specify that enrollment would be complete by the end of summer.

"I remember pointing out that we presented this at the executive committee, and people didn't seem to be very concerned," John recalled. "And Bob said, 'First priority: do it.'"

On Monday morning, John Curd assembled the members of the SWAT team and told them that completing enrollment before the end of summer was the company's absolute, number-one, top priority. They were heavy with fatigue and had a hard time imagining that they could work harder than they already were. But Curd, having just arrived, brought fresh blood to the effort. They went through the list of sites and figured out what it would take to finish enrollment by September 21, the first day of autumn. The team told Bob and Don that the clinics would need about $1-million worth of outreach materials and advertising money, and the request was approved.

Even more important, John Curd inspired the worn-out staff with his unflagging conviction that they could get it done. He went on a road trip of his own, throwing dinners for doctors and nurses in dozens of cities, giving talks, emphasizing that the clinic staff and volunteers were the most important people in the search for an AIDS vaccine. "To enroll a study like this, you have to get in people's hearts and minds. You can sit here in San Francisco and want to do this, but ultimately what you have to do is go out to your investigators and participants and interact with them, and get into their hearts and minds. Because they fill the study."

In each city, John talked with a core group of four or five clinic staff, the people who explained the trial to potential volunteers, gave the shots, and collected all the thousands of bits of information that would eventually be analyzed and sent to the FDA. He also met some of the thousands of people who stepped forward to be screened, some of whom would be turned away because they didn't fit the enrollment criteria. He was reminded that a trial like this doesn't need dozens and dozens of people who work for VaxGen. "What you need are great sites and a motivated community."

Back in California, VaxGen was now headquartered in suburban Brisbane, just off Route 101, on the second floor of an office building shaped like an irregular chunk of black glass. On either side of the main reception desk, sandblasted glass doors lead into the two wings of the building. Every week, the latest enrollment total was posted on these doors, outside John Curd's office, and on walls throughout the company. Employees might not have known the current price of VaxGen's stock, but they could not escape knowing where enrollment stood.

"We lived and died on those numbers," John Curd said. He told the SWAT team that an efficacy trial is like the Queen Mary: it's big and builds steam slowly, then it goes full speed ahead, and then it has to be brought in for a gentle landing that doesn't overshoot the goal. The campaign picked up speed as he predicted: By the end of August, 150 to 200 new participants were entering the study every week. And when they passed the 4,000 mark in August, he said, "We realized 'We're gonna do this!' And people started to feel incredibly good about what we had accomplished."

By September 21, fifty-eight sites in the United States, the Netherlands, and Puerto Rico had finished their enrollments. Three Canadian sites, in Vancouver, Toronto, and Montreal, were given several weeks to fill about 300 slots set aside for them. John had visited these sites and had no doubt that they would make the goal. And when the last shot was given, every dose of vaccine allocated to the domestic trial would be used up. The Queen Mary did not overshoot its berth.

●

John Curd invited everyone in the company to his house for a party. On the evening of Saturday, October 9, some sixty VaxGen employees, dressed up for the occasion, flowed through the doors of John's gracious Mediterranean-style home in the wooded, monied suburb of Hillsborough. They had come to celebrate VaxGen's three major accomplishments for 1999. The first was the completion of Phil Berman's new laboratory, a facility equipped to develop new antigens and process nearly half a million blood samples from the domestic and international studies. The second was the successful IPO. And the third, of course, was fully enrolling the U.S. trial.

"Everyone in the company was personally involved in at least one of those things, if not two or three," John said. There was plenty of food and drink and fellowship, with a few ceremonial remarks from Don. The members of the SWAT team, decked out in snappy white sailor hats, presented John with an officer's cap identifying him as captain of the Queen Mary. Circulating among his guests, John thought about the underlying reason for their presence. "They want to do something about the epidemic. It's either affected them personally, or their families, and they really care about this. There's a sense of great pride in doing something that people didn't think could get done. But this is not about VaxGen and not about the trial. For most people here, this is about the epidemic."

Not everyone, of course, thought that VaxGen's endeavors were so noble. Even as the party goers stood around the pool, eating and drinking in style, some of the talk concerned a sensational article published only one week earlier, in the London *Sunday Times*. Writer Brian Deer accused VaxGen of engaging in financial malfeasance and influence peddling in Bangkok, aimed at exploiting Thai junkies as guinea pigs. The story asserted that the company needed the Thais because "a parallel trial among gay men at American clinics is having problems finding and keeping volunteers, owing to skepticism towards the venture." Finally, the writer speculated that immunization with the B/E vaccine, instead of protecting Thai volunteers, might actually make them more susceptible to infection.

People who had cooperated with Deer, during the several days he spent interviewing at VaxGen, were understandably distressed. When he approached the company, no one had realized that the *Sunday Times* was the holocaust denier of the AIDS pandemic. In 1993, the scientific journal *Nature* attacked the newspaper for a series of articles claiming that HIV did not cause AIDS and that the African epidemic was a hoax. The editors of *Nature*, along with outraged British health officials, accused the *Sunday Times* of betraying the public trust and misleading its several million readers.

Although VaxGen's enemies would no doubt circulate the article, the fact was that not many Americans read London's scandalous Sunday broadsheets. Phil Berman shrugged off the attack as "another cheap shot." VaxGen had more important things to think about than press coverage in England.

Bob Nowinski had scheduled a conference call for the board of directors on Sunday, the day after John Curd's party. The topic was a new proposal from Vulcan Ventures, Paul Allen's biotech investment group. Vulcan had bought into VaxGen just before the June IPO and now was interested in investing another $25 million in the company. This would increase Allen's stake from 8 percent to 22 percent and would give VaxGen a lot more capital to work with. Part of the money would be invested in research, so that Phil could put more people to work on a clade C vaccine for Africa.

Bob spent weekends with his children in Seattle, and on this occasion had a houseguest as well. Shortly before the conference call, his guest was struck by an asthma attack so severe that he rushed her to a nearby hospital. He ran the board meeting from a public phone outside the ER, and it did not take long for the board to approve the sale of $25 million of common stock to Allen. Don's response to the deal was "if Paul Allen wants Jimi Hendrix played at shareholders meetings, that would be fine."

When Bob came down to Brisbane later that week, he threw his own party for VaxGen's employees. He saw enrollment of the U.S. trial as the moment "when people began to believe they could exceed what they thought they could do." Pulling together and meeting the deadline "levitated the company," he said. The board had set aside about 60,000 shares of stock for employees, and Bob distributed them to everyone. There was food and drink and lots of praise for a job well done.

●

In reality, of course, the fat lady was nowhere near ready to sing.

Don and Marlene were still working closely with their colleagues in Bangkok, trying to keep enrollment moving in the seventeen BMA drug clinics. The data-management operation and the laboratory in Bangkok also required lots of attention. Meanwhile, at Phil Berman's capacious new lab at Oyster Point, a few miles south of VaxGen's Brisbane headquarters, thousands of samples arrived for testing every week.

"There's a ton of work to be done," John Curd said after the celebrations had quieted down. The minute the domestic trial was filled, he began creating a regulatory department from scratch. This meant hiring experts and developing systems for supplying the voluminous information the FDA demanded before it would consider approving the vaccine for commercial use. As soon as the clinical trial indicated that the vaccine was efficacious, even if it was only moderately protective, they would file. The broad topics covered by their submission would be the trustworthiness of the clinical data and VaxGen's capacity to produce large quantities of consistently high-grade vaccine for sale.

Although these might not sound like demanding requirements, Don and John both knew how much work it would take to fulfill them. Both men had been through this before. In the precomputer era, "an FDA submission filled more than an average-sized room with stacks of paper," Don said. Although technology may have turned hundreds of pounds of paper into a short stack of floppy disks, all the FDA's questions still had to be answered.

The Bangkok trial enrolled its 2,500th volunteer on August 31, 2000, nearly a full year after the U.S. study was filled. VaxGen now had 7,900 people actively participating in clinical trials on two continents. This number far exceeded the sum of participants in all the HIV vaccine trials that NIH had sponsored since 1988, when it first tested MicroGeneSys gp160 and the vaccinia vectors made at Oncogen, a company founded by Bob Nowinski.

In part because VaxGen had been regarded so lightly by NIH officials and other elite scientists, its achievement radically altered the climate for future efficacy trials. "People who used to say, 'We're not ready, this can't be done, it's too hard,' now say, 'Well, we can do this, because VaxGen could do it. If VaxGen could do it, we can do it,'" John Curd said. The Thai trial was also going to make it harder for others to hang back, claiming that political and ethical complexity made international experiments impossible. "We've enrolled a trial in the developing world. It's been done. It wasn't easy, but it's a fact now. It's like somebody walking on the moon. It's been done."

What everyone at VaxGen really wanted to know, of course, was whether vaccination was protecting individual volunteers against AIDS.

The first chance to learn anything about efficacy would come in November 2001, when the twelve-member Data and Safety Monitoring Board would convene in VaxGen's main conference room. At this point, twenty-four months of data would be available, and it would be time for the "interim analysis" specified by the research protocol.

On the shiny conference table would be reams of printouts prepared by the company. Using codes that only they possessed, the DSMB would examine the data and be able to tell whether immunized people were less likely to become infected than people who'd been injected with saline solution. No one in the company could unlock these secrets.

Don knew that on this day, waiting for the DSMB analysis would be "a harrowing experience." If the members were certain that the vaccine was effective, they could halt the trial early and VaxGen could begin filing for approval. This would happen only if the DSMB was sure that the rate of infection in vaccinated individuals was at least 30-percent lower than in those injected with placebo. In order to be mathematically certain, there would have to be 40-percent to 60-percent fewer infections in the immunized group. There is a margin of uncertainty in clinical trials, just as in political exit polls. And DSMB members, unlike television broadcasters, will not announce a result unless they are certain it falls outside the margin of error.

If there was statistical uncertainty about the vaccine's efficacy, the DSMB would thank the VaxGen researchers for their help, urge them to carry on, and walk away. They would come back twelve months later, when the three-year trial had run its full course, and break the code once more. Nearly twenty years earlier, Don had worked on a hepatitis B vaccine trial that yielded an answer only at the very end. He didn't relish the thought of going through that again.

In the unlikely event that the DSMB did stop the study in November 2001, John Curd's new regulatory team would not really be ready to file for approval. But this wouldn't matter. "For the first week or two, we'll just party. I think none of us will leave work for two days." Then they would start work on the filing, with plenty of help from the FDA. Only a highly effective vaccine would justify stopping the trial, and he was sure the FDA "would bend over backwards" to speed approval of such a product.

Realistically, Curd expected the vaccine to be moderately effective, and to require three years of testing before its benefits emerge in November 2002. Not even Don, gp120's most passionate advocate, predicted that AIDSVAX B/B™ or B/E™ would be a home run. If gp120 vaccines protect some people but not others, "then we have to hope that the assay systems are sharp enough to show correlates of protection, so that we can clearly see why this occurred." In the past, partially effective vaccines have been used to slow the spread of disease, while scientists worked to develop better ones. Jonas Salk's polio vaccine saved thousands of lives before the more efficacious Sabin vaccine became available. And although AIDS is an unprecedented disease in many ways, many experts predict that the first AIDS vaccine will be good and the second better, with an excellent one somewhere down the road.

It is also possible, of course, that the vaccine will fail completely. "That would be the worst situation. Not that we haven't done a great thing. This needed to be done, it had to be done, and we're doing it as it should be done. It will advance the field no matter what. If this vaccine doesn't work, we move on to the next idea," Don said. "Who knows?"

ACKNOWLEDGMENTS

S CIENCE HAS BEEN DESCRIBED as "a special kind of storytelling, with no right or wrong answers, just better and better stories." The stories in this book came from patient and generous people who laid aside their work to tell me about their personal adventures and to explain the scientific, economic, and political complications of the vaccine quest. Some talked to me for hours at a time, repeatedly, and still had the energy to respond to phone calls and e-mails spread over months or years. While many of these people show up as characters in this book, some do not. Yet every one enriched my understanding of the vaccine story, and I hope they feel their time was well spent.

The people who talked with me also shared all sorts of official documents, correspondence, and ephemera with me. I am especially grateful to Patricia Fast, Margaret "Peggy" Johnston, and John McNeil, who not only filed reams of documents but also could put their hands on relevant items. And everyone who is interested in the history of AIDS vaccine research owes special thanks to Claudia Goad, a National Institutes of Health staff member who unearthed the verbatim transcript of the pivotal June 16, 1994, meeting of the AIDS Research Advisory Committee. Although I had been told repeatedly that this transcript did not exist, Ms. Goad found it for me. It was later posted on the Web by Bruce Weniger.

My own research was greatly enhanced by the acute and perceptive searches done by Martha Downs, who repeatedly found sources and information I had not thought to ask for. Also pitching in on research was James Jarrett, who is special to me in many ways. Once the manuscript was written, scientific review was provided by Dr. Larry Loomis-Price, whose wide-ranging knowledge of biology and vaccine research was invaluable as I revised my work. Any errors that may have slipped into print are solely my responsibility.

Support from several private foundations made it possible for me to spend four years on this book. In early 1997, a grant from the Albert B. Sabin Vaccine Foundation saw me through the first rounds of interviews; since then, the unflagging enthusiasm of H. R. "Shep" Shepherd, chairman of the Sabin Foundation, has fueled this project in countless ways. Shep made me a research fellow of the Sabin Vaccine Institute, introduced me to people, sent me books I ought to read, invited me to conferences, and was my rabbi when my spirits flagged.

The Leonard Silk Journalism Award kept me going at a later stage, when the book was well underway but resources were running low. The family and friends of *New York Times* reporter and columnist Leonard Silk created this award in his memory, which makes it a tremendous honor for any journalist to receive. It is ably administered by the staff of The Century Foundation, who have been encouraging all the way. Additional support for the final laps came from the Friendship Fund, led by Ellen Tully, which awarded me a grant in 1999 and generously renewed it the following year. Finally, I gratefully acknowledge the backing of my mother, Leatrice S. Magic of Dunnellon, Florida, who never once suggested that I forget about the book and get a real job.

The hospitality of friends also helped make possible the extensive travel required by this project. I'm especially grateful to Barbara and Wallace Waterfall in Washington, D.C.; Jim and Anne Clune in Seattle; Katie Baer, Ina Jane Wundram, and Daphna Gregg and David Gibson in Atlanta; and the Bobos of San Francisco—Kit Cameron and Peter Vaccaro, Marilyn and Steve Johnston, Judith Horstmann, and Carol Henderson.

The Henry M. Jackson Foundation facilitated travel to Thailand in 1997, and to Uganda two years later, by inviting me to meetings in those key locations. And my 1999 trip to Thailand was made possible by the adventurous spirit of Kit Boggio, who agreed to let a near-stranger share her accommodations for two weeks. During that same trip, all manner of advice and assistance was provided by Peter Lange of the Research Institute for Health Sciences in Chiang Mai, and by Bruce Merrell of the Armed Forces Research Institute of the Medical Sciences in Bangkok. Each of these gentlemen provided me with a temporary base of operations far from home, and Bruce hooked me up with Julie's Taxi—truly the best of Bangkok.

None of these adventures would have occurred without the efforts of my agent, Jill Kneerim, and the excellent team at the Hill & Barlow Literary Agency. The perceptive editing of Sarah Larson helped shape the proposal, and advice from attorney Zick Rubin eased my relations with the biotechnology world.

At PublicAffairs, I'm grateful to Peter Osnos for his faith in the book, to editor Geoff Shandler for guiding me through the early stages, and to editor Lisa Kaufman for stepping in and seeing it through. Lisa's warmth, wit, and insistence that I simplify the science were invaluable.

Cheerleading, goading, and reality testing has been provided by my wonderful writers' group in Boston: Nancy Day, Anne Driscoll, Florence Graves, Phyllis Karas, Melissa Ludtke, Carolyn Toll Oppenheim, and Judy Stoia. I also appreciate the efforts of Cliff Barnett of Hollywood, California, who served as a "test reader" for the manuscript.

And finally, love and profound thanks to the two people who've been most intimately involved with this project from start to finish. Meriwether Rhodes held my hand and was the first to read every page of every draft. And although I gave birth to this book, Daphna Gregg was the indispensable midwife. I cannot imagine a better author's editor than my friend Daphna.

DIRECTORY OF CHARACTERS, GOVERNMENT AGENCIES, AND OTHER ENTITIES

CAST OF CHARACTERS

Ammann, Arthur. Pediatric infectious disease expert who was one of the first to study HIV infection in infants and children. He left the University of California-San Francisco in the mid-1980s to head AIDS-related clinical trials for Genentech, but soon returned to the nonprofit world.

Axelrod, David. Physician-researcher who served as New York State's Health Commissioner for twelve years, before being felled by a massive stroke in early 1991. He was known as a public-health crusader and a powerful advocate for people with AIDS, substance abusers, and others often excluded from the health-care system. He backed the creation of Virogenetics, a biotechnology company founded to pursue new vaccine technologies, and served on its board of directors until he was disabled. He died in 1994.

Baltimore, David. Winner of the 1975 Nobel Prize in medicine for his codiscovery of reverse transcriptase, the enzyme that retroviruses use to integrate their genome into host DNA. In late 1996, NIH Director Harold Varmus asked him to lead the AIDS Vaccine Research Committee, an advisory group that has promoted basic science related to vaccine research and development. In 1999, the AVRC also became the scientific advisory board to NIH's new intramural Vaccine Research Center. Unofficially, Baltimore has also influenced corporate decisions concerning AIDS vaccine research.

Barnett, Susan. A molecular biologist and a leading designer and developer of DNA vaccines at Chiron. In 2000, her team was awarded a major vaccine development grant by the National Institutes of Health (NIH).

Baxter, George. A New Jersey–based attorney who represented plaintiffs in product liability cases, including those involving the screening of donated blood for HIV. In 1995, he brokered the connection between Don Francis and Bob Nowinski that led to the founding of VaxGen; in 2000, he joined the company as its in-house counsel.

Berman, Philip (Phil). A molecular biologist who joined Genentech in 1982 and became that company's primary designer of protein subunit vaccines. He first developed a gp160 vaccine that was scrapped after it failed to protect chimps against HIV challenge, then a gp120 that entered human trials in 1991. He became the chief scientist at VaxGen, a Genentech spin-off company, and in 1996 he designed two new bivalent vaccines for HIV. Both are in Phase III testing, one in the United States and one in Thailand.

Beyrer, Chris. A physician and public-health researcher who spent six years based in Chiang Mai and is an expert on the epidemiology of AIDS in Thailand and other countries in Southeast Asia. A faculty member at Johns Hopkins School of Public Health, he is the author of *War in the Blood: Sex, Politics, and AIDS in Southeast Asia.*

Bhamarapravati, Natth. An American-trained Thai physician and vaccine researcher who was president of Mahidol University from 1979 to 1991. Subsequently, he became head of the Center for Vaccine Development at Mahidol's Salaya campus and took a leading role in setting vaccine policy through Thailand's National AIDS Commission; also serves on numerous international committees on vaccines for AIDS and other diseases.

Birx, Deborah (Debbi). An immunologist and army officer who joined the Division of Retrovirology at Walter Reed Army Institute of Research in 1988, where she later became deputy chief of Robert Redfield's department of retrovirology research. She became chief of that department in 1994, and in 1996 succeeded Don Burke as director of the division. She attained the rank of colonel in 1997.

Bolognesi, Dani. A Duke University virologist who chaired the Vaccine Working Group (VWG) and headed the central immunology laboratory for the AIDS Vaccine Evaluation Group (AVEG). In March 1999, he left Duke to become CEO of Trimeris, a biotech company he had helped found. The company's lead product is a novel anti-HIV drug.

Boswell, Neil. A physician and air force major who was stationed at Wilford Hall Air Force Base in San Antonio in 1992, when he filed scientific misconduct charges against Robert Redfield. In 1993, after those charges were dismissed, Boswell was hired by Don Burke to be deputy director of the Division of Retrovirology at WRAIR.

Boyer, Herbert (Herb). A University of California-San Francisco professor who, along with Stanford University's Stanley Cohen, pioneered the technique of gene splicing, which is the basis for genetically engineered drugs. Boyer and Robert Swanson cofounded Genentech in 1976, and in 1990 Boyer returned to academia.

Bradac, James. A longtime government virologist who is in charge of the viral diversity program for the NIH Division of AIDS.

Brown, Arthur. An infectious disease physician and epidemiologist who has been in Bangkok at AFRIMS, the Armed Forces Research Institute of the Medical Sciences, longer than any other American scientist. Brown worked first on malaria vaccines, then on HIV research, and eventually became chief of retrovirology for the U.S. Army component at AFRIMS.

Burke, Donald. After six years as a virologist in Thailand, Burke came to Walter Reed Army Institute of Research in 1984 as chief of virology. In 1988, he started the Division of Retrovirology, which he led until he was asked to step down in 1996. In 1997, he retired from the army as a colonel, becoming director of the Center for Immunization Research at Johns Hopkins School of Public Health. When Mary Lou Clements-Mann was killed in late 1998, he succeeded her as principal investigator on the Center's major grants and contracts.

Caley, Ian. A British virologist who in 1993 spliced an HIV gene into a live-vector vaccine made from attenuated Venezuelan equine encephalitis (VEE). At the time, he was a graduate student in the laboratory of Robert E. Johnston at the University of North Carolina. He is now a scientist at AlphaVax in Durham, NC.

Capon, Dan. A molecular biologist at Genentech who cloned and sequenced HIV_{LAI}, a lab-adapted strain of the AIDS virus.

Chernow, Marlene. A clinical trials expert who worked at Genentech from 1990 to 1997, when she joined VaxGen as the new company's third employee. There, she has been involved in regulatory filings in the United States and Thailand and was instrumental in coordinating the Phase III trial of VaxGen's bivalent B/E vaccine in Bangkok.

Chiu, Joseph. An American physician who first went to Thailand in 1981, where he provided medical care to refugees from Laos. In 1991, he set up an AIDS counseling and training center in Chiang Mai and in 1994–1999 worked on HIV vaccine research in northern Thailand.

Chulabhorn, Princess. One of several scientifically sophisticated members of the Thai royal family, she earned a doctorate in organic chemistry in 1985. She established the Chulabhorn Research Institute in 1987 and uses her influence to promote public health and biomedical research. In 1990, she sponsored Thailand's first major AIDS conference.

Clements-Mann, Mary Lou. Founder of the Immunization Research Center at Johns Hopkins University, Clements was one of the most productive clinical researchers in vaccinology. She led one of the NIH-sponsored AIDS Vaccine Evaluation Units and was an important adviser on HIV vaccine research to NIH, WHO, and foreign governments.

She married Jonathan Mann in 1996, and the two died in September 1998 in the crash of Swissair Flight No. 111 off Nova Scotia.

Cohen, Stanley. A Stanford University researcher, Cohen collaborated with Herb Boyer in the landmark gene-splicing experiment that gave birth to genetic engineering.

Corey, Lawrence. A professor of laboratory medicine and microbiology at the University of Washington, in 1988 Corey conducted the first clinical trial of an HIV vaccine in the United States. He went on to chair the AIDS Vaccine Evaluation Group, the clinical trials network backed by the NIH. When that system was replaced by the HIV Vaccine Trials Network (HVTN) in 2000, he was the nongovernment scientist charged with running tax-supported trials of AIDS vaccines.

Crewdson, John. Pulitzer Prize–winning investigative reporter for the *Chicago Tribune*, best known for his 1989 article on controversies surrounding the discovery of the AIDS virus. He wrote a high-impact news story about clinical trials of the gp120 vaccines in May 1994.

Culliton, Barbara J. Washington-based journalist who was news editor of *Science* and deputy editor of *Nature*. Founder of *Nature Genetics* and *Nature Medicine*.

Curd, John G. Harvard-trained physician who left academic medicine in 1991 to run clinical trials for Genentech. He was vice president of clinical development for Genentech when he left the company to join VaxGen in May 1999. At VaxGen, he headed clinical trial and regulatory affairs, prior to leaving the company in early 2001.

Davis, Nancy. A molecular biologist and virologist who in 1988 assembled the first genetically engineered vaccine against Venezuelan equine encephalitis; originally intended to protect military personnel against VEE when they are deployed in South America, this vaccine became the basis for experimental live-vector vaccines against HIV, influenza, and other diseases. She and Robert Johnston are research partners at the University of North Carolina, and along with Jonathan Smith, they founded AlphaVax, a biotechnology company in Durham, NC.

Deer, Brian. British journalist who wrote a sensational account of VaxGen's Phase III vaccine trial in Bangkok. The article appeared in the *Sunday Times* (London), a broadsheet known for its iconoclastic views of the AIDS pandemic.

Delaney, Martin. A prominent AIDS treatment activist from San Francisco, he left a management consulting career to found Project Inform. He went from being an adversary of government agencies to an insider, serving on many prominent advisory committees and wielding considerable influence within the NIH and FDA. In 1994, he was a member of the AIDS Research Advisory Committee (ARAC) and an opponent of expanding clinical trials for the gp120 vaccines.

Dekker, Cornelia (Corey). Vice president for clinical research at Chiron in 1994; supervisor of Anne-Marie Duliege.

Dina, Dino. A retrovirologist who was president of Chiron Biocine, the vaccine division at Chiron, he collaborated with Kathy Steimer and Paul Luciw in their early work on HIV. Dina left Chiron in 1997.

Douglas, Gordon. Infectious-disease physician and researcher who became president of Merck Vaccines in 1991, after a distinguished career in academic medicine. He retired from Merck in 1999 and in 2000 joined the NIH Vaccine Research Center as director of strategic planning.

Duliege, Anne-Marie. A French physician who worked briefly on HIV clinical trials at Genentech before joining Chiron in 1992 to head clinical trials for the gp120 vaccine. She oversaw gp120 trials in the United States and Thailand, and even after Chiron withdrew its support in early 1998, she continued tying up loose ends.

Emini, Emilio. A microbiologist and director of HIV biology and immunology at Merck, Emini was in charge of developing a protease inhibitor to treat AIDS until 1997, when he supplanted Margaret Liu as leader of Merck's HIV vaccine program.

Essex, Myron (Max). Originally trained as a veterinarian and virologist, he joined Robert Gallo in the early hunt for the AIDS virus. His laboratory at the Harvard School of Public Health has been engaged in HIV research ever since, mainly on African strains and related primate viruses. As professor of virology and chairman of the Harvard AIDS Institute, Essex wields considerable influence in international AIDS research. His lab first identified the gp120 surface feature of HIV, and he has long favored clinical testing as part of an empirical approach to vaccine development.

Excler, Jean-Louis. A French pediatrician and public-health physician who joined Pasteur Mérieux Connaught in 1990, responsible for negotiating clinical testing of ALVAC-HIV™ in the United States and France. In 1998, he left PMC and joined the clinical trials group at Walter Reed Army Institute of Research in Rockville, MD.

Fast, Patricia (Pat). A pediatrician who also held a Ph.D. in immunology, Fast joined the AIDS program at NIH in 1989 to coordinate vaccine trials, becoming associate director for vaccine and prevention research of DAIDS (Division of AIDS) in 1992. She left NIH for the private sector in late 1997, and in 2001 moved to the International AIDS Vaccine Initiative.

Fauci, Anthony (Tony). Director of the NIH's National Institute of Allergy and Infectious Diseases since 1984, Fauci administers the largest AIDS research budget in the federal government. He also leads an active immunology research laboratory and sees patients. His political and media savvy have made him the government's point man on the epidemic under four different presidents so far. Fauci was elected to the National Academy of Sciences in 1992.

Felgner, Philip (Phil). While director of gene therapy at Vical, a California biotechnology company, Felgner discovered naked DNA's potential as a vaccine against AIDS and other infectious diseases. Vical licensed this technology to Merck for further development.

Fields, Bernard (Bernie). An American physician and virology researcher who chaired the microbiology and molecular genetics program at Harvard Medical School. He became a major force in setting AIDS research policy during the last years of his life, after he had been diagnosed with pancreatic cancer. In early 1994, illness caused him to turn down the opportunity to be the first director of the NIH Office of AIDS Research. He died in January 1995.

Francis, Donald (Don). As a public-health officer at CDC's Atlanta headquarters in the early 1980s, Francis was an outspoken proponent of AIDS testing and safe-sex practices among homosexuals. After alienating his superiors at CDC, he transferred to the San Francisco area in 1985 and in 1987 was made famous by Randy Shilts's portrait of him in *And the Band Played On*. After retiring from the Public Health Service, Francis joined Genentech 1993. In 1995, he used the gp120 vaccine that Genentech had disowned to found a new company, VaxGen. In 1998, Francis launched the world's first efficacy trial of an HIV vaccine.

Gallo, Robert (Bob). A researcher at the NIH's National Cancer Institute, Gallo and French researcher Luc Montagnier both announced in 1983 that they had found the virus that causes AIDS. Their competing claims spawned an international battle over profits from diagnostic tests, as well as a scientific fraud investigation against Gallo. Eventually cleared of wrongdoing, Gallo left NIH in 1995 to head the Institute of Human Virology at the University of Maryland.

Gayle, Helene D. Public-health physician and director of the National Center for HIV/AIDS, Sexually Transmitted Diseases, and Tuberculosis Prevention at the Centers for Disease Control and Prevention in Atlanta. The CDC's small HIV vaccine research program is part of her Center.

Goeddel, Dave. A virologist and head of microbiology research at Genentech, Goeddel and Denny Kleid won a hotly contested race to clone the gene for human insulin. This was Genentech's first big discovery. Goeddel was a major force in the company's aggressive, "clone-or-die" culture. He left Genentech to form his own company, Tularik.

Gregory, Tim. Head of process development at Genentech, Gregory set up systems for making large quantities of gp120 vaccines in mammalian cells. He remained with Genentech when VaxGen was launched, but he still works with Phil Berman on vaccine manufacture.

Haase, Ashley. A physician-researcher whose ties to NIH go back to his training as a fellow in Tony Fauci's laboratory, Haase heads the microbiology department at the University of Minnesota Medical School. He chaired the NIAID AIDS Research Advisory Committee from 1993 to 1996, and in April 1994 he was acting chair of the Vaccine Working Group meeting. These were pivotal meetings in the history of the gp120 vaccines, and they arrived at opposite recommendations.

Haigwood, Nancy. A molecular biologist who specialized in gene expression systems, she was responsible for producing Chiron's gp120 vaccine. She was co-leader of the vaccine project with Kathy Steimer, before leaving Chiron in 1992 to join Bristol-Myers Squibb in Seattle. There, she pursued her interest in primate models for vaccine testing. When that company abandoned HIV vaccine work in late 1996, Haigwood moved to the Seattle Biomedical Research Institute, where she continues working on vaccines for AIDS.

Hansen, Lori. A microbiologist who did research on antiviral and anticancer drugs before joining Chiron in 1995, where she became a research project manager. In this capacity, she was the administrative coordinator for Chiron's gp120 vaccines from 1995 through 1999.

Heckler, Margaret. Secretary of the Department of Health and Human Services (DHHS) from 1983 to 1985, Heckler announced Bob Gallo's discovery of the AIDS virus at a 1984 press conference and at Gallo's suggestion predicted that a vaccine would be ready in two years. At the first international AIDS conference in 1985, her off-the-cuff remarks about protecting "the general public" against AIDS, which seemed to imply that homosexuals were not part of society at large, outraged activists.

Heilman, Carole. Career NIH employee who began as an intramural virology researcher but soon switched to extramural vaccine research, including clinical testing of the acellular pertussis vaccine, an important childhood immunization. She was the executive staff member for the AIDS Vaccine Research Committee, where she worked closely with David Baltimore. She headed the HIV vaccine research program in the Division of AIDS from November 1997 to July 1998, leaving when she was named director of NIAID's Division of Microbiology and Infectious Diseases.

Hendrix, Craig. Infectious disease physician who was a coinvestigator in the Defense Department's clinical trials of MicroGeneSys gp160 as a therapeutic vaccine. While stationed at Wilford Hall Air Force Base in San Antonio, Major Hendrix asked that Lieutenant Colonel Robert Redfield be investigated for scientific misconduct.

Heyward, William. Physician-epidemiologist who coordinated international AIDS activities for the U.S. Centers for Disease Control in the early days of the epidemic and who ran AIDS programs in both Africa and Thailand. In 1998, he became chief of CDC's first official vaccine unit and was instrumental in securing CDC support for VaxGen's U.S. efficacy trial. He was investigated for conflict of interest in early 2000, when he became VaxGen's vice president after retiring from the public health service.

Hilleman, Maurice. Director of Virus and Cell Biology at Merck from 1957 to 1984, and since then head of Merck's charitable foundation. The dean of American vaccinology, Hilleman is responsible for developing more successful vaccines than any other single researcher. He was an early backer of DNA vaccines and encouraged Merck to license that technology. He has been influential in advising the National Institutes of Health on vaccine science and policy since the beginning of the HIV epidemic.

Ho, David. Director of the Aaron Diamond AIDS Research Center in New York, this physician and virology researcher was named *Time* magazine's 1996 Man of the Year. He was forty-four years old and had gained fame for his work on multidrug "cocktails" for treating AIDS. He was previously known mainly for findings about the dynamics of HIV infection in humans. Once famous, Ho began to dabble in the politics of international vaccine trials.

Hodel, Derek. A prominent AIDS treatment activist from New York, in 1994 he served as a community representative on the Vaccine Working Group. With foundation support, he led a study of the social, ethical, and political dimensions of HIV vaccine trials proposed for the United States. He presented material from this effort at meetings of the VWG and the AIDS Research Advisory Committee in 1994.

Hu, Shiu-Lok. A molecular biologist who got in on the ground floor of biotechnology in 1981; invented the vaccinia-based product that in 1988 became the first AIDS vaccine tested in humans in the United States. After Bristol-Myers Squibb shut down his vaccine research program in 1997, he turned his part-time faculty position at the University of Washington into a full-time research career; he continues to work on animal models for AIDS and vaccines.

Jermano, John A. Originally trained as a nurse, he cared for AIDS patients at the NIH Clinical Center before going back to school for a Master of Public Health degree. He worked on clinical-trials research at NIH, consulting firms, and in biotechnology before joining VaxGen in 1998. He organized the launch of VaxGen's domestic Phase III study and oversaw its operation until he resigned in early 2001.

Johnston, Margaret (Peggy). With a Ph.D. in immunology and experience in laboratory research and medical-school teaching, Johnston first joined the AIDS program at NIH in 1987. She was deputy director of the Division of AIDS when she left NIH to launch the scientific programs of the International AIDS Vaccine Initiative (IAVI) in early 1997. In mid-1998, she returned to NIH as associate director of NIAID and head of vaccine and prevention research for DAIDS.

Johnston, Robert E. (Bob). A Texas-born virologist who has spent his whole professional life working with alphaviruses, he is a professor microbiology and immunology at the University of North Carolina. He is the visionary behind the live-vector vaccines based on Venezuelan equine encephalitis and a founder, along with Nancy Davis and Jonathan Smith, of AlphaVax, a biotechnology company in Durham, NC.

Johnston, Stephen. In 1992, he published an article in *Nature* reporting that he had invented a "gene gun" that used high pressure to force naked DNA through the skin. He was one of the pioneering researchers on DNA vaccines, although he has focused more on the gene-gun technology than on vaccine design.

Khamboonruang, Chirasak. Thai physician and researcher in Chiang Mai, director of the Research Institute for Health Sciences and member of the faculty at Chiang Mai University Medical School.

Killen, John Y. (Jack). Physician who became deputy director of the Division of AIDS in 1987; previously managed clinical trials at the National Cancer Institute and was medical director of a gay medical clinic in Washington, DC. He was the director of DAIDS from 1993 to 2000, and his final major project was a controversial reorganization the NIH-sponsored network for testing HIV vaccines.

Kitayaporn, Dwip. A research epidemiologist on the faculty at Mahidol University in Bangkok, as well as on the staff of the HIV/AIDS Collaboration, a joint project of the U.S. Centers for Disease Control and Prevention and the Ministry of Public Health of Thailand.

Kleid, Dennis (Denny). A virologist at Genentech, Kleid collaborated with Dave Goeddel to clone the gene for human insulin. Kleid was instrumental in attracting Jack Obijeski to the biotech company.

Klein, Michel. French physician and immunology researcher who worked on HIV vaccines at Connaught before that company merged with Pasteur Mérieux in 1990. He became PMC's vice president for research in 1993, which gave him oversight for all the company's AIDS vaccine research.

Koff, Wayne. A molecular biologist, Koff was the first project officer for AIDS vaccines at NIH's NIAID. In 1988, he was promoted to branch chief for vaccine research and development in the newly created DAIDS. Frustrated with the bureaucracy at NIH, Koff left in 1992 to work for United Biomedical, Inc. In 1998, Koff replaced Peggy Johnston as vice president for scientific affairs at the International AIDS Vaccine Initiative.

Koprowski, Hilary. A Polish-born physician and researcher who came to the United States in 1944, Koprowski developed polio vaccines for Lederle Laboratories. In 1957, he became director of the Wistar Institute in Philadelphia, and it was there that he promoted the career of DNA vaccine designer David Weiner. He is now on the faculty at Thomas Jefferson University in Philadelphia.

Kourilsky, Philip. Paris-based director of corporate research for Pasteur Mérieux Connaught in the mid-1990s, who then left the company to head the Pasteur Institute.

LaRosa, John. Primary author of 1990 article in *Science* that convinced Phil Berman to re-engineer Genentech's HIV vaccine, so that it would emulate the surface protein on a viral strain that seemed to elicit a broader range of antibodies. LaRosa was a vaccine researcher at Repligen Corporation in Cambridge, MA, at the time.

Lasky, Larry. A molecular biologist at Genentech, Lasky worked with Phil Berman on an experimental herpes vaccine. He was briefly involved in the design of protein subunit vaccines against AIDS.

Levine, Arnold. Highly respected Princeton University molecular biologist who in 1994 was chosen to lead the NIH AIDS Research Program Evaluation Task Force of the Office of AIDS Research Advisory Council. The group quickly became known as the Levine committee, and in March 1996 its recommendations were released in the massive Levine report. Among other things, this report recommended a complete restructuring of the government's HIV-vaccine research efforts.

Levinson, Arthur D. Molecular biologist who was part of the original "clone-or-die" culture in the early days of Genentech. He went on to become the company's chief scientist, and a critic of the gp120 vaccine concept, before being promoted to CEO in 1995. Defying predictions that a scientist could not be a good manager, he proved immensely successful as a corporate executive.

Levy, Jay. A virologist at the University of California-San Francisco who, like Gallo and Montagnier, isolated a retrovirus in AIDS patients. He called his discovery ARV (AIDS-associated retrovirus). He worked with Paul Luciw at Chiron on the sequencing and cloning of this virus. Levy continues to be an active HIV researcher at UCSF.

Liu, Margaret. As a relative newcomer to Merck's prestigious virus and cell department, Liu was charged with looking for promising new technologies emerging from biotech companies. When Vical approached Merck with its naked DNA vaccines, she was quick to see their potential while others were skeptical. Liu developed Merck's DNA vaccine for influenza and did preclinical work on an HIV product. She left Merck in 1997 to fill an upgraded version of Kathy Steimer's old job at Chiron. In early 2000, she left Chiron and became an adviser on vaccines to the World Health Organization and the Bill and Melinda Gates Foundation, as well as a consultant to corporations.

Luciw, Paul. A specialist in retroviruses, Luciw joined Chiron in 1982. He and Kathy Steimer were among the first to grow the AIDS virus successfully in the laboratory, and Luciw was the first to clone and sequence the virus. Essentially not a corporate type, Luciw joined the faculty at the University of California-Davis in 1986. There, he is a leading researcher on the use of animal models in vaccine testing and development.

Lynch, Nicole. Although her job title was director of public relations for VaxGen, Lynch also played a major role in recruiting volunteers for the company's Phase III trial in the United States. She decamped for business school in 2001.

Mann, Jonathan M. As a physician and epidemiologist, Mann played a prominent role in the AIDS pandemic from its earliest days to his untimely death in September 1998, when he and his second wife, vaccine expert Mary Lou Clements-Mann, were killed in a plane crash off Nova Scotia. From CDC, where he was among the first to study AIDS in Africa, Mann became the first director of the Global Programme on AIDS (the forerunner of UNAIDS). He later taught at the Harvard School of Public Health, then became dean of a new school of public health at Allegheny University in Philadelphia.

Mastro, Timothy D. A U.S. Centers for Disease Control epidemiologist and physician who became director of CDC's Bangkok operations in 1993. There, he ran the HIV/AIDS Collaboration, which has been instrumental in describing the molecular epidemiology of the disease in Thailand and Southeast Asia. He returned to CDC headquarters in Atlanta in 2000 to direct the HIV vaccine research program there.

Mathieson, Bonnie. With a Ph.D. in immunology and experience in basic science research at NIH, Mathieson was hired by Wayne Koff in 1988 to work on NIAID's infant AIDS vaccine program. In mid-1995, she moved from DAIDS to the NIH Office of AIDS Research. Her first assignment at OAR was to staff the research and writing of the Levine report, which criticized NIH's lackluster performance in HIV vaccine research and called for an overhaul.

McCutchan, Francine. A civilian molecular biologist employed by the Henry M. Jackson Foundation, McCutchan did pioneering work on classifying HIV viral subtypes according to their genetic sequences. She remains one of the leading researchers on HIV evolution and genetic diversity.

McElrath, Juliana. An infectious disease physician and AIDS researcher at the University of Washington's Fred Hutchinson Cancer Research Center in Seattle; director of the AIDS Vaccine Evaluation Unit at UW; and expert on T-cell responses to HIV infection.

McNeil, John. An army preventive medicine physician and epidemiologist, he helped test the army's HIV screening system while stationed at Fort Dix, New Jersey, in 1985. In 1986, he went to Walter Reed Army Institute of Research, where he studied the epidemiology of HIV infection among active-duty personnel and prospective recruits. In 1991, he began working in Thailand to set up an infrastructure for HIV vaccine testing, and in 1993, he became chief of HIV vaccine development for WRAIR. In 1998, he attained the rank of colonel.

Montagnier, Luc. He was a virologist at the Institut Pasteur in France when he and Bob Gallo each announced that they had discovered the virus that causes AIDS. Montagnier called his virus LAV (lymphadenopathy-associated virus) after the chronically swollen lymph nodes exhibited by many AIDS patients. After much controversy in the press and scientific community, most scientists now credit Montagnier with being the first to identify the virus now called HIV.

Moore, John P. British-trained biochemist who came to the Aaron Diamond AIDS Research Center in New York in 1992. As a senior investigator there, his research has focused on HIV envelope proteins: their structure, function, and the immune system's response to them. He has been an outspoken critic of protein subunit vaccines such as gp120 and gp160, and of many facets of NIH's vaccine research program. He left ADARC in 2000.

Nowinski, Robert C. (Bob). New York–born retrovirologist and entrepreneur who moved to Seattle and founded three biotech companies between 1981 and 1992. Along the way, his hardball business methods earned him the nickname "No-Lose-Ski." Oncogen, a spin-off of his first company, developed the vaccinia-based HIV vaccine invented by Shiu-Lok Hu. In 1995, he and Don Francis cofounded VaxGen, and in June 1998, the company launched the world's first AIDS vaccine efficacy trials. Citing health reasons, Nowinski stepped down as VaxGen CEO and chairman in December 2000.

Obijeski, John F. (Jack). A major cheerleader for AIDS vaccine research at Genentech, Obijeski began his career as a self-described "gumshoe" virologist at the Centers for Disease Control. He worked on vaccines against rabies, herpes, and HIV at Genentech and helped introduce his CDC friend Don Francis to the company.

Olmsted, Robert A. (Bob). A microbiologist who trained under Robert E. Johnston and earned his Ph.D. from North Carolina State University in 1985. He was a postdoctoral fellow at NIH, then spent seven years as a research scientist at Pharmacia & Upjohn. When Johnston founded AlphaVax, Olmsted returned to North Carolina to become research director for the new biotech.

Panetta, Leon. President Bill Clinton's chief of staff during his second term, 1996–2000.

Panicali, Dennis. A molecular biologist who joined Enzo Paoletti's lab at the New York State Health Department in 1977 and left in 1985; coinventor of several vaccinia-based vaccines. He later became president and CEO of Therion Biologics, a Massachusetts-based biotech company that has worked on several experimental HIV vaccines but has not yet brought a product to clinical trials. This may still happen, thanks to a 2001 grant from the International AIDS Vaccine Initiative.

Paoletti, Enzo. Born in Italy and raised in Buffalo, this classic virologist trained at NIH before coming to the New York State Health Department in 1974. He and Dennis Panicali developed early live-vector vaccines that used vaccinia to deliver genes from other infectious agents; later, he sparked the launch of Virogenetics, a biotech company meant to commercialize those products. The company was backed by Institut Mérieux, later called Pasteur Mérieux Connaught, and Paoletti led the research program until he and the French company had an unpleasant parting in 1995.

Paul, William (Bill). Chief of the laboratory of immunology at the National Institute of Allergy and Infectious Diseases since 1970, Paul served as the first director of the NIH Office of AIDS Research from 1994 to 1997. As OAR director, he significantly increased federal spending on HIV vaccine research. He currently heads the laboratory of immunology at NIAID.

Penhoet, Edward. He was a member of the biochemistry faculty at the University of California-Berkeley when he and William Rutter, who was at UC–San Francisco, teamed up to found Chiron Corporation. He was a pioneer in the field of genetic engineering and served as CEO of Chiron until 1998, when he returned to UC–Berkeley as dean of the School of Public Health.

Phanuphak, Praphan. An American-trained physician who diagnosed Thailand's first official AIDS case in 1984, and who led the country's first HIV vaccine trial (without official approval from the government) in 1994. He heads the AIDS program at the Royal Thai Red Cross in Bangkok.

Plotkin, Stanley. One of the best-known figures in the vaccine world, he invented the rubella vaccine and wrote more than 500 research articles and a score of important textbooks. In 1990, after decades on the University of Pennsylvania faculty, Plotkin left academia to become medical and scientific director of Pasteur Mérieux Connaught. Although he was officially retired in 1998, he still calls the shots at Aventis Pasteur, PMC's newest corporate incarnation.

Raab, Kirk. Controversial CEO of Genentech from 1985 to 1995, a period of great growth leavened with criticism that the company's sales tactics were so aggressive as to be unethical. He was a great supporter of Don Francis and the gp120 vaccine until he was forced out in 1995, after it was discovered that he had floated a large personal loan from the pharmaceutical company that owned most of Genentech.

Radke, Kathryn. An animal retrovirologist who went to graduate school with Kathy Steimer, she is a longtime faculty member at the University of California-Davis. Radke introduced Steimer and Martin Wilson, who became Steimer's husband, and remained close friends with the couple.

Redfield, Robert (Bob). As an infectious disease physician at Walter Reed Medical Center, Redfield saw AIDS patients from the early days of the epidemic. He was the first to identify heterosexual contact as a means of HIV transmission, and he more than anyone shaped the army's humane policies toward infected soldiers. He studied therapeutic HIV vaccines from 1986 until 1994, and this research was the subject of a scientific misconduct investigation in 1992–1993. He was cleared of all charges and retired from the army as a colonel in 1996. Redfield joined Bob Gallo at the Institute of Human Virology at the University of Maryland, where he is director of clinical care and research. He still treats AIDS patients.

Rhodes, Gary. Previously an immunology researcher at Scripps Clinic, Rhodes was hired by Vical to determine whether naked DNA could elicit immune responses that could protect animals against infectious agents. He pioneered the model influenza vaccine that was tested in mice, and which convinced Merck to license Vical's DNA vaccine technology. Rhodes left Vical in 1994 to join the faculty at the University of California-Davis. He and Paul Luciw are in the same department and sometimes collaborate on vaccine testing in primate models.

Robinson, Harriet. A pioneering researcher on DNA vaccines, Robinson made her first experimental vaccines in 1988 when she was at the University of Massachusetts. She worked on vaccines for influenza, then HIV. In 1998, she moved to Emory University in Atlanta, where she collaborates with both the Yerkes Regional Primate Center and the Centers for Disease Control on HIV vaccine research.

Rutter, William (Bill). A biochemist and pioneering researcher on the hepatitis B virus, Rutter co-founded Chiron Corporation with Ed Penhoet. His hepatitis B research paved the way to Chiron's first successful product, a protein subunit vaccine against hepatitis B that was licensed to Merck for manufacture. Rutter remains president of Chiron, where he has been a tenacious proponent of HIV vaccine research.

Salk, Jonas. (1914–1995) An early pioneer in vaccine research, Salk's polio vaccine—which was made from killed virus—was approved by the FDA in 1955. He founded the Salk Institute for Biological Studies and later started a biotech company, Immune Response Corporation, to develop and test a therapeutic AIDS vaccine called Remune™. IRC continued to test Remune™ after Salk's death and in 2000 was accused of trying to suppress negative findings about its effectiveness.

Schultz, Alan. The in-house expert at Division of AIDS on the use of primates as animal models for studying HIV and AIDS vaccines. He left DAIDS in 1999 to become a scientific officer for the International AIDS Vaccine Initiative.

Shalala, Donna. A university administrator who served as U.S. secretary of health and human services during both Clinton administrations.

Shannon, James. An outspoken, dynamic kidney doctor from New York City, Shannon was appointed director of the National Institutes of Health in 1955. Shannon changed the character of the NIH by shifting its focus away from public health issues and toward basic laboratory science. Although he retired in 1968, he is still regarded as the most influential NIH director in history.

Sinangil, Faruk. A Turkish-born virologist who trained at Columbia University before being hired by Kathy Steimer at Chiron. He worked with her on preclinical studies of the gp120 vaccine; once clinical trials were underway, he was her closest collaborator on the assays used to measure the product's immunologic effects.

Sirisopana, Narongrid. A physician and epidemiologist who was an officer with the Royal Thai Army component of AFRIMS in Bangkok, and John McNeil's collaborator in establishing a national HIV screening system for military conscripts.

Smith, Jonathan. A virologist who went to graduate school with Robert Johnston at the University of Texas, he is a leading infectious disease and vaccine researcher at U.S. Army Medical Research Institute of Infectious Diseases (USAMRIID); he and Johnston teamed up in 1986 to work on a live attenuated vaccine for Venezuelan equine encephalitis, which gave rise to experimental VEE-based vaccines for HIV and other diseases. Along with Johnston and Nancy Davis, he is a cofounder of AlphaVax, a biotech company in Durham, NC.

Snow, William. A San Francisco-based writer and consultant who was one of the first HIV-infected activists to take up the cause of preventive vaccine research and development. One of the founders of the AIDS Vaccine Advocacy Coalition, a respected watchdog group, and a member of numerous NIH advisory committees. Snow was the only nonscientist chosen to serve on the AIDS Vaccine Research Committee, led by David Baltimore.

Steimer, Kathelyn (Kathy). A retrovirologist who also had postgraduate training in immunology, Steimer joined Chiron in 1983. She and Paul Luciw were among the first to successfully culture HIV in the laboratory, and after Luciw cloned and sequenced the virus, she designed Chiron's gp120 vaccine. In 1993, she was the first to report that this vaccine did not elicit antibodies against HIV isolated newly infected patients. This discouraging result was a major factor in Tony Fauci's decision not to go forward with large-scale testing of gp120 vaccines in 1994. She was working on other HIV vaccine strategies when she died of cancer in November 1996.

Swanson, Robert. A venture capitalist with undergraduate training in science and an MBA, Swanson cofounded Genentech with Herb Boyer in 1976. He encouraged scientists to work long hours in a highly competitive environment and to blow off steam at Friday beer busts, where he would sometimes dress in outlandish costumes. Swanson died of brain cancer, at age fifty-two, in late 1999.

Tartaglia, James (Jim). A molecular biologist hired at Virogenetics in 1986; worked on vaccinia vectors and on the newer delivery systems based on canarypox. He became research director at Virogenetics following Enzo Paoletti's departure in 1995 and was later promoted to vice president of research at Pasteur Mérieux Connaught; today, he holds that position at Aventis Pasteur. He refined the original canarypox vectors so that they incorporate more HIV genes and are somewhat easier to manufacture.

Thongchoroen, Prasert. A physician who served as president of Mahidol University during the early 1990s, then became an emeritus professor of medicine at Mahidol's highly regarded Siriraj Hospital in Bangkok. There, he heads one of the four HIV vaccine-testing sites that constitute the Thai AIDS Vaccine Evaluation Group.

Ungpakorn, Jon. A half-British, politically connected physicist turned HIV activist. He was appointed to lead independent monitoring of risk-reduction counseling provided during the Phase III VaxGen study in Bangkok.

Valenzuela, Pablo. A dominant scientific force at Chiron from the moment of its founding, Valenzuela discovered how to make yeast cells produce hepatitis B antigen, which made possible a vaccine against the hepatitis B virus. He hired Kathy Steimer, Paul Luciw, and many other important researchers. He is still a senior research executive with the company.

Vanichseni, Supak. A Thai physician who received her graduate training at the London School of Public Health, then returned to Bangkok and was instrumental in establishing the city's network of drug-treatment clinics. In 1988, she initiated the first surveys of HIV infection among injection drug users in Bangkok and was instrumental in preparing for vaccine trials among that population. After retiring from the Bangkok Metropolitan Administration, she joined the staff of VaxGen's collaboration with the BMA.

Varmus, Harold. Varmus shared the 1989 Nobel Prize for medicine with Michael Bishop for their work on cancer-causing viruses. He was appointed director of the National Institutes of Health in 1993, resigning in late 1999 to become president of Memorial Sloan Kettering Cancer Institute. Varmus was primarily interested in basic science research, and NIH did not push clinical trials of AIDS vaccines during his administration. Only after President Clinton publicly announced the creation of an HIV Vaccine Research Center did Varmus manifest much interest in the development and testing of HIV vaccines.

Virani-Ketter, Nzeera. Born in Uganda and trained as a physician in the United States, Virani-Ketter worked on HIV vaccine trials for the Department of Defense and the NIH Division of AIDS. She was VaxGen's first medical director, and during her brief tenure there in 1998, she laid the groundwork for efficacy testing in the United States and Thailand.

Volvovitz, Frank. President of MicroGeneSys, the Connecticut biotech company that made a gp160 vaccine in the mid-1980s. He became notorious for hiring former Senator Russell Long to promote his product on Capitol Hill and for using press releases to report scientific results that had not been peer reviewed.

Watkins, Mark. A Philadelphia physician who treats AIDS patients, and is gay himself, Watkins was the first volunteer immunized in the first HIV vaccine efficacy trial in the United States. He received his initial shot, while television cameras recorded the moment, on June 23, 1998, at the Philadelphia FIGHT clinic in Center City.

Watson, James. Having shared the 1962 Nobel prize for discovering the double helix shape of the DNA molecule, Watson became director of Cold Spring Harbor Laboratory in 1968. He built the Long Island institution into a major force in genetics research and molecular biology. Although he turned day-to-day administration of the laboratory over to a successor in 1993, Watson remains president of the laboratory and of the Watson School for Biological Sciences. From 1988 until 1992, Watson was the first (and most controversial) director of the NIH National Center for Human Genome Research.

Weiner, David (Dave). While an assistant professor of pathology at the University of Pennsylvania, Weiner began working on a DNA vaccine for AIDS that used a local anesthetic to enhance the body's immune response. Hilary Koprowski, director of the Wistar Institute, boosted Weiner's career and helped him find a corporate partner for his idea. His was the first DNA vaccine tested in healthy volunteers.

Weniger, Bruce G. Longtime physician and epidemiologist with the Centers for Disease Control, who started CDC's AIDS research program in Thailand and coauthored one of the earliest descriptions of that country's fast-growing epidemic. He was appointed to the President's Advisory Council on HIV and AIDS in 1995 and in January 1997 challenged NIH's approach to HIV vaccine development on the op-ed page of the *New York Times*.

Willis, Loretta. A longtime senior technician in the laboratory of Robert Johnston and Nancy Davis at the University of North Carolina; teamed with Davis to assemble the first live-attenuated vaccine against Venezuelan equine encephalitis.

Wilson, Martin. A British-born neuroscientist on the faculty at the University of California-Davis, Wilson was introduced to Kathy Steimer by Kathryn Radke, a mutual friend. Wilson and Steimer married in 1989 and adopted a daughter the following year.

Wolff, Jon. Wolff was a postdoc at the University of California-San Diego when he met Phil Felgner of Vical. After moving to the University of Wisconsin, he and Felgner collaborated on a series of animal experiments that led to the serendipitous discovery that naked DNA might be useful as a vaccine.

Zagury, Daniel. A researcher at the Université Pierre et Marie Curie in Paris, Zagury conducted the first human trial of an AIDS vaccine in 1986. He first tested the vaccine on himself without any ill effects, then immunized eighteen children in Zaire. Although he obtained the Zairean government's permission, his failure to get parental permission scandalized the international science community.

Zolla-Pazner, Susan. A professor at New York University and scientific director of HIV/AIDS research at the N.Y. Veterans Administration Hospital, she has been studying the immune system's response to HIV since the earliest days of the epidemic. In 1994, she was a member of the Vaccine Working Group and the AIDS Research Advisory Committee.

UNITED STATES GOVERNMENT AGENCIES

Armed Forces Research Institute of the Medical Sciences (AFRIMS). Founded in 1959, this is the largest of the U.S. Army's overseas biomedical research laboratories. Located in Bangkok, it is operated as a joint command of the U.S. and Royal Thai Armies. It played a key role in clinical trials of vaccines for hepatitis A and Japanese encephalitis virus and is the base of operations for HIV research in Thailand and the rest of Southeast Asia.

Centers for Disease Control and Prevention (CDC). This is the federal agency responsible for tracking outbreaks of disease to determine their cause, means of spread, risk factors, and impact on the public. The agency collaborates with local, county, and state public-health departments and each year compiles statistics on the major causes of illness and death in the United States by age, sex, and race. In the early 1980s, CDC was the lead federal agency on AIDS in the United States and subsequently in Africa and Southeast Asia. The NIH soon shouldered CDC aside and began to garner the bulk of federal funding for AIDS research. Although CDC continues to count AIDS-related illnesses and deaths, its research has focused mainly on epidemiology and behavioral prevention strategies. In 1998, the CDC established an HIV Vaccine Unit for the first time. In 1999, CDC announced that it would spend $8 million helping VaxGen with the groundbreaking efficacy trial that the company launched the previous year.

Department of Health and Human Services (DHHS). Nearly all civilian health activities in the federal government are under the enormous, cumbersome umbrella of DHHS. It has eight agencies (including the Centers for Disease Control, Food and Drug Administration, and National Institutes of Health) and four operating divisions. The secretary of DHHS is nominated by the president and must be approved by Congress. As a result, DHHS is immersed in Washington politics, which naturally influences the kinds of research and policy initiatives pursued by its agencies and divisions. Washington, DC, is the center for DHHS administrative operations.

Division of AIDS (DAIDS). A division of NIH's National Institute of Allergy and Infectious Diseases (NIAID), DAIDS was created in 1988. Extramural funding for AIDS vaccine research is administered by this division.

Food and Drug Administration (FDA). Billing itself as "The Nation's Foremost Consumer Protection Agency," the FDA oversees the safety of drugs, biologics, foods, cosmetics, medical devices, products that emit radiation, and farm animal feed and drugs. (In 1970, the Environmental Protection Agency assumed responsibility for pesticides.) The FDA is headquartered in Rockville, Maryland.

National Cancer Institute (NCI). Established in 1937, NCI was the first disease-specific research entity created at the National Institutes of Health. Bob Gallo was based at NCI when he discovered the AIDS virus, and during the early years of the epidemic, it battled the NIAID for money and influence in AIDS research. The NIAID prevailed, although some HIV research still goes on at NCI.

National Institute of Allergy and Infectious Diseases (NIAID). Part of the NIH, NIAID conducts intramural research and funds extramural investigations of diseases that involve the human immune system, from hay fever to AIDS. Anthony Fauci has been director of NIAID since 1984, and it has grown dramatically during his administration NIAID created the Division of AIDS (DAIDS) in 1988. It administers 75 percent of all NIH spending on AIDS.

National Institutes of Health (NIH). NIH is not only the largest agency within DHHS but also the world's largest and richest government medical-research institution. It has a 318-acre campus in Bethesda, Maryland, as well as a number of off-site facilities. NIH's total budget exceeded $15 billion in 1999, which is spread across twenty-five institutes and centers. In 1999, NIH awarded $181 million in contracts and grants to public- and private-sector researchers working on HIV vaccines. This is more than the rest of the world—taking into account other governments, corporations, and private funding sources—spent on HIV vaccine research during the same period. NIH, created by Congress in 1930, grew out of the U.S. Public Health Service.

Office of AIDS Research (OAR) Congress created the OAR in late 1993, badgered into doing so by AIDS activists, who complained that there was no orderly process for managing AIDS-related spending within the National Institutes of Health. The Office is accountable only to the NIH director and makes recommendations about what the scientific agenda for AIDS research should be. OAR also has a discretionary fund that it can use to stimulate research of its choosing.

U.S. Army Medical Research Institute of Infectious Diseases (USAMRIID). A military research facility with programs including infectious disease, vaccine research and development, and biological warfare. Located at Fort Detrich in Frederick, Maryland.

U.S. Public Health Service (PHS). The PHS is a personnel system for commissioning health officers who are on call twenty-four hours a day, seven days a week, in case they are needed for health emergencies. They are a uniformed service and can be designated as military personnel by the president in the event of a national emergency. The majority of PHS personnel are assigned to DHHS agencies (such as CDC, FDA, and NIH), although some are assigned to other agencies such as the Bureau of Prisons. The surgeon general serves as nominal head of the PHS.

Walter Reed Army Institute of Research (WRAIR). The Defense Department's lead agency for infectious disease research, WRAIR is the largest laboratory within the U.S. Army Medical Research and Material Command. One of WRAIR's central missions is to produce vaccines needed to keep American service personnel healthy no matter where they are deployed. WRAIR enters into partnerships with companies and academic investigators to develop and test HIV vaccines and since 1991 has been working with government agencies in Thailand to prepare for vaccine testing in that country. Funding has always been tight for WRAIR, which has never had an AIDS research budget that exceeded $40 million.

OTHER ENTITIES: BIOTECHS, PHARMACEUTICAL COMPANIES, AND PRIVATE LABORATORIES

AlphaVax. A biotechnology company formed in January 1998 to develop live-vector vaccines based on modified Venezuelan equine encephalitis virus. The founders are Robert Johnston, Nancy Davis, and Jonathan Smith. Start-up funding came from a licensing agreement with Wyeth, and in October 1998, the International AIDS Vaccine Initiative made one of its first major vaccine development grants to AlphaVax. IAVI is backing development of a clade C vaccine for testing in South Africa.

American Home Products. One of the largest health care and pharmaceutical companies in the world, Wyeth-Ayerst Laboratories is one of its divisions, and Wyeth-Lederle Vaccines is a business unit of that division. Purchased Apollon in May 1998.

Amgen. Originally located in Massachusetts, where AIDS was one of its core interests, Amgen later moved to California and gained notoriety for its work on experimental drugs for Alzheimer's disease.

Apollon. A spin-off from Centocor, Apollon was founded in 1992 by venture capitalist Michael Wall and Vince Zurawski, who left his executive position with Centocor to become Apollon's CEO. The company was based in Malvern, Pennsylvania, and its initial emphasis was on antisense molecules, a type of genetically engineered drug. In 1994, with encouragement from Wistar Institute director Hilary Koprowski, the company licensed David Weiner's DNA vaccine technology from the University of Pennsylvania. Several versions of the company's HIV vaccines have been in clinical trials since 1995. In May 1998, Apollon ceased to exist when it was acquired by Wyeth-Lederle Vaccines, a part of American Home Products.

Aventis Pasteur. The most recent incarnation of the venerable French vaccine company Institut Mérieux, Aventis Pasteur is part of Aventis S.A., formed when Rhône-Poulenc (owner of PMC) merged with Hoechst in December 1999. Along the way, Institut Mérieux became Pasteur Mérieux Serums & Vaccines in 1989 but soon was renamed Pasteur Mérieux Connaught. By any name, this company is the largest vaccine manufacturer in the world, selling about 1 billion doses of its products each year.

Biocine. The vaccine division of Chiron from 1991 to 1997, known first as the Biocine Company, then as Chiron Biocine Research.

Bristol-Myers Squibb. The fifth-largest drug company in the world, which was temporarily engaged in HIV vaccine research in the early 1990s but currently has no program for AIDS vaccine development.

Centocor. A major biotech company located in Malvern, Pennsylvania, Centocor was cofounded in 1979 by Hilary Koprowski, Director of Philadelphia's Wistar Institute. The company specializes in therapeutic and diagnostic products.

Cetus. An Emeryville, California, biotech company that was acquired by Chiron in 1989.

Chiron Corporation. A biotech company founded in 1981 by William Rutter and Edward Penholt, Chiron made history by inventing the first genetically engineered vaccine. This breakthrough vaccine against hepatitis B was licensed to Merck. Today, the company's product lines include diagnostic and screening tests, vaccines, and biologics such as interleukin-2, a drug that is being tested against AIDS. Chiron is headquartered in Emeryville, California.

Ciba-Geigy. A multinational pharmaceutical company with headquarters in Switzerland; owns a major interest in Chiron.

Cold Spring Harbor Laboratory. A not-for-profit research facility located at Cold Spring Harbor, Long Island, NY, the institute was established in 1890 by the Brooklyn Institute of Arts and Sciences. Research is focused on basic science and genetics. A graduate school of biological sciences was added in the 1990s and named after Nobel laureate James Watson, who was director of the facility from 1968 until 1993. Watson remains active in the running of the laboratory today.

Eli Lilly & Company. A major pharmaceutical company based in Indianapolis, Indiana. Among its products is recombinant human insulin for diabetics (developed by Genentech).

Genentech. A biotech company headquartered in South San Francisco, Genentech was founded in 1976 by Herbert Boyer and Robert Swanson. The company has focused mainly on treatments for disease rather than on preventive vaccines. Breakthrough products include genetically engineered human insulin; synthetic human growth hormone; t-PA, the famous clot-busting drug used to treat heart-attack victims; and Herceptin, a drug for treating metastatic breast cancer.

Genenvax. The proposed name for the Genentech spin-off that Don Francis and

Robert C. Nowinski founded to advance gp120 vaccines into efficacy trials. Legal action by Apollon caused this name to be abandoned, because it was too close to Genevax™, Apollon's trademarked name for its DNA vaccine against HIV.

Genetic Systems, Inc. Founded in 1981 by biotech entrepreneur Robert C. Nowinski, Genetic Systems developed one of the first HIV tests in a collaboration with the Pasteur Institute in France. Bristol-Myers Squibb acquired the company in 1986.

Genetics Institute. A biotechnology company based in Cambridge, Massachusetts.

Immune Response Corporation. Jonas Salk founded this company in 1987 as a way to raise money for his research on a therapeutic vaccine for AIDS, which he was sure could turn the disease into a chronic, nonlethal infection. He took investors on a roller-coaster ride fueled by rosy predictions and sobering experimental results. The FDA approved a Phase II trial of Remune™ in 1995, and Salk died soon after that. The product's benefits remain controversial, and in 2000, the company was accused of trying to suppress negative findings from clinical trials.

Institut Mérieux. Formed in 1897 by Marcel Mérieux, a colleague of Louis Pasteur, Institut Mérieux specialized in applied immunology, including vaccines. In 1985, it joined forces with the Pasteur Institute to form Pasteur Mérieux Serums & Vaccines; in 1989, this company acquired Connaught Laboratories of Canada. Now the largest vaccine maker in the world, Pasteur Mérieux Connaught became a wholly owned subsidiary of the Rhône-Poulenc Group in 1994. In 1999, PMC was renamed Aventis Pasteur after Rhône-Poulenc and Hoechst merged to form Aventis S.A.

Merck & Company. A leading pharmaceutical company that is often referred to as "America's most admired corporation." Merck's home base is Whitehouse Station, New Jersey, and its Merck Research Laboratory in West Point, Pennsylvania, is the largest corporate research institution in the United States. Merck is one of the world's largest manufacturers of preventive vaccines, and its DNA vaccine for influenza was one of the first genetic vaccines tested in humans.

MicroGeneSys. Connecticut-based biotech company that manufactured a gp160 vaccine that was tested in healthy volunteers by the NIH beginning in 1986, and in HIV-infected patients by Walter Reed Army Institute of Research starting in 1989. The company became very controversial for its aggressive use of lobbyists and willingness to publicize preliminary results.

Oncogen. A 1985 spin-off of Seattle-based Genetic Systems, Inc., created to develop novel diagnostic and therapeutic products for cancer. In 1986, both Genetic Systems and Oncogen were acquired by Bristol-Myers Squibb.

Pasteur Mérieux Connaught. The world's largest vaccine manufacturer, created in 1989 when Pasteur Mérieux Serums & Vaccines bought Canada's Connaught Laboratories. In 1994, PMC became a wholly owned subsidiary of the Rhône-Poulenc Group; in 1999, it was renamed Aventis Pasteur when Rhône-Poulenc merged its life-science businesses with Hoechst to form Aventis S.A.

Pharmacia & Upjohn. A major pharmaceutical company headquartered in Kalamazoo, Michigan.

Salk Institute for Biological Studies. An independent not-for-profit research facility, the Salk Institute was founded in 1960 by Jonas Salk. Its major focuses are genetic engineering and neuroscience, and one of its most famous researchers is Francis Crick, who shared the Nobel Prize with James Watson for discovering the shape of DNA. The institute is located in La Jolla, California.

Sandoz. A multinational pharmaceutical company headquartered in Switzerland.

Syntex. A pharmaceutical company in Palo Alto, California, that is best known for developing the world's first oral contraceptive.

TransGene. A small biotech company based in Strasbourg, France; developed an HIV gp160 protein subunit vaccine that was licensed by Pasteur Mérieux Connaught.

United Biomedical, Inc. Located on Long Island, this small biomedical company developed several peptide vaccines against HIV that were tested by the NIH between 1993 and 1996. Wayne Koff, the first branch chief for vaccine research and development at DAIDS, joined the company in 1992. The company is no longer in business, and Koff has moved on.

VaxGen. In 1995, Don Francis and Seattle entrepreneur Robert C. Nowinski founded this company to develop gp120 vaccines against HIV. In June 1998, VaxGen launched the world's first HIV vaccine-efficacy trial in the United States; in February 1999, the Thai component of this study began among IV drug users in Bangkok. Both test bivalent products, which incorporate antigens from two types of virus. AIDSVAX B/B™ was designed for domestic use, AIDSVAX B/E™ for Thailand.

Viagene. A San Diego–based biotech company focused on developing alphavirus vectors for gene therapy and immunization. Acquired by Chiron in October 1994.

Vical. Founded in 1988 by a group of AIDS researchers at UC-San Diego, the initial focus of this biotech company was to develop AZT-like drugs for treating AIDS. Instead, Vical discovered and patented immunization using naked DNA, then licensed certain aspects of this technology to Merck for development. The company remains in San Diego, where it still develops plasmids for delivering genetic material to human cells.

Virogenetics. Originally founded by the New York State Health Department as a vehicle for commercializing live-vector vaccines invented by two state research scientists, Enzo Paoletti and Dennis Panicali. It operated on a shoestring until 1986, when Institut Mérieux purchased 51 percent of the company for $4 million, spread over three years. Three years later, the French company increased its holdings to 80 percent. Virogenetics' early vaccinia-based vaccines gave way to a series of canarypox vectors, including ALVAC-HIV™.

The Wistar Institute. Founded in 1892, Wistar was the first independent medical-research facility in the United States and was named after a prominent Philadelphia physician, Caspar Wistar.

Wyeth-Ayerst Laboratories. This company, based in Pearl River, NY, is a research division of American Home Products.

Wyeth-Lederle Vaccines and Pediatrics. A major developer and manufacturer of vaccines, this business unit of Wyeth-Ayerst Laboratories is also based in Pearl River, NY. In 1998, it licensed several VEE-based vaccines from AlphaVax and acquired Apollon, which was commercializing naked DNA vaccines developed by David Weiner at the University of Pennsylvania. It also licenses HIV peptide vaccines invented at Duke University.

INTERVIEWS

All quotations in this book come from my interviews, unless otherwise noted, and so does information that is not covered by source notes.

I reported this story over a four-year period beginning in January 1997 and during that time tape-recorded 175 interviews, most of them in person, in the United States and Thailand. Dates and locations are listed below, and when no site is given, the conversation was by telephone. Brief, informal conversations have not been included.

Rafi Ahmed—December 10, 1999, Atlanta, GA

Missie Allen—December 14, 1999, Research Triangle Park, NC

David Anderson—March 20, 1997, Seattle, WA

Larry Arthur—March 13, 1997, Frederick, MD

Susan Barnett—January 25, 1997, Washington, DC; March 24, 1997, Emeryville, CA; January 26, 1998, Emeryville, CA

Steve Bende—December 1, 1998

Philip Berman—January 27, 1998, South San Francisco, CA; May 26, 1999; June 26, 2000, Brisbane, CA

Chris Beyrer—September 24, 1998, Rockville, MD

Natth Bhamarapravati—February 18, 1999, Salaya, Thailand

Deborah Birx—March 11, 1997, Rockville, MD; October 18, 1999

Kit Boggio—October 27, 1998, Oakland, CA

Arthur Brown—February 15, 1999, Bangkok, Thailand

Donald Burke—May 4, 1999, Bethesda, MD

Jo Chaddic—February 8, 1999, Bangkok, Thailand

David Chernoff—March 24, 1997, Emeryville, CA

Marlene Chernow—June 26 and 28, 2000, Brisbane, CA

Joseph Chiu—February 10, 1999, Chiang Mai, Thailand

Richard Ciccarelli—October 22, 1999

Mary-Lou Clements-Mann—March 15, 1998, Washington, DC

Lawrence Corey—October 6, 1999, Dedham, MA; November 8, 1999

John Crewdson—April 20, 2000

Barbara Culliton—May 1, 2000

John Curd—June 7, 2000; November 29, 2000

Nancy Davis—December 13, 1999, Chapel Hill, NC; January 7, 10, and 13, 2000

Gordon Douglas—July 22, 1997

Thomas Dubensky—October 23, 1998, Emeryville, CA

Anne-Marie Duliege—April 16, 1997; January 26, 1998, Emeryville, CA

Niles Eaton—March 19, 1997, Seattle, WA

Emilio Emini—July 14, 1997

Jean Louis Excler—April 17, 1997, Boston, MA; August 25, 1998, Baltimore, MD

Patricia Fast—February 20 and May 13, 1997, both in Rockville, MD; July 26, 1998

Anthony Fauci—May 6, 1997, Bethesda, MD

Philip Felgner—August 2, 1999

Don Francis—March 26, 1997, San Francisco, CA; June 26 and 27, 2000, Brisbane, CA

Garance Franke-Ruta—May 8, 1997, Cambridge, MA

Robert Gallo—March 12, 1997, Baltimore, MD

Chris Galloway—March 19, 1997, Seattle, WA

Murray Gardner—October 20, 1998, Davis, CA

Timothy Gregory—January 27, 1998, South San Francisco, CA

Ashley Haase—May 5, 1997, Bethesda, MD

Nancy Haigwood—March 20, 1997, Seattle, WA; April 6, 1998; June 16, 1999

Lori Hansen—October 27, 1998, Emeryville, CA

Mark Harrington—March 7, 2000

Peter Hawley—April 28, 2000

Barton Haynes—December 15, 1999, Durham, NC

Carole Heilman—March 17, 1997; February 3, 1998, Rockville, MD

William Heyward—November 20, 1998

Keith Higgins—October 23, 1998, Emeryville, CA

Rodney Hoff—March 10, 1998

David Hone—March 12, 1997, Baltimore, MD

Shiu-Lok Hu—March 20, 1997, Seattle, WA

John Jermano—June 28, 2000, Brisbane, CA

Margaret I. (Peggy) Johnston—January 23, 1997, Washington, DC; February 18, 1997; May 5, 1997, Bethesda, MD; September 15, 1997, Baltimore, MD; March 16, 1998, Washington, DC; September 28, 1998

Robert Johnston—December 13, 1999, Chapel Hill, NC

Jack Killen—March 13, 2000

Dwip Kitayaporn—February 16, 1999, Nonthaburi, Thailand

Michel Klein—August 29, 1999, Baltimore, MD

Julie Klinger—March 24, 1997, Emeryville, CA

Wayne Koff—August 30, 1999, Baltimore, MD

Diana Lee—October 23, 1998, Emeryville, CA

Jay Levy—March 26, 1997, San Francisco, CA

George Lewis—March 12, 1997, Baltimore, MD

Margaret Liu—July 9, 1997; January 26, 1998, Emeryville, CA; October 22, 1998, Emeryville, CA; July 12, 1999; September 7, 2000

Larry Loomis-Price—January 18, 1998; September 24, 1998, Rockville, MD

Paul Luciw—October 19 and 21, 1998, both in Davis, CA

Timothy Mastro—February 16, 1999, Nonthaburi, Thailand

Bonnie Mathieson—February 19, 1997, Bethesda, MD; August 23 and 25, 1998, both in Baltimore, MD; August 26, 1999, Baltimore, MD

Juliana McElrath—March 19, 1997, Seattle, WA

John McNeil—March 13, 1997, Rockville, MD; March 16, 1998, Rockville, MD; September 24, 1998, Rockville, MD; June 18, 1999; October 16, 1999

Kate McQueen—November 30, 1998

Matthew Meldorf—March 19, 1997, Seattle, WA

David Montefiori—December 15, 1999, Durham, NC; March 8, 2000

John Moore—July 16, 1998, New York, NY

William Morton—March 20, 1997, Seattle, WA

Gary Nabel—July 19, 1999

Neal Nathanson—July 15, 1998

Kenrad Nelson—February 10, 1999, Chiang Mai, Thailand

Robert Nowinski—July 20, 2000, New York, NY

Jack Nunberg—August 23, 1998, Baltimore, MD

John Obijeski—October 22, 1998, South San Francisco, CA

Robert Olmsted—December 14, 1999, Durham, NC

Dennis Panicali—January 25, 1999, Cambridge, MA; January 17, 2000

Enzo Paoletti—January 19, 2000, Delmar, NY; January 31, 2000

William Paul— May 27, 1997; April 24, 2000

Edward Penhoet—October 22, 1998, Emeryville, CA

Stanley Plotkin—March 8, 2000

Punnee Pitisuttithum—February 8, 1999, Bangkok, Thailand

Kathryn Radke—October 19, 1998, Davis, CA

Robert Redfield—August 24 and 25, 1998, both in Baltimore, MD

Gary Rhodes—October 21, 1998, Davis, CA; June 22, 1999

Harriet Robinson—December 10, 1999, Atlanta, GA

Zeda Rosenberg—June 12, 1998; April 20, 2000

William Rutter—June 29, 2000, Emeryville, CA

Alan Schultz—November 25, 1998; June 16, 1999

Steve Self—January 19, 1999

David Serwadda—May 5, 1999, Bethesda, MD

Gene Shearer—February 19, 1997, Bethesda, MD

Faruk Sinangil—March 24, 1997, Emeryville, CA; January 26, 1998, Emeryville, CA

William Snow—March 25, 1997, San Francisco, CA; June 9 and 10, 1998; February 21, 2000

Harry Steimer—October 20, 1998, West Sacramento, CA

Jim Stephens—October 27, 1998, Emeryville, CA

Pravan Suntharasamai—February 8, 1999, Bangkok, Thailand

James Tartaglia—January 20, 2000

Edmund Tramont—March 17, 1997

Jeff Ulmer—October 23, 1998, Emeryville, CA

Gary Van Nest—March 24, 1997, Emeryville, CA

Supak Vanichseni—February 17, 1999, Bangkok, Thailand

Mary Clare Walker—September 28, 1998; September 28, 1999

David Weiner—March 3 and 4, 1997, Philadelphia, PA; April 9, 1997, Dedham, MA; August 24, 1998, Baltimore, MD; August 4, 1999

Kent Weinhold—December 15, 1999, Durham, NC

Martin Wilson—January 24, 1998, Benicia, CA; October 20, 1998, Davis, CA

Peter Young—December 14, 1999, Durham, NC

Susan Zolla-Pazner—May 6, 1997, Bethesda, MD; August 24, 1998, Baltimore, MD; March 3, 2000

NOTES

1. WHISTLING PAST THE GRAVEYARD

PAGE

6: In 1981, the same year ... CDC reported five cases in Los Angeles in the June 5 issue of *Morbidity and Mortality Weekly Report,* and subsequently twenty-six more cases, twenty in New York City and six in San Francisco, in the July 3 issue.

7: They practiced recombinant DNA . . . The discovery and rise of recombinant DNA technology is described in Martin Kenney, *Biotechnology: The University-Industrial Complex* (New Haven: Yale University Press, 1986).

7: At the top of their list . . . Chiron was the first to clone the hepatitis C virus and, in 1990, the first to receive FDA approval for a test for the virus.

7: Making vaccine this way . . . The history of Merck's hepatitis B vaccines appears in Louis Galambos, with Jane Eliot Sewell, *Networks of Innovation: Vaccine Development at Merck, Sharp & Dohme, and Mulford, 1885–1995* (Cambridge: Cambridge University Press, 1995), 183–196.

7: He figured out ... Ibid., 199.

7: The yeast cells cranked out . . . Pablo Valenzuela et al., "Synthesis and Assembly of Hepatitis B Virus Surface Antigen Particles in Yeast," *Nature* 298:347–350.

8: This precedent-setting . . . Galambos, with Sewell, *Networks of Innovation,* 196–206.

8: Now recombinant DNA ... In fact, this technology has changed the development of therapeutic drugs as well. For an overview, see Philip Leder and Patricia Thomas, "Making Drugs from DNA," *Harvard Health Letter,* Special Supplement, July 1994.

9: Old-guard academic . . . The uneasiness that academics felt toward the application of "pure science" to commercial ends is described in Robert Teitelman's *Gene Dreams: Wall Street, Academia, and the Rise of Technology* (New York: Basic Books, 1989), 14–17.

11: The first generation . . . On the first day of publicly offered stocks, shares in one biotech company jumped from $35 to $89 a share in twenty minutes. See Linda Marsa, *Prescription for Profits: How the Pharmaceutical Industry Bankrolled the Unholy Marriage Between Science and Business* (New York: Scribner, 1997), 100–101.

11: The *New York Times* wrote ... Lawrence K. Altman, "AIDS Now Seen as a Worldwide Health Problem," *New York Times,* November 29, 1983.

11: San Francisco was hit . . . Steven Epstein, *Impure Science: AIDS, Activism, and the Politics of Knowledge* (Berkeley: University of California Press, 1996), 45–79.

12: AIDS was an ugly . . . Randy Shilts, *And the Band Played On: Politics, People, and the AIDS Epidemic* (New York: St. Martin's Press, 1987), 34–50.

12: The human catastrophe . . . Ibid., 354–357.

13: In 1983, the French . . . Both reports appeared in the May 20, 1983, issue of *Science*. See Robert C. Gallo et al., "Isolation of Human T-Cell Leukemia Virus in Acquired Immune Deficiency Syndrome (AIDS)," 220:865–867; F. Barre-Sinoussi et al., "Isolation of a T-Lymphotrophic Retrovirus from a Patient at Risk for Acquired Immunodeficiency Syndrome (AIDS)," 220:868–870.

13: He called his ARV . . . Jay A. Levy et al., "Isolation of Lymphocytic Retroviruses from San Francisco Patients with AIDS," *Science*, August 24, 1984 (225):840–842.

13: Most life forms . . . Bruce Alberts et al., *The Molecular Biology of the Cell*, 3rd ed. (New York: Garland Publishing, 1994), 98–102.

14: Retroviruses have an even stranger . . . Ibid., 282–284.

14: Links to leukemia . . . Laurie Garrett, *The Coming Plague: Newly Emerging Diseases in a World out of Balance* (New York: Farrar Straus Giroux, 1994), 227–233.

14: Gallo called these retroviruses . . . Ibid., 229.

14: The human toll of AIDS . . . Jonathan Mann and Daniel Tarantola, eds., *AIDS in the World II* (New York: Oxford University Press, 1996), 12.

16: The government had already . . . Shilts, *And the Band Played On*, 455.

17: Finally, in early June . . . *Chiron Corp v. Abbott Laboratories* (22300/4), U.S. District of California/Northern District, 1995, deposition of Paul Luciw, 257.

18: The disease was rampaging . . . Shilts, *And the Band Played On*, 445–447.

18: There was widespread panic . . Ibid., 457–458.

19: Stripped down to its basics . . . Eli Benjamini, Geoffrey Sunshine, and Sidney Leskowitz, *Immunology: A Short Course*, 3rd ed. (New York: Wiley-Liss, 1996), 1.

20: Paul cloned . . . His report appeared in December (P. A. Luciw et al., "Molecular Cloning of AIDS-Associated Retrovirus," *Nature* 312 [1984]:760–763). Jay Levy's findings were published the previous August (J. A. Levy et al., "Isolation of Lymphocytopathic Retroviruses from San Francisco Patients with AIDS," *Science*, August 24, 1984 [225]:840–842).

21: In April 1984, Secretary . . . Shilts, *And the Band Played On*, 450–451.

21: Gallo pulled . . . Author interview.

21: Largely on the strength . . . Marsa, *Prescription for Profits*, 184–186.

22: Kathy's mission . . . gp120 was discovered by Max Essex in 1985. Ibid., 184.

2. ARE WE NOT MEN? WE ARE GENENTECH

PAGE

28: Their upset victory . . . The race to clone the insulin gene is colorfully described in Stephen S. Hall, *Invisible Frontiers* (New York: Atlantic Monthly Press, 1987).

28: Genentech was more like . . . Ibid., 232; Marsa, *Prescription for Profits*, 206–207; author interviews.

29: These findings suggested . . . Hall, *Invisible Frontiers*, 61–63.

29: And work it did . . . S. Cohen et al., "Construction of Biologically Functional Bacterial Plasmids In Vitro," *Proceedings of the National Academy of Sciences (PNAS)* 70 (November 1973):3240–3244.

30: It was an improbable . . . Marsa, *Prescription for Profits*, 85–91.

30: Although this exact . . . Hall, *Invisible Frontiers*, 82–85.

30: In September 1978, Genentech . . . Ibid., 266–267.

30: The technology for making . . . Marsa, *Prescription for Profits*, 93.

31: Although the company . . . Ibid., 94, 100.

31: In whatever spare time . . . Hall, *Invisible Frontiers*, 199.

31: In a 1979 talk . . . Quoted in Hall, *Invisible Frontiers*, 277.

34: When the Boyer-Cohen . . . Marsa, *Prescription for Profits*, 59, 99–100.

35: Unlike Chiron's founders . . . Ibid., 87.

36: Drag queens . . . Author's notes from the Atlanta AIDS Conference, 1985. Also see Shilts, *And the Band Played On*, 548.

36: At the World Congress Center . . . By March 1985, over 9,000 confirmed cases had been reported to the CDC, more than 4,300 of whom had died. In his opening remarks at the conference, James Curran, Director of CDC's AIDS Task Force, estimated that between 500,000 and 1 million people were infected. For many years, criticism was leveled at the CDC for exaggerating the numbers, but actually the "head count" was conservative. Part of the confusion stems from the terminology: CDC counted AIDS cases, not HIV infection. People with AIDS have severe, recurrent, and often fatal complications of HIV infection; in contrast, HIV infection doesn't necessarily lead to AIDS and, in fact, many individuals have remained symptom-free for years. Furthermore, there is simply no way to determine how many are unknowingly infected.

Still another reason for underestimations was that the criteria for diagnosing AIDS changed several times. Originally called GRID (gay-related immune deficiency) on the assumption that only homosexuals were affected, the first guidelines essentially excluded everyone else. And since there was no reliable test at that time, diagnosis was predicated on the appearance of Kaposi's sarcoma (a type of cancer), *Pneumocystis carinii* pneumonia, or other "opportunistic" infections caused by common organisms that don't usually cause illness. The AIDS case definition changed as the disease was recognized in IV drug users and hemophiliacs (in 1983), heterosexuals and transfusion recipients (1984), and infants (1987).

The Harvard-based Global AIDS Policy Coalition, which has tracked the HIV/AIDS pandemic worldwide, estimates that by 1985, nearly 2 million people in sub-Saharan Africa had been infected with HIV versus about 310,000 in the United States (Mann and Tarantola, *AIDS in the World II*, 12).

37: In a 1985 cartoon . . . Jules Feiffer, untitled cartoon, Universal Press Syndicate, 1985.

37: We must conquer it . . . Ann Giudici Fettner with Pat Thomas, "Big Doings in Hotlanta," *New York Native*, April 1985.

37: In a flash . . . Shilts, *And the Band Played On*, 554–555, and author's notes from conference.

37: Gay leaders were mad . . . Ibid., 548–550.

38: A real sore point . . . Ibid., 524–525.

38: The transfer was approved . . . Ibid., 550–551.

38: At the time, Francis . . . Ibid., 549.

40. The animals mounted . . . Harvey J. Alter et al., "Transmission of HTLV-III Infection from Human Plasma to Chimpanzees: An Animal Model for AIDS," *Science*, November 2, 1984 (226): 549–552; Flossie Wong-Staal and Robert C. Gallo, "The Family of Human T-Lymphotrophic Leukemia Viruses: HTLV-I as the Cause of Adult T Cell Leukemia and HTLV-III as the Cause of Acquired Immunodeficiency Syndrome," *Blood* 65 (February 1985):253–263.

42: As a result, vaccine research . . . Marsa, *Prescription for Profits*, 47–48, and Roy Porter, *Of Greatest Benefit to Mankind* (New York: W. W. Norton, 1997), 633, 685.

42: Healthy people, on the other hand . . . Christine Grady, *The Search for an AIDS Vaccine* (Bloomington: Indiana University Press, 1995), 19–20.

43: There was also an increasing . . . Between 1985 and 1986, the number of HIV-infected people in sub-Saharan Africa nearly doubled, from 1.9 to 2.8 million. Much of this was attributable to an increasing number of infants who acquired the infection before, during, or shortly after birth (Mann and Tarantola, *AIDS in the World II*, 13, 273–276).

43: Genentech's own experience . . . Marsa, *Prescription for Profits*, 207–209.

43: Of this amount, industry analysts . . . Ibid., 202.

43: In the *New York Times* . . . Philip M. Boffey, "Campaign to Find Drugs for Fighting AIDS Is Intensified," *New York Times*, February 14, 1988.

44: If the patient's system . . . Ibid.

44: This virus was not easily . . . Epstein, *Impure Science*, 212, and author interviews.

48: Unlike people, however . . . A. M. Shultz and Shiu-Lok Hu, "Primate Models for HIV Vaccines," *AIDS* 7 (supp. 1) (1993):S161–S170.

48: After infection, the virus doesn't . . . Ibid.

48: Elsewhere, researchers had discovered . . . J. LaRosa, J. P. Dande, and K. Weinhold, "Conserved Sequence and Structural Elements in the HIV-1 Principal Neutralizing Determinant," *Science* 249 (1990):932.

48: Other experiments showed . . . K. K. Murthy et al., "Active and Passive Immunization Against HIV Type A Infection in Chimpanzees," *AIDS Research and Human Retroviruses 1998,* 14 (supp. 3):S271–S276.

3. NAKED CAME THE DNA

PAGE

51: Just for a lark . . . A group of *Newsday* reporters masqueraded as Penelope Ashe, "a demure Long Island housewife," to write *Naked Came the Stranger* (New York: Lyle Stuart, 1969).

52: A plasmid, also referred to . . . Kenney, *Biotechnology,* 23; Philip Felgner, "Nonviral Strategies for Gene Therapy," *Scientific American,* June 1997; and David B. Weiner and Ronald C. Kennedy, "Genetic Vaccines," *Scientific American,* July 1999.

53: Already doctors were reporting . . . *Physicians' Desk Reference* lists toxic effects for AZT, later renamed "zidovudine," including blood-cell abnormalities, gastrointestinal problems, headache, and malaise. Some of these were downplayed in the rush to approve a treatment for AIDS. See Bruce Nussbaum, *Good Intentions: How Big Business and the Medical Establishment Are Corrupting the Fight Against AIDS* (New York: Penguin Books, 1990).

53: AIDS cases in the United States . . . Centers for Disease Control, AIDS Weekly Surveillance Report—United States, December 28, 1987; Centers for Disease Control, HIV/AIDS Surveillance, January 1989.

53: They based this reasoning on earlier . . . Felgner, "Nonviral Strategies for Gene Therapy," and author interviews.

54: Vical was a tiny company . . . Author interviews. Salk's Immune Response Corporation made a vaccine, Remune™, that was tested as a treatment for HIV-infected patients. Lengthy accounts of Salk's vaccine work can be found in Marsa, *Prescription for Profits,* and in Elinor Burkett, *The Gravest Show on Earth: America in the Age of AIDS* (New York: Picador USA, 1996).

56: Just before Christmas . . . An abbreviated version of this story appears in Mark Caldwell, "The Dream Vaccine," *Discover* (September 1997):86.

57: If they did nail down . . . Author interviews; Felgner, "Nonviral Strategies for Gene Therapy"; Felgner personal communication. Vical filed its first application for a patent related to naked DNA on March 23, 1989, and made claims for both protein expression and immunization.

57: Nancy was willing . . . Felgner personal communication; author interviews.

57: Chiron was riding high . . . "Is Chiron on the Verge of a Biotech Breakthrough?" *Business Week,* June 4, 1990; Marilyn Chase, "Demand for MS Drug May Help Chiron Corp. Emerge from the Pack," *Wall Street Journal,* September 1, 1993.

58: By now Vical had set up . . . The absence of an ideal small animal model for studying AIDS and the limitations of various primate models have frequently been described. For example, Barney S. Graham and Peter F. Wright, "Candidate AIDS Vaccines," *New England Journal of Medicine*, November 16, 1995 (333):1331–1339; Alan Schultz and Shiu-Lok Hu, "Primate models for HIV Vaccines," *AIDS* 7 (supp. 1) (1993).

60: It was early 1989 . . . Author interviews. For Hilary Koprowski's accomplishments, see Koprowski and Michael Oldstone, eds., *Microbe Hunters: Then and Now* (Bloomington, IL: Medi-Ed Press, 1996), 9, 141–152.

61: For genetic engineers, the first . . . The many roles of plasmids in the wild and in the laboratory are described in standard biology texts, including Bruce Alberts et al., *The Molecular Biology of the Cell*, 3rd ed. (New York: Garland, 1994).

63: Once it became apparent . . . Felgner personal communication and author interviews.

63: Beautifully situated in farm country . . . Fact sheet on Merck Research Laboratory from corporate public affairs; author interviews.

64: The most famous and imposing . . . Galambos, with Sewell, *Networks of Innovation*; author observations and interviews.

64: Emilio Emini, a stocky New Yorker . . . Author interviews and Emini's curriculum vitae, 1997, supplied by Merck public affairs.

64: HIV-specific protease is . . . Malorye Allison, "Combating HIV in the Nineties," *Harvard Health Letter*, September 1991.

65: Margaret Liu, one year younger . . . Author observations and interviews; Liu's curriculum vitae.

66: Just as cities need both . . . Benjamini, Sunshine, and Leskowitz, *Immunology*, chaps. 1, 9, 10.

66: Once it became clear . . . Graham and Wright, "Candidate AIDS Vaccines," 1331; author interviews.

67: Although many vaccines elicit . . . Author interviews. Mechanisms of action are discussed in W. Michael McDonnell and Frederick K. Askari, "DNA Vaccines," *New England Journal of Medicine*, January 4, 1996 (331):42–45, and Weiner and Kennedy, "Genetic Vaccines."

68: Six months after . . . According to personal communication from Felgner, the agreement for the proof of principle experiment was negotiated in October 1990, but not signed until June 1, 1991.

69: It took most of 1991 . . . Vical submitted its first six-month report to Merck, showing protection of mice against influenza in the California lab, on January 1, 1992, according to personal communication from Felgner.

70: No matter who conducted . . . Jeffrey Ulmer et al., "Heterologous Protective Immunity to Influenza A by Intramuscular Injection of DNA Encoding a Conserved Viral Protein," *Science* 259 (1993):1745–1749.

70: At about the same time . . . Merck 1996 Annual Report, 28–29. Larry Armstrong "Besting AIDS and the Drug Giants," *Business Week*, June 9, 1997.

71: Meanwhile, on the Penn campus . . . J. A. Wolff et al., "Direct Gene Transfer into Mouse Muscle In Vivo," *Science* 247 (1990):1465–1468; author interviews.

71: About the same time, he noticed . . . The University of Pennsylvania filed for numerous patents related to Weiner's DNA vaccines, and many of them specify bupivacaine or related agents as a means for facilitating cellular uptake of genes. Issued U.S. Patent No. 5,593,972 is an example.

73: By January 1992 . . . Weiner and Kennedy, "Genetic Vaccines," 53; author interviews.

73: During the 1980s . . . Author interviews and observations.

75: In 1992, however, . . . In author interviews, there is consensus that this was the watershed event in the acceptance of DNA vaccines as a legitimate technology.

75: Johnston had just published . . . D. Tang, M. DeVit, and S. A. Johnston, "Genetic Immunization Is a Simple Method for Eliciting an Immune Response," *Nature* 356 (August 1992):152–154; author interviews.

76: Dave Weiner stood . . . Author interviews; program from American Society for Microbiology.

76: In the March 19, 1993 . . . Ulmer et al., "Heterologous Protective Immunity to Influenza A by Intramuscular Injection of DNA Encoding a Conserved Viral Protein"; author interviews.

76: In April, Dave . . . Bin Wang et al., "Gene Inoculation Generates Immune Responses Against HIV-1," *PNAS* 90 (1993):4156–4160.

4. WHERE THE LIVE THINGS ARE

PAGE

77: In addition to the thousands . . . Viruses are presently grouped into 3,600 species, 164 genera, and 71 families. (Several viruses have not yet been classified because difficulties growing them in the laboratory have prohibited sufficient study of their characteristics. In addition, the discovery of several previously unknown viruses over the past two decades suggests that more genera and families may be added to the lexicon.) HIV belongs to the *Retroviridae* family, *lentivirinae* genus. See Samuel Baron, ed., *Medical Microbiology*, 4th ed. (Galveston: University of Texas Medical Branch at Galveston, 1996), 536, 540–541.

77: These are the mass murderers . . . From the standpoint of ensuring a species' survival, it might seem suicidal for a virus to kill its host, but this potential risk is balanced by the ease of transmission from one person to another.

78: Once a virus gets inside . . . Baron, *Medical Microbiology*, 543–545.

79: When Enzo took over . . . Vaccinia is a member of *Poxviridae orthopoxvirus* ("pox" means "pustule-producing," and "ortho" means "true").

80: At this point, most heterosexuals . . . Genital herpes is painful and embarrassing, but not life-threatening. In the late 1970s and early 1980s, it was considered an epidemic in the United States among heterosexuals, with as many as 500,000 new cases diagnosed annually. See Ann Giudici Fettner and William A. Check, *The Truth About AIDS: Evolution of an Epidemic,* rev. ed. (New York: Holt, Rinehart and Winston, 1985), 19.

83: To reduce the odds . . . Stephen S. Hall, *Invisible Frontiers: The Race to Synthesize a Human Gene* (New York: Atlantic Monthly Press, 1987), 114.

85: Their starting point . . . In 1966, the World Health Organization launched a global campaign to eradicate smallpox through mass immunization with vaccinia, surveillance, and isolating existing cases to prevent spread. The last diagnosed case was in 1977, and WHO declared that smallpox was completely eradicated worldwide in 1980. See D. A. Henderson, "Smallpox Eradication," in *Microbe Hunters: Then and Now,* ed. Koprowski and Oldstone, 39–43.

86: Within a few months, health . . . Virogenetics was established under Health Research Inc., a nonprofit corporation set up by the State Health Department in the 1950s. See "New York State Weighs Venture to Market Vaccine," *New York Times,* October 30, 1982.

87: In 1982 and 1983, he and Dennis . . . Dennis Panicali and Enzo Paoletti, "Construction of Poxviruses as Cloning Vectors: Insertion of the Thymidine Kinase Gene from Herpes Simplex Virus into the DNA of Infectious Vaccinia Virus," *PNAS* 79 (1982):4927–4931. Dennis Panicali et al., "Construction of Live Vaccines by Using Genetically Engineered Poxviruses: Biological Activity of Recombinant Vaccinia Virus Expressing Influenza Virus Hemagglutinin," *PNAS* 80 (1983):5364–5368. Enzo Paoletti et al., "Construction of Live Vaccines Using Genetically Engineered Poxviruses: Biological Activity of Vaccinia Virus Recombinants Expressing the Hepatitis B Virus Surface Antigen and the Herpes Simplex Virus Glycoprotein E," *PNAS* 81 (1984):193–197.

87: By 1985, they had reported . . . Marion E. Perkus et al., "Recombinant Vaccinia Virus: Immunization Against Multiple Pathogens," *Science* 229 (1985):981–984.

89: It was in Madison . . . Shiu-Lok Hu's publications prior to 1979 are entirely concerned with bacteriophage research.

91: They knew that in 1986 . . . The investigator was Daniel Zagury, and the questionable trial took place in Zaire. Grady, *The Search for an AIDS Vaccine,* 101–102.

91: He published a preliminary . . . S.-L. Hu, S. G. Kosowski, and J. M. Dalrymple, "Expression of AIDS Virus Envelope Gene in Recombinant Vaccinia Viruses," *Nature* 320 (1986):537–540, and S. Chakrabarti et al., "Expression of the HTLV-III Envelope Gene by a Recombinant Vaccinia Virus," *Nature* 320 (1986):535–537.

91: A page-one story . . . Harold M. Schmeck, "AIDS Researchers Begin Testing New Version of Smallpox Vaccine," *New York Times,* April 10, 1986.

92: One was to minimize . . . L. Corey et al., "A Trial of Topical Acyclovir in Genital Herpes Simplex Infections," *New England Journal of Medicine* 306 (1982):1313–1319.

93: Meetings in Washington followed . . . Shiu-Lok Hu, personal communication.

94: And occasionally vaccinia-based . . . *Vaccinium necrosum* (tissue death around the vaccination site) can occur in people with immune deficiencies, and systemic spread of vaccinia can occur in patients with eczema or other serious skin conditions. The rarest and most severe complication is postvaccinial encephalitis, an inflammation of the brain that can result in death. See Phyllis B. Moses, "Vaccinia Virus: Reinventing the Wheel," *Bioscience* 36 (3) (March 1986):149.

95: On the contrary, he had . . . Charles Mérieux's accomplishments included a vaccine for hoof-and-mouth disease in cattle and, in collaboration with Hilary Koprowski, a safer rabies vaccine for humans. One of his greatest contributions was establishing a center that trained professionals to manage public-health emergencies, especially in developing countries. He died at age ninety-four in January 2001.

96: One of his postdocs . . . J. Taylor et al., "Fowlpox Virus Based Recombinant Vaccines," in *Technological Advances in Virus Development: UCLA Symposia on Molecular and Cellular Biology, New Series,* ed. L. Lasky (New York: Alan R. Liss, 1988), 84:321–334.

97: Jim Tartaglia focused . . . M. E. Perkus and E. Paoletti, "Recombinant Virus as Vaccination Carrier of Heterologous Antigens," in *Concepts in Vaccine Development,* ed. Stefan H.E. Kaufmann (Berlin, New York: de Gruyter, 1996), 382–383.

97: WHO also estimated . . . F. Fenner et al., *Smallpox and Its Eradication* (Geneva: World Health Organization, 1988).

98: In an audit released . . . According to a news report, the audit cited Paoletti for being offered a $12,000 payment "before state legislation was passed allowing employees to receive outside income for scientific discoveries made as part of their state employment" (Jeannie H. Cross, "Audit Blasts Health Officials for Conflicts of Interest, Cheating State," UPI, December 27, 1989). The U.S. Congress passed legislation in 1980 that allowed academic institutions and scientists to benefit financially from faculty inventions, including those supported by federal funds. It did not, however, address possible conflict-of-interest issues of partnerships between research and industry.

98: Although Connaught's HIV work . . . The company was working on a recombinant gp160 protein, on synthetic peptides, and on pseudovirions—synthetic HIV-like particles.

99: In fact, Axelrod died . . . "Axelrod stricken while in Washington," UPI, February 26, 1991; Robert D. McFadden, "David Axelrod, Health Chief Under Cuomo, Is Dead at 59," *New York Times,* July 5, 1994.

100: He wanted Virogenetics . . . Refer to Chapter 3 for an explanation of cellular and humoral immune responses.

104: He and Jonathan Smith . . . Diseases caused by alphaviruses occur in tropical and semitropical regions because they are transmitted to humans and other vertebrates by mosquitoes. See Perkus and Paoletti, "Recombinant Virus as Vaccination Carrier of Heterologous Antigens," 401.

107: One reason was that alphavirus . . . P. Liljestrom and H. Garoff, "A New Generation of Animal Cell Expression Vectors Based on the Semliki Forest Virus Replicon," *Bio/Technology* 9 (1991):1356–1361.

109: Nancy, meanwhile, had been . . . These results were presented at scientific meetings, including the 1994 Annual Meeting of the American Society for Microbiology and Keystone Symposia on Molecular and Cellular Biology: Molecular Aspects of Viral Immunity in 1995.

5. TROUBLE IN THE IVORY TOWER

PAGE

114: A Hollywood movie . . . Edward Shorter, *The Health Century: A Companion to the PBS Television Series* (New York: Doubleday, 1987), 6–13.

115: Before any kind . . . Lawrence W. Davenport, "Regulatory Considerations in Vaccine Design," in *Vaccine Design: The Subunit and Adjuvant Approach*, ed. Michael Powell and Mark Newman (New York: Plenum Press, 1995), 81–96.

115: Each stage of testing . . . Patricia Fast et al., "Clinical Considerations in Vaccine Trials with Special Reference to Candidate HIV Vaccines," in *Vaccine Design*, ed. Powell and Newman, 97–124; Donald Francis, "Laboratory Empiricism, Clinical Design, and Social Value: The Rough Road Toward Vaccine Development," in *Vaccine Design*, ed. Powell and Newman, 135–139.

116: Nothing in their formal . . . Author interviews. Impact of activists described in Nussbaum, *Good Intentions*, 1990.

116: On public television . . . Shorter, *The Health Century*, xiv.

117: In 1987, U.S. government support . . . Ibid., 1–20, and Paul Starr, *The Social Transformation of American Medicine* (New York: Basic Books, 1982), 340.

117: In 1937, it became . . . Ibid., 340–343.

117: The real impact . . . Ibid., 340.

117: The NIH assumed . . . Shorter, *The Health Century*, 20; Starr, *The Social Transformation of American Medicine*, 340.

117: World War II changed . . . Shorter, *The Health Century*, 41–46.

117: Once the war was . . . Ibid., 58, 72, 73.

118: When Shannon taught . . . Ibid., 53–54, 58–60.

118: When virologist Robert Gallo . . . Robert Gallo, *Virus Hunting: AIDS, Cancer, and the Human Retrovirus* (New York: Basic Books, 1991), 30.

118: Although Shannon talked . . . Ibid., 31; Shorter, *The Health Century*, 76.

119: Basic science, the attempt . . . Shorter, *The Health Century*, 73–74.

119: Unprecedented wealth . . . Ibid., 205; author interviews.

119: Although the War . . . Gallo, *Virus Hunting*, 38–39

119: The 1987 PBS series . . . Shorter, *The Health Century*, 95–100.

120: An entirely different view . . . Shilts, *And the Band Played On*, 596, 600–601; author observations.

120: News of the rubber gloves . . . "Hundreds at AIDS Talks Protest Reagan Policy," *Boston Globe*, June 6, 1987.

121: Only 24 hours . . . Shilts, *And the Band Played On*, 590–596.

121: No matter how . . . Anthony Fauci, "The AIDS Paradigm: Scientific and Policy Lessons for the 21st Century," lecture at Annual Meeting of the Institute of Human Virology, August 30, 1999.

121: On a table . . . Author's observation.

122: At the conference . . . Abstracts, Third International Conference on AIDS, June 1–6, 1987; miscellaneous news coverage of same; author notes.

122: During one session . . . Grady, *The Search for an AIDS Vaccine*, 101–102; author notes.

122: By the time . . . Shorter, *The Health Century*, 20.

123: Few of the Institute's . . . Fauci, August 1999 lecture.

123: When AIDS surfaced . . . Shorter, *The Health Century*, 95–100; Shilts, *And the Band Played On*, 366; Laurie Garrett, *The Coming Plague* (New York: Farrar Straus Giroux, 1994), 283–316.

124: Part of Fauci's portfolio . . . Author interviews. The 1996 report was *Confronting AIDS*, released by the National Academy of Sciences' Institute of Medicine.

127: Over the course of one year . . . Author's notes: During my 52 weeks as a volunteer in a Phase 1 HIV vaccine trial at the National Institutes of Health, blood samples collected at each of my 17 visits were subjected to as many as 23 separate laboratory tests. My participation in this study generated more than 300 test results; a trial with 15 participants would yield 4,500. In 1994, the Division of AIDS Trial Design Team drafted a protocol that would require 30–40 tests per participant during a 30-month study, or 300,000–400,000 tests for 10,000 volunteers.

127: Towering uncertainties . . . Barney S. Graham and Peter F. Wright, "Candidate AIDS Vaccines," *New England Journal of Medicine*, November 16, 1995 (333): 1331–1339.

129: In June 1989 . . . Patricia Thomas, "The Montreal Conference: Warnings of Things to Come," *Medical World News*, July 24, 1989, 40–49.

130: Back in his office . . . The history of the Human Genome Project is well told in the *New York Times*'s special edition of Science Times, June 27, 2000. The government-funded sequencing effort was launched in 1987 and completed in June 2000, at a cost of $250 million.

131: Kathy Steimer and Nancy Haigwood . . . Kathy Steimer's datebook for 1990; author interviews.

131: Kathy and Nancy had heard . . . AIDS Vaccine Evaluation Group (AVEG) Protocol Activity Overview Chart, April 1997. This was the recruitment experience for AVEG 003, 003A, and 003B, clinical trials of a recombinant gp160 vaccine made by MicroGeneSys, a Connecticut biotech company.

133: After 001 was scrapped . . . Ibid.; author interviews.

133: By taking the authority . . . Epstein, *Impure Science*, 284–287; author interviews.

134: The vaccine selection committee . . . Grady, *The Search for an AIDS Vaccine*, 108–109; author interviews.

134: Biotech company scientists . . . Burkett, *The Gravest Show on Earth*, 38–39.

134: His valedictory comments . . . Gordon Ada, Wayne Koff, and John Petricciani, "The Next Steps in HIV Vaccine Development," *AIDS Research and Human Retroviruses* 8 (8) (1992):1317–1319.

135: Although 1992 was . . . NIAID biographical fact sheet (1997); Joan Stephenson, "Fighting Infectious Disease Threats via Research: A Talk with Anthony S. Fauci," *Journal of the American Medical Association*, January 17, 1996 (275):173–174; author interviews.

135: And work he did . . . Fauci, August 1999 lecture; Burkett, *The Gravest Show on Earth*, 272; Stephenson, "Fighting Infectious Disease Threats"; author interviews.

136: And so was Margaret "Peggy" Johnston . . . Rick Weiss, "AIDS Prevention as Global Mission: Vaccine Hunter Mixes Science, Diplomacy," *Washington Post*, August 19, 1999; author interviews.

136: Another manifestation . . . Starr, *The Social Transformation of American Medicine*, 343–344.

138: Study sections are . . . "Report of the NIH AIDS Research Program Evaluation Working Group of the Office of AIDS Research Advisory Council," March 1996. This comprehensive review of AIDS research, usually called the Levine Report, criticizes the handling of AIDS-related grant proposals, especially those for vaccine research.

138: In fiscal year 1993 . . . Stan Katzman, NIH Office of AIDS Research, personal communication, September 13, 1999.

139: Kathy Steimer, for example . . . Steimer curriculum vitae.

140: When Wayne resigned . . . AVEG Protocol Activity Overview Chart, April 1997; Table 1, AIDS Vaccine Candidates Studied by the AVEG, May 1, 1997; author interviews.

140: It took twelve months . . . Jon Cohen, "Trials Set in High-Risk Populations," *Science*, December 11, 1992 (258):1729; author interviews.

140: During the fiscal year . . . FY 1994, Katzman personal communication.

140: As early as February . . . DAIDS, "Guidelines for Entry of HIV Vaccines into Efficacy Trials in Uninfected Volunteers, Draft B," February 15, 1993; "DAIDS Vaccine Briefing," March 23, 1993; DAIDS, "A Phase III Trial to Evaluate the Efficacy of Candidate HIV Vaccine(s), Draft," April 1, 1993.

141: In September, DAIDS . . . DAIDS, "Guidelines of Clinical and Research Data Which Will Facilitate the Decision-Making Process for Entry of Candidate Vaccines into Pivotal Phase III Efficacy Trials," September 1993.

142: In the absence of . . . Carl Veith Hanson, "Measuring Vaccine-Induced HIV Neutralization: Report of a Workshop," *AIDS Research and Human Retroviruses* 10 (1994):645–648; author interviews.

142: In the early 1990s . . . E. S. Daar et al., "High Concentrations of Recombinant CD4

Are Required to Neutralize Primary Human Immunodeficiency Virus Type 1 Isolates," *PNAS* 87 (1990):6547.

142: No one knew . . . Hanson, "Measuring Vaccine-Induced HIV Neutralization," 645–646.

144: While the whole . . . DAIDS, "Talking Points on HIV Vaccine Efficacy Trials for NCVDG, 1993," meeting; draft dated October 19, 1993; draft dated October 25, 1993; author interviews.

6. SOLDIERS AT WAR

PAGE

145: Harder to imagine . . . Douglas Starr, *Blood: An Epic History of Medicine and Commerce* (New York: Alfred A. Knopf, 1998), 360.

146: Like other educated . . . Frank Fenner, "History of Smallpox," in *Microbe Hunters: Then and Now*, ed. Koprowski and Oldstone, 31–34. Lord Jeffrey Amherst ordered the use of smallpox-contaminated blankets as biowarfare, a command decision that prompted the town of Amherst, Massachusetts, to consider shedding his name in 2000. See David Arnold, "Another Look at History Spurs Drive to Rename Amherst," *Boston Globe*, March 6, 2000.

146: More than two centuries . . . U.S. Army Medical Research and Materiel Command, Walter Reed Army Institute of Research, *Entering a 2nd Century of Research for the Soldier*, 1997; author interviews.

147: When AIDS hit . . . The interest of military researchers is reflected in the scientific program for the International Conference on AIDS, April 14–17, 1985.

148: Lt. Col. Robert Redfield's . . . Scientific Program, International Conference on AIDS, 1985, 66; author interviews.

148: Many in the audience . . . Fettner and Check, *The Truth About AIDS*, 198–200; Epstein, *Impure Science*, 51–54.

150: As Redfield showed . . . Randy Shilts, *Conduct Unbecoming: Gays and Lesbians in the U.S. Military* (New York: St. Martin's Press, 1993), 480–485. For coverage of army versus navy response to HIV, see Paul Smith, "Army, Navy Differ in Policies on Homosexual AIDS Patients," *Army Times*, August 26, 1985.

150: Because top army . . . Robert R. Redfield, D. C. Wright, and Edmund C. Tramont, "The Walter Reed Staging Classification for HTLV-III, LAV Infection," *New England Journal of Medicine* 314 (1986):131–132.

151: Although the generals . . . Donald S. Burke's curriculum vitae, January 1999; author interviews.

152: In October 1985 . . . Shilts, *Conduct Unbecoming*, 549; J. F. Brundage et al., "Tracking the Spread of the HIV Infection Epidemic Among Young Adults in the United States: Results of the First Four Years of Screening Among Civilian Applicants for U.S. Military Service," *Journal of AIDS* 3 (1990):1168–1180.

152: Back at Walter Reed . . . Shilts, *Conduct Unbecoming,* 546; author interviews.

153: Redfield and a handful . . . Burkett, *The Gravest Show on Earth,* 116–119.

154: In March 1988 . . . Deborah L. Birx's curriculum vitae, 1999; author interviews.

158: Six months into the trial . . . Richard A. Knox, "Vaccine Seen Promising in Early Stages of AIDS," *Boston Globe,* October 17, 1989.

160: Bangkok's first AIDS case . . . Chris Beyrer, *War in the Blood: Sex, Politics, and AIDS in Southeast Asia* (London: Zed Books, 1998), 20–21.

161: Back in Rockville . . . Francine E. McCutchan et al., "Genetic Variants of HIV-1 in Thailand," *AIDS Research and Human Retroviruses* 8 (1992):1887–1895; Beyrer, *War in the Blood,* 29; author interviews.

162: In the wake of these . . . Beyrer, *War in the Blood,* 26–29; Phyllida Brown, "Sex and Drugs Spread Different Types of HIV," *New Scientist,* July 25, 1992:6; author interviews.

163: For decades, vaccine development . . . "U.S. Military HIV Research Program: Leading the Battle Against HIV," public relations booklet, n.d., 18; author interviews.

163: In fact, everything about . . . John G. McNeil et al., "Direct Measurement of Human Immunodeficiency Virus Seroconversions in a Serially Tested Population of Young Adults in the United States Army, October 1985 to October 1987," *New England Journal of Medicine,* June 15, 1989 (320):1581–1585; author interviews.

166: The statistics were chilling . . . Beyrer, *War in the Blood,* 24–29; author interviews.

166: When Tramont left . . . Don Burke's curriculum vitae; author interviews.

167: Burke channeled much . . . Shilts, *Conduct Unbecoming,* 547; author interviews.

168: No matter how dark . . . Malcolm Gladwell, "A Divergent Strategy in the War on AIDS: Vaccines Can Help Body Win, Some Say," *Washington Post,* July 20, 1992.

169: "What we've shown . . . Richard A. Knox, "Researcher Urges Early Use of Imperfect AIDS Vaccines," *Boston Globe,* July 22, 1992; Phyllida Brown, "Protein Therapy 'Stimulates Antibodies,'" *New Scientist,* August 1, 1992:8.

170: Redfield's Amsterdam glory . . . Jon Cohen, "Army Investigates Researcher's Report of Clinical Trial Data," *Science,* November 6, 1992 (258):883.

171: Meanwhile, the Phase II . . . Gladwell, "A Divergent Strategy in the War on AIDS: Vaccines Can Help Body Win, Some Say"; Barry Meier, "Scientists Assail Congress on Bill for Money to Test an AIDS Drug," *New York Times,* October 26, 1992; author interviews.

172: On September 16 . . . Jon Cohen, "Congress Plays Doctor; How Come Capitol Hill Is Choosing a New AIDS Vaccine?" *Washington Post,* November 1, 1992; author interviews.

172: Hostile stories about . . . "Key Lobbyist Wins AIDS Vaccine Trials," Associated Press, *New York Times,* October 20, 1992. Jessica Mathews, "Pork-Barrel Research," *Washington Post,* November 2, 1992.

173: His intramural troubles . . . Jon Cohen, "Army Investigates Researcher's Report of Clinical Trial Data," *Science,* November 6, 1992 (258):883; author interviews.

173: The *Science* story was . . . CNN broadcast the story on November 5, 1992; CBS Evening News on November 11, 1992; author interviews.

175: Chris Beyrer, however, knew . . . Beyrer, *War in the Blood*, ix; author interviews.

176: Thailand was a hotbed . . . Ibid., 32–33; author interviews.

176: Back in Rockville . . . John McNeil's curriculum vitae; author interviews.

178: None of this unglamorous . . . Hundreds of news stories tracked this convoluted story. Among them were: Jon Cohen, "NIH Panel OK's Vaccine Test—in a New Form," *Science*, December 4, 1992 (258):1569; Colin Macilwain, "MicroGeneSys Drops Out of NIH Trial for AIDS Vaccine," *Nature*, March 25, 1993 (362):277; Sally Squires, "Army to Test AIDS Drug Despite Objections; NIH and FDA Urged That Clinical Trial Include Other Therapeutic Vaccines," *Washington Post*, April 7, 1993; Sally Squires, "Bowing to Pressure, Defense Dept. Agrees to Drop AIDS Vaccine Test," *Washington Post*, April 15, 1993; John Schwartz, "Pentagon Drops Plan to Test an AIDS Vaccine; Health Officials Had Opposed Single-Drug Trial," *Washington Post*, January 23, 1994; author interviews.

181: In fact, John McNeil wrote . . . John McNeil, "Proposal for *Your Organization*—Military Medical Consortium for Applied Retroviral Research Cooperative Research, Development, Testing and Evaluation of HIV-1 Prophylactic Vaccines: Thailand," June 1993 draft; author interviews.

183: Back in the states . . . In an October 11, 1993, letter to Don Burke, Kathy Steimer wrote: "We are moving forward with our efforts to produce the Thai E gp120 and it is my hope that I, along with Anne-Marie Duliege, will be able to convince our management that it is truly a rational strategy to work toward future efficacy trials in Thailand." On November 17, 1993, Kathy's assistant, Michael Gill, faxed Don Burke and John McNeil an agenda for their upcoming visit on November 22–23. In addition to a seminar and luncheon with scientists and managers, they were to have dinner with Bill Rutter and other top executives.

7. NOTHING VENTURED, NOTHING GAINED

PAGE

187: There would be bad weather . . . All Phil's past predictions are available at www.groundhog.org.

188: Already, the disease had killed . . . Centers for Disease Control, "HIV/AIDS Surveillance Report: U.S. HIV and AIDS Cases Reported Through December 1993," year-end ed., vol. 5, no. 4, March 1994.

188: The case definition was expanded . . . Epstein, *Impure Science*, 289.

188: Now that women were . . . Centers for Disease Control, "HIV/AIDS Surveillance Report . . . Through December 1993."

188: The global shadow . . . Mann and Tarantola, *AIDS in the World II*, 12.

189: As a result, random changes . . . Douglas D. Richman, "HIV Therapeutics," *Science*, June 28, 1996 (272):1887.

193: At Johns Hopkins University . . . Mary Lou Clements-Mann and her husband, pioneering AIDS researcher Jonathan Mann, died in the September 2, 1998, crash of Swissair Flight 111 off the coast of Nova Scotia. Her distinguished career as a vaccine researcher was summarized in many publications at that time. See Wolfgang Saxon, "Mary Lou Clements-Mann, 51, an Expert on AIDS Vaccines," *New York Times*, September 4, 1998; AIDS Vaccine Advocacy Coalition, "In Memory," September 15, 1998, press release.

193: An ideal AIDS vaccine . . . Mary Lou Clements, "Historical Perspectives on Vaccine Development," notes for presentation at VWG meeting, April 21–22, 1994.

194: Maurice Hilleman . . . Galambos, with Sewell, *Networks of Innovation*, 79–181.

195: In 600 adult volunteers . . . NIAID, DAIDS, HIV Vaccine Working Group, April 21–22, 1994, Meeting Summary, draft, May 1994.

197: After the group heard Kathy's report . . . Peggy Johnston, note to Tony Fauci, through acting director, DAIDS, October 18, 1993.

197: In November, one of Kathy's . . . Depakote, manufactured by Abbott Laboratories, is the trade name for divalproex sodium. Sometimes used to tame the manic phases of bipolar disorder, the drug is mainly prescribed for the control of epileptic seizures (*Physicians' Desk Reference*, 50th ed. [Montvale, NJ: Medical Economics Company, 1996]).

199: A multiyear ranking . . . "AIDS Research: Which Institutions Are Most Productive and Influential?" *Scientist*, October 18, 1993 (7):14.

199: The company was so confident . . . NIAID, DAIDS, HIV Vaccine Working Group, April 21–22, 1994, Meeting Summary, draft, May 25, 1994.

201: In 1990, Phil Berman . . . These experiments are described in Chapter 2.

201: Others in the room . . . NIAID, DAIDS, HIV Vaccine Working Group, April 21–22, 1994, Meeting Summary, draft, May 25, 1994.

202: Chiron's gp120, in contrast . . . MF59 is an oil-and-water emulsion containing squalene; by mid-1994, it had been safely used in clinical trials of experimental vaccines against herpes simplex and influenza viruses, as well as HIV. Its safety profile was part of the Chiron Biocine presentation at this meeting.

203: More than 90 percent of infections . . . In fact, the Global AIDS Policy Coalition estimated that by the end of 1985, 92 percent of all adults, 97 percent of all women, and 98 percent of all children living with HIV/AIDS were in the developing world (Mann and Tarantola, *AIDS in the World II*), 21.

207: Four months earlier . . . Carl V. Hanson, "Meeting Report: Measuring Vaccine-Induced HIV Neutralization: Report of a Workshop," *AIDS Research and Human Retroviruses* 10 (6) (1994):645–648.

207: Although all the assays . . . Ibid.; and Thomas J. Matthews, "Tenth Anniversary Perspective on AIDS: Dilemma of Neutralization Resistance of HIV-1 Field Isolates and Vaccine Development," *AIDS Research and Human Retroviruses* 10 (6) (1994):631–632.

208: "The only certainty . . . Hanson, "Meeting Report," 648.

8. MAY IS THE CRUELEST MONTH

213: The first detonation was . . . Bernard N. Fields. "AIDS: Time to Turn to Basic Science," *Nature*, May 12, 1994 (369):95–96.

215: Fields had spent . . . "In Memoriam: Bernard Fields: Scientist, Mentor, Visionary," *Focus: News from Harvard Medical, Dental and Public Health Schools*, February 3, 1995:1.

215: Congress had created . . . See Chapter 3.

216: Finally, Varmus asked . . . Jon Cohen, "New AIDS Chief Takes Charge," *Science*, March 11, 1994 (263):1364–1366.

217: Culliton invited Fields . . . Personal communication.

217: On May 12, when Bernie Fields's . . . Gina Kolata, "Saying Strategy to Find Cure for AIDS Has Gone Awry, Researchers Seek Redirection," *New York Times*, May 12, 1994.

220: On May 13, DAIDS sent drafts . . . DAIDS, "Trial Design Team," draft, May 3, 1994.

223: As an alternative . . . Genentech, Inc., "Design Proposal for a Large Simple Efficacy Trial of HIV Preventative Vaccines," May 19, 1994.

224: DAIDS asked the trial sites . . . Patricia Fast, "Subject: AIDS Vaccine Trial News," memo, June 2, 1994.

224: The previous day, they had been . . . The EMMES Corporation, "AIDS Vaccine Evaluation Group: Suggested Informed Consent for Participation," redline version: "Proposed Protocol 016A Consent Form," May 20, 1994.

225: They could resume recruitment . . . NIH letter to principal investigators, June 1, 1994; Patricia Fast memo, June 2, 1994.

229: An aftershock came . . . David Brown and Benjamin Weiser, "HIV Infections Cast Pall over Expanding Vaccine Experiments," *Washington Post*, May 30, 1994

229: In recent years, the company's . . . Linda Marsa, *Prescription for Profits: How the Pharmaceutical Industry Bankrolled the Unholy Marriage Between Science and Business* (New York: Scribner, 1997), 199–222.

230: By noon on Tuesday . . . Unsigned draft of letter to Anthony Fauci, June 1, 1994.

231: Although he had won . . . John Crewdson, "The Great AIDS Quest," *Chicago Tribune*, special section, November 19, 1989.

232: All this dragged on . . . Burkett, *The Gravest Show on Earth*, 40–47.

235: In 1992, shortly before Chris . . . Chaiyos Kunanusont and Vipa Thiamchai, "Lessons from HIV Vaccine Development in Thailand," handout prepared for

Harvard AIDS Institute workshop on HIV vaccines for developing countries, October 1999.

236: In the 1980s, thousands . . . These studies were sponsored by the U.S. Department of Defense and field-tested products made by U.S. companies.

238: The final version of the letter . . . THAIVEG letter to Anthony Fauci, June 13, 1994.

239: Young investigators followed the lead . . . Anthony Fauci, "The AIDS Paradigm: Scientific and Policy Lessons for the 21st Century," lecture at annual meeting of the Institute of Human Virology, Baltimore, August 30, 1999, author's transcript.

240: Fauci's actions and accomplishments . . . Michael Maccoby, "Narcissistic Leaders: The Incredible Pros, the Inevitable Cons," *Harvard Business Review* (January–February 2000):69–77. Although the term "narcissism" often conjures up negative images, Maccoby points out that some of the most inspirational leaders and innovators throughout history have been productive narcissists. (He gives many examples, among the best known: Napoleon Bonaparte, Thomas Edison, Henry Ford, Mahatma Gandhi, Franklin D. Roosevelt, Winston Churchill, John F. Kennedy, Mao Tse-tung, Bill Clinton, Bill Gates, and Steve Jobs.)

241: In early May . . . See two articles by Jon Cohen: "The HIV Vaccine Paradox," *Science,* May 20, 1994 (264):1072, and "Will Media Reports KO Upcoming Real-life Trials?" *Science,* June 17, 1994 (264):1660.

241: Looking back, during . . . Author interview.

9. DEATH IN THE AFTERNOON

PAGE

243: In addition to author interviews, the main source for this chapter was a verbatim transcript of the meeting prepared for internal use at the National Institute of Allergy and Infectious Diseases. It was supposedly destroyed after an official meeting summary had been written. However, a copy was located and provided to me by NIAID staff member Claudia Goad. Page numbers cited here correspond to a double-spaced printout of the transcript. An electronic version of this document is available at www.aids.harvard.edu/resources/NIH_documents/index.html.

244: Three dozen members . . . NIAID Council–ARAC official seating chart, June 1994; Jesse Green, "Who Put the Lid on gp120?" *New York Times Magazine,* March 26, 1995.

246: The room exploded with light . . . ARAC transcript, 29; Green, "Who Put the Lid on gp120?" 56.

246: On this occasion, two members . . . ARAC transcript, 2–3.

248: Fauci told the group . . . Ibid., 29–39. "Opening Statement of Anthony S. Fauci, M.D., Director, NIAID, NIH, to AIDS Research Advisory Committee (ARAC), NIAID, June 17, 1994, Bethesda, Maryland," prepared text distributed at meeting.

248: Jack Killen came back to the microphone . . . ARAC transcript, 39–42.

250: Some participants in that earlier . . . Ibid., 42–53.

250: "Ashley's summary of the meeting . . . Ibid., 56–58.

252: Pat Fast was next in the lineup . . . Ibid., 77–93. "Clinical Research Update, June 17, 1994, Patricia Fast, M.D., Ph.D., Division of AIDS, NIAID," handout distributed at meeting.

253: The next presentations . . . ARAC transcript, 93–103. "HIV Vaccine Trial Design, July 17, 1994, Rod Hoff, D.Sc., MPH, Division of AIDS, NIAID," handout distributed at meeting.

253: Uninfected gay men and IV drug . . . ARAC transcript, 114–125. "Vaccine Feasibility Research, June 17, 1994, Amy R. Sheon, MPH, Division of AIDS, NIAID," handout distributed at meeting.

253: The next speaker on the agenda . . . ARAC transcript, 128–139.

254: Six presentations had rushed past . . . Ibid., 145. The transcriptionist noted the time of recess as 12:19 P.M.

254: Even people who disagree . . . Ibid., 146–157.

255: Francis was a hard act to follow . . . Ibid., 157–164 (Dino Dina's remarks) and 164–167 (Anne-Marie Duliege).

255: Without taking a beat . . . Ibid., 167.

256: Burke, who was still . . . Ibid., 167–186; Green, "Who Put the Lid on gp120?" 56.

257: The minute that Haase called for . . . ARAC transcript, 186–227; Green, "Who Put the Lid on gp120?" 56–57.

258: During a short afternoon break . . . ARAC transcript, 227–255.

258: Finally, when the clock . . . Ibid., 255–256.

258: Haase's first efforts to draft . . . Ibid., 256–271.

258: "Do I hear a call to vote?" . . . Ibid., 271–287.

258: In the end, the proposed . . . Ibid., 281.

259: "What I am going to do now . . . Ibid., 281–292 (adjournment time noted on p. 292).

259: As soon as it was over . . . Lawrence K. Altman, "Panel Rejects Wider Testing to Develop AIDS Vaccine," *New York Times*, June 18, 1994.

259: The minute the meeting was . . . Green, "Who Put the Lid on gp120?" 57; author interviews.

10. THE BIG CHILL

PAGE

265: Her main ally . . . See Chapter 6 for a discussion of clade E and Kathy's commitment to making a vaccine for Thailand.

266: In late 1992, NIH officials . . . Jon Cohen, "Trials Set in High-Risk Populations," *Science*, December 11, 1992 (258):1729. The first Phase I test of ALVAC vCP125 and Chiron Biocine's SF2 gp120 was AVEG 012A, a clinical trial that began in May 1993.

267: After all, corporate executives . . . This story is told in Chapter 2.

269: WHO convened vaccine experts . . . The WHO Global Programme on AIDS, "Meeting on Scientific and Public Health Rationale for HIV Vaccine Efficacy Trials," Geneva, October 13–14, 1994, list of participants.

269: After two days of discussion . . . WHO Global Programme on AIDS, "Expert Group Concludes Vaccine Trials Can Go Forward," note to correspondents, October 14, 1994.

269: Genentech's total revenues . . . "Genentech Annual Report, 1996," online version, chart showing revenues for 1994, 1995, 1996.

271: Leading the study . . . Corey chaired AVEG 022, which began enrolling volunteers in May 1995.

271: In addition to research . . . Biocine's vaccines included DPT (diphtheria/pertussis/tetanus), MMR (measles/mumps/rubella), cholera, polio, influenza, meningococcus, and a genetically engineered pertussis vaccine called Acelluvax ("Chiron Annual Report, 1994").

274: This 1986 transaction . . . Joan O'C. Hamilton, "Jealousy, Money, Power: A Biotech Marriage Breaks Up," *Business Week,* July 21, 1986.

274: Three years later . . . Nowinski's new company, ICOS, got off to a running start. He raised $33 million, at the time a record for a biotech start-up, with 10 percent of that coming from Microsoft's Bill Gates. See Greg Heberlein, "Biotech's New ICOS Starts Big," *Seattle Times,* July 3, 1990; author interviews.

274: By 1991, he was no longer . . . Karen Milburn, "Management Shakeup at Biotech Star ICOS," *Seattle Times,* September 28, 1991; author interviews.

274: He had started yet another . . . The company was PathoGenesis Corp.

276: Troy had fallen . . . Leslie Eaton, "Desperate in 1995, a Small City's Fortunes Rebound Sharply," *New York Times,* August 28, 2000; author interviews.

277: The ANRS agreement . . . "Pasteur Mérieux-Connaught Signs a Research Agreement with the ANRS," Canada NewsWire, April 6, 1995.

279: Kathy brought a stack . . . For an update on the dismal prognosis for patients with this type of cancer, see Desmond N. Carney and Heine H. Hansen, "Editorial: Non-Small-Cell Lung Cancer—Stalemate or Progress?" *New England Journal of Medicine,* October 26, 2000 (343):1261–1263.

281: A few months earlier, controversial . . . Lawrence M. Fisher, "Genentech: Survivor Strutting Its Stuff," *New York Times,* October 1, 2000.

281: A short news item . . . "Investors Sought for AIDS Vaccine Trials," *Science,* March 1, 1996 (271):1237.

282: A later article . . . Diane Gershon, "Genentech Sheds gp120 Vaccine," *Nature Medicine* 2 (April 1996):370.

283: For 1996 alone, the death toll . . . WHO/UNAIDS statistics released on November 27, 1996. See Lawrence K. Altman, "U.N. Reports 3 Million New HIV Cases Worldwide for '96," *New York Times,* November 27, 1996.

283: As grim as these numbers were . . . Lawrence K. Altman, "The Doctor's World: Discussing Possible AIDS Cure Raises Hope, Anger and Question: What Exactly

Is Meant by 'Cure'?" *New York Times*, July 16, 1996; Sarah Richardson, "Crushing HIV," *Discover* (January 1997):27. Although the antiviral cocktails penetrated the public consciousness in July, in fact the first positive results had been presented in January 1996, during a smaller retrovirus conference in Washington.

284: They began treatment immediately . . . Christine Gorman, "Man of the Year: The Disease Detective," *Time,* December 30, 1996–January 6, 1997.

284: Ho's presentation touched off . . . Ibid.

284: "The AIDS Dream Team" . . . Anne-Christine D'Adesky, *Out,* February 1997.

284: Eventually the publicity . . . Hillary J. Johnson, "Dr. David Ho and the Lazarus Equation," *Rolling Stone,* March 6, 1997.

284: At the Vancouver conference . . . Stephen Fried, "Cocktail Hour," *Washington Post Magazine,* May 18, 1997; author interviews.

287: Fauci not only said . . . Altman, "The Doctor's World: Combination Strategy Reinvigorates Search for an AIDS Vaccine," *New York Times,* February 26, 1996.

292: On Saturday, November 16 . . . "Kathelyn Sue Steimer, 48, AIDS Researcher," *New York Times,* November 24, 1996.

11. THE VIRUS MUST BE LAUGHING AT US

PAGE

293: The title of this chapter is lifted from a remark made by vaccine researcher James Tartaglia, during a January 2000 interview. Years ago, he expected that developing an AIDS vaccine would be much less complicated—in economic and political terms—that it has turned out to be. Looking back over what's actually happened, Tartaglia said, "The virus is probably laughing at us."

295: In August 1994 . . . John R. Mascola, John G. McNeil, and Donald S. Burke, "AIDS Vaccines: Are We Ready for Human Efficacy Trials?" *Journal of the American Medical Association,* August 10, 1994 (272):488–489.

295: One place he delivered his impassioned . . . WHO Global Programme on AIDS, "Expert Group Concludes Vaccine Trials Can Go Forward," note to correspondents, October 14, 1994; Lawrence K. Altman, "After Setback, First AIDS Vaccine Trials Are Planned; Even a Weak Vaccine Would Help Slow the Epidemic," *New York Times,* November 29, 1994; author interviews.

296: In early 1996, WRAIR and MicroGeneSys . . . Gina Kolata, "Maker of an AIDS Vaccine Says Test Found No Benefit," *New York Times,* April 19, 1996; author interviews.

297: Consider the NIH Office of . . . Jon Cohen, "New AIDS Chief Takes Charge," *Science,* March 11, 1994 (263):1364.

298: In order to change the status quo . . . National Institutes of Health, "NIH Plan to Implement Recommendations of the NIH AIDS Research Program Evaluation Task Force," August 1997; author interviews.

298: More than 100 scientists . . . Levine Committee, "Report of the NIH AIDS Research Program Evaluation Working Group," March 13, 1996; author interviews.

298: John Moore, for example . . . Levine Committee, "Vaccine Research and Development Area Review Panel, Findings and Recommendations," March 13, 1996; Anne-Christine D'Adesky, "The AIDS Dream Team," *Out* 70 (February 1997); author interviews.

298: For nine months . . . Levine Committee, "Vaccine ARP," 7 and Appendix A.

299: The vaccine ARP echoed . . . Ibid., 2.

299: The propagation of new . . . Ibid., 3–4.

299: "The entire vaccine research effort . . . Levine Committee, "Working Group Report," 10; author interviews.

300: In a memo to Killen, Pat Fast . . . Patricia Fast, "Note to Jack Killen," n.d., probably March–April 1995; author interviews.

300: Less than one month . . . Stu Borman, "Criteria May Speed AIDS Vaccine Development," *Chemical and Engineering News,* February 19, 1996:9; author interviews.

300: When Tony Fauci ruminates aloud . . . Anthony Fauci, "The AIDS Paradigm: Scientific and Policy Lessons for the 21st Century," lecture at Annual Meeting of the Institute of Human Virology, August 30, 1999.

302: Most Western doctors . . . David D. Celentano et al., "Preventive Intervention to Reduce Sexually Transmitted Infections: A Field Trial in the Royal Thai Army," *Archives of Internal Medicine* 160 (4) (February 28, 2000):535–540; author interviews.

303: The trouble with success . . . Beyrer, *War in the Blood,* 119–123.

303: After long negotiations . . . AFRIMS-RIHES Vaccine Evaluation Group (ARVEG), "ARVEG V6P17 Protocol: Recruitment and Safety Data," n.d., probably late 1996–early 1997.

304: By February 1995, Burke . . . Gilbert Lewthwaite, "Dozens of 'Nondefense' Pentagon Programs Fall Under Scrutiny," *Baltimore Sun,* February 3, 1995; author interviews.

305: Although Burke says he didn't . . . Dana Priest, "'Non-Defense' Projects Targeted; Pentagon Supports Some, Not All, Against GOP Attack," *Washington Post,* February 10, 1995; White House Press Office, "Text of a Letter from White House Chief of Staff Leon Panetta to Defense Secretary William J. Perry," February 10, 1995; author interviews.

308: Drug cocktails had since become . . . David Sanford, "Back to the Future: One Man's AIDS Tale Shows How Quickly Epidemic Has Turned," *Wall Street Journal,* November 8, 1996; Andrew Sullivan, "When Plagues End: Notes on the Twilight of an Epidemic," *New York Times Magazine,* November 10, 1996; author interviews.

309: Bill Paul used the December 3 . . . Steve Sternberg, "A Shot in the Dark: Prototypes Attack Virus on All Fronts," *USA Today,* May 22, 1997; author interviews.

309: In contrast, there was intense media . . . Warren Leary, "Nobel Laureate to Head Panel Pushing for AIDS Vaccine," *New York Times*, December 13, 1996; "MIT Laureate to Head AIDS Vaccine Search," Reuters, *Boston Globe*, December 13, 1996; Gary Taubes, "Busting the Fraud-Busters," *Discover* (January 1997):76; Anne-Christine D'Adesky, "Dr. Baltimore's Vaccine Dreams," *Out* (April 1997):33.

310: The Levine report recommended . . . Levine Committee, "Working Group Report," 10; AIDS Vaccine Research Committee roster, fall 1997; author interviews.

311: The second began shortly after . . . AIDS Vaccine Evaluation Group, "Outline of Protocol 202"; author interviews.

311: "A newcomer to vaccine . . . Bruce G. Weniger and Max Essex, "Clearing the Way for an AIDS Vaccine," *New York Times*, January 4, 1997.

312: He and several Thai collaborators . . . Bruce Weniger, K. Limpakarnjanarat, K. Ungchusak, "The Epidemiology of HIV Infection and AIDS in Thailand," *AIDS* 5 (1991):S71–S85; author interviews.

312: Max Essex was a retrovirologist . . . Garrett, *The Coming Plague*, 353–354, 358, 371–374, 587; author interviews.

313: NIH Director Varmus . . . Letters to the editor from Harold Varmus and Steven S. Witkin, *New York Times*, January 11, 1997.

313: In a January 22 interview . . . David Baltimore, interviewed by Christopher Lydon on *The Connection*, WBUR, January 22, 1997, author's notes.

314: This NCVDG meeting was different . . . Conference on Advances in AIDS Vaccine Development, Ninth Annual Meeting of the NCVDG for AIDS, May 4–7, 1997, program book; author's notes.

315: He told the NCVDG meeting . . . Anthony Fauci, "Introductory Remarks, NCVDG, May 4, 1997," author's transcript.

316: When David Baltimore stepped up . . . David Baltimore, "Fighting with HIV While It Fights Back," presentation at NCVDG, May 4, 1997, author's transcript; author notes and interviews.

317: Ten days later, headlines . . . Richard Saltus, "MIT Laureate to Lead Caltech," *Boston Globe*, May 14, 1997.

318: On the morning of May 18, 1997 . . . William J. Clinton, "Commencement Address at Morgan State University," White House Press Office, May 18, 1997.

318: Critics were standing by . . . Alison Mitchell, "Clinton Calls for AIDS Vaccine as Goal," *New York Times*, May 19, 1997; Sonya Ross, "Clinton Targets an AIDS Vaccine Date," *Boston Globe*, May 19, 1997.

318: One week after the Morgan State speech . . . Thomas H. Maugh, Marlene Cimons, and John-Thor Dahlburg, "Can Clinton Kick Quest for AIDS Vaccine into Gear?" *Los Angeles Times*, May 25, 1997.

319: An editorial in the *San Francisco Chronicle* . . . "Editorial: A Vaccine for AIDS—a New Goal for Science," and Charles Petit, "AIDS Experts Dubious About 10-Year Target," *San Francisco Chronicle*, May 20, 1997.

320: They had come for a workshop . . . "Workshop on Cellular and Humoral Immunity," Chiang Mai, Thailand, October 20–22, 1997, agenda and directory of participants; author notes.

320: The festive atmosphere changed . . . Author's notes on presentations by Sudapol Issaragrisil, of Mahidol University, and Thira Sirisanthana, Chiang Mai University.

322: John McNeil had been working . . . John McNeil' slide, "U.S. Department of Defense HIV Vaccine Development: Thailand"; author notes and interviews.

322: A strong supporter of the army's efforts . . . Peggy Johnston, "HIV Vaccines—International Efforts," presentation at Chiang Mai workshop, author's notes; author interviews.

324: On May 18, 1998 . . . AIDS Vaccine Advocacy Coalition, *9 Years and Counting: Will We Have an AIDS Vaccine by 2007?"* (San Francisco: AVAC, May 1998); author interviews.

325: His illustrated lecture laid out . . . Jack Killen's handouts distributed at AIDS Research Advisory Committee meeting, June 2, 1998, Bethesda. Nussbaum's *Good Intentions* is a critical history of AIDS drug testing.

325: In 1998, Baltimore not only . . . M.A.J. McKenna, "AIDS Scientists Regroup," *Atlanta Journal and Constitution,* February 1, 1998.

12. THE NEXT GENERATION

328: At Merck, Margaret Liu . . . Lisa Seacrist, "A Dose of DNA to Fight Influenza Virus," *Science News,* June 3, 1995 (343); author interviews.

329: He and Apollon were now . . . "$4.2 Million for Apollon AIDS Vaccine," SCRIP No. 1967, October 18, 1994, 16; author interviews.

330: By the summer of 1995 . . . Lisa Bain, "Therapeutic AIDS Vaccine Vlinical Trial Begins at Penn," press release from University of Pennsylvania Medical Center, June 16, 1995; author interviews.

331: In the final months of the year . . . Karen Bernstein, "1995 Was a Very Fine Year: Performance Pays Off," *BioCentury,* January 2, 1996; author interviews.

331: Frustrated by the NIH peer-review system . . . The project title was "Attenuated VEE Vaccine Vectors Expressing HIV Immunogens," September 1, 1994–August 31, 1999.

332: The beauty of VEE was . . . Nancy Davis, K. Brown, and Robert Johnston, "A Viral Vaccine Vector That Expresses Foreign Genes in Lymph Nodes and Protects Against Mucosal Challenge," *Journal of Virology* 70:3781–3787; author interviews.

333: They had made two different VEE . . . Nancy Davis et al., "Attenuating Mutations in the E2 Glycoprotein Gene of Venezuelan Equine Encephalitis Virus: Construction of Single and Multiple Mutants in a Full-Length cDNA Clone," *Virology* 183

(1991):20–31; P. Pushko et al., "Replicon-Helper Systems from Attenuated Venezuelan Equine Encephalitis Virus: Expression of Heterologous Genes In Vitro and Immunization Against Heterologous Pathogens In Vivo," *Virology* 239 (1997):389–401; author interviews.

334: By April 1995, Ian knew ... Nancy Davis, personal communications; author interviews.

335: Her team made a tremendous ... John J. Donnelly et al., "Preclinical Efficacy of a Prototype DNA Vaccine: Enhanced Protection Against Antigenic Drift in Influenza Virus," *Nature Medicine* 1 (6) (June 1995):583–587.

335: Although Emini was not actively ... Emilio A. Emini, "Hurdles in the Path to an HIV-1 Vaccine," *Scientific American Science and Medicine* (May–June 1995):38–47.

336: This was a milestone ... John Travis, "DNA Vaccine Set to Tackle HIV Infection," *Science News*, February 17, 1996:100; author interviews.

337: Soon after the FDA approved ... NIAID began recruiting volunteers for study number 96-1-0050 in mid-March 1997.

337: In particular, he cited ... Jean Boyer et al., "Protection of Chimpanzees from High-Dose Heterologous HIV-1 Challenge by DNA Vaccination," *Nature Medicine* 3 (5) (May 1997):1–7.

338: Fauci's comments reflected this ... Lawrence K. Altman, "Vaccine Protects Two Chimps from AIDS," *New York Times*, April 30, 1997; author interviews.

338: Chiron Biocine had become ... Diane Gershon, "Chiron Buys Hoechst Vaccine Interest," *Nature Medicine* 2 (4) (April 1996).

342: Bob was able to engage ... David Strow, "AlphaVax Touts New Model for Biotech Firms," *Triangle Business Journal*, February 27, 1998. The attorney was Fred Hutchinson and the launch specialist was Sherry Reynolds, who also served as the company's first president.

343: On May 21, 1997, R. Gordon Douglas ... "May 21, 1997, Remarks of R. Gordon Douglas, MD, President, Merck Vaccines, Merck & Co., Inc., Congressional Task Force on International HIV/AIDS, Briefing on AIDS Vaccines," Merck Public Affairs.

343: Douglas was the very model ... R. Gordon Douglas biographical sketch, Merck Public Affairs, 1997.

343: Even politicians with ... Larry Armstrong, "Besting AIDS and the Drug Giants," *Business Week*, June 9, 1997.

344: And when Mary Lou Clements-Mann ... Clements-Mann presented results from the Merck flu vaccine trial at an American Society for Virology meeting in Vancouver, B.C., in July 1997.

345: She and other researchers ... Gary Taubes, "Immunology: Salvation in a Snippet of DNA?" *Science*, December 5, 1997; David Gold and Sam Avrett, "HIV DNA Vaccines Move Slowly into Clinical Trials," *IAVI Report* 3 (July–September 1998):1; author interviews.

346: Like the view, Margaret's professional horizons ... "An Interview with Margaret Liu," *IAVI Report* 3 (July–September 1998):1; author interviews.

348: Within months, however, the St. Louis manufacturing facility . . . "Chiron Announces Plans to Close St. Louis, Missouri, Manufacturing Site," Chiron press release, March 5, 1998; author interviews.

348: On the research front . . . AIDS Vaccine Advocacy Coalition, *8 Years and Counting* (Washington, DC: AVAC, May 1999), 39; author interviews.

349: They had periodic infusions . . . "Price Waterhouse LLP Venture Capital Survey, Second Quarter 1996," published August 19, 1996, *Mercury Center-San Jose Mercury News.*

349: Grasping at straws . . . "Apollon, Inc. Is Another Early-Stage Biotech Company Jumping on the IPO Bandwagon . . . " *Genetic Engineering News*, November 1, 1997:25; "Apollon Will Offer 2.5 Mil Shares, with Proceeds Being Used for Research and Development," *Going Public: The IPO Reporter*, November 24, 1997 (21):10; author interviews.

349: Eventually, in May 1998 . . . "American Home Products Buys Biotechnology Concern," Bloomberg News, *New York Times*, May 12, 1998; author interviews.

350: The Thai component . . . "The Progress of Phase I, II and III Clinical Trials of Candidate HIV Vaccines in Thailand as of February 9, 1999," prepared by Vipa Thiamchai, AIDS Vaccine Coordinating Unit, AIDS Division, CDC, MOPH, Thailand; author interviews..

352: The reckoning began . . . Agenda for Thai HIV Vaccine Scientific Subcommittee meeting, February 11–13, 1998, Siam City; author interviews.

353: Back in North Carolina . . . David Ranii, "Company Sets Sights on Vaccines," *Raleigh News and Observer*, January 22, 1998; author interviews.

355: Fortunately, Bob came up with . . . Robert Olmsted's curriculum vitae, AlphaVax biographic sketch; author interviews.

355: Monkeys were immunized . . . M. Hevey et al., "Marburg Virus Vaccines Based upon Alphavirus Replicons Protect Guinea Pigs and Nonhuman Primates," *Virology* 251 (1998):28–37.

13. THE CATBIRD SEAT

PAGE

362: This happened with oral contraceptives . . . Loretta McLaughlin, *The Pill, John Rock, and the Church: The Biography of a Revolution* (Boston: Little, Brown and Company, 1982). In Puerto Rico, there were religious and economic barriers to the sale of birth control pills in the country where the first large field studies had been carried out. Like AIDS, contraception was a medical issue complicated by moral attitudes.

362: In 1996, one of these . . . Timothy D. Mastro and Isabelle de Vincenzi, "Probabilities of Sexual HIV-1 Transmission," *AIDS* 10 (1996):S75–S82.

363:   In early 1997, the vaccine world . . . Jon Cohen, "Looking for Leads in HIV's Battle with Immune System," *Science*, May 23, 1997 (276):1196–1197.

364:   Ho and Wolinsky . . . Steven M. Wolinsky and David D. Ho, letter to Praphan Phanuphak, dated April 4, 1997, with transmittal memo from Praphan to Dr. Kachit Choopanya, deputy governor of Bankok, dated April 18, 1997.

364:   In a speech during a medical conference . . . Aphaluck Bhatiasevi, "Researcher Warns over Vaccine Trials," *Bangkok Post*, May 17, 1997.

365:   In July 1997, the panel . . . Barry R. Bloom and José Esparza, letter to Professor Natth Bhamarapravati, dated July 28, 1997, with comments from the thirteen panelists attached.

368:   By the end of the day . . . Lawrence K. Altman, "FDA Authorizes First Full Testing for HIV Vaccine. Results Due in 4 Years. Experiment Will Be Conducted on Volunteers in Thailand and in North America," *New York Times*, June 4, 1998.

370:   These trials had been conducted . . . This debate was kicked off by two articles in a single prestigious journal, but soon spread. Marcia Angell, "The Ethics of Clinical Research in the Third World," *New England Journal of Medicine*, September 18, 1997 (337):847–849. Angell, acting editor of *NEJM* at the time, compared placebo-controlled studies to the infamous Tuskegee Study of Untreated Syphilis, sponsored by the U.S. Public Health Service from 1932 to 1972, in which impoverished African-American men with syphilis were observed to determine the "natural history" of the disease, even after penicillin had proved effective and had become widely available. A second article accused the WHO, NIH, and CDC of violating their own regulations and ethics codes. See Peter Lurie and Sidney M. Wolfe, "Unethical Trials of Interventions to Reduce Perinatal Transmission of the Human Immunodeficiency Virus in Developing Countries," *NEJM* September 18, 1997 (337):853–856.

Media coverage of this debate was intense. For example, see Sheryl Gay Stolberg, "U.S. AIDS Research in Poor Nations Raises an Outcry. Some Call It Unethical. Comparisons with a Syphilis Study Arise Because Some Do Not Get Therapy," *New York Times*, September 18, 1997. Two days later, a rebuttal appeared in the *Times* Op-Ed section: Joseph Saba and Arthur Ammann, "A Cultural Divide on AIDS Research: American Values, African Realities," *New York Times*, September 20, 1997. The authors, a research specialist for the UNAIDS and the president of the American Foundation for AIDS Research, denounced the comparison with Tuskegee as "inflammatory and wrong" and said the *NEJM* articles demonstrated "a lack of understanding of the medical needs of developing countries."

Other big names weighed in as well. The October 2, 1997, *New England Journal of Medicine* carried a letter from Harold Varmus, director of NIH, and David Satcher, director of CDC, also charging that comparisons with the Tuskegee study were unwarranted. They emphasized that host-country scientists had helped design the AIDS studies and that government authorities had signed off on them in advance. Varmus and Satcher quoted the chairman of the AIDS Research Committee in one of the study countries, who wrote: "These are Ugandan studies conducted by Ugandan investigators on Ugandans. It is not NIH . . . but Ugandans conducting their study on their people for the good of their people." See Harold Varmus and David Satcher, "Ethical Complexities of Conducting Research in Developing Countries," *New England Journal of Medicine*, October 2, 1997 (337):1003–1005.

The fallout from the debate was considerable. David Ho and Catherine Wilfert, the journal's chief advisers on AIDS, resigned from the *NEJM* board in protest against Angell's editorial. Dr. Wilfert called the September editorial "bad policy" and "a grievous misuse of the journal's power." See Lawrence K. Altman, "AIDS Experts Leave Journal After Studies Are Criticized," *New York Times*, October 15, 1997. The following February, CDC suspended the placebo arm of the maternal-infant transmission study that had caused all the uproar. See Editor's Note in correspondence section, *New England Journal of Medicine*, March 19, 1998 (338):841.

370: He believed this could be accomplished . . . Francis summarized these standards at the June 6, 1997, meeting of the FDA Advisory Committee on Vaccines and Related Biological Products. They are expressed in the Declaration of Helsinki, issued in 1964 by the World Medical Association, which outlines the conduct that should guide human experimentation. It states that the well-being of subjects should be the first priority (not the needs of science or society), that subjects give their informed consent of their own free will, that all subjects be assured of the best proven tests and treatments, and that placebos are permissible only when no proven test or therapy exists (World Medical Association Declaration of Helsinki, adopted by the Eighteenth World Medical Assembly, Helsinki, 1964; revision adopted by the Forty-eighth World Medical Assembly, Republic of South Africa, 1996).

375: Inside this issue of the journal . . . Moises Agosto et al., letter to the editor, *Science*, May 8, 1998 (280):803

375: Mann was famous . . . Meredith Wadman, "Ex-UN AIDS Chief Is Blasted for Remarks on Vaccine Strategy," *Nature*, April 9, 1998 (392):527–528. Author's notes on President's Council on HIV and AIDS meeting, March 15, 1998, Washington, DC.

375: This impression was reinforced . . . Jean-Paul Levy, letter to the editor, *Science*, May 8, 1998 (280):803.

377: Although he doubted . . . Altman, "FDA Authorizes First Full Testing for HIV Vaccine"; Ralph T. King, "FDA Allows Large-Scale Trial of AIDS Vaccine," *Wall Street Journal*, June 3, 1998.

378: "But we're not going to . . . Huntly Collins, "Trials of AIDS Vaccine Get Started in Phila. It's the First Vaccine to Undergo Large-Scale Testing. Researchers Don't Give It Much Chance," *Philadelphia Inquirer*, June 24, 1998.

378: Every reporter's Rolodex . . . Ibid.; Ann Schrader, "Major Test Next for HIV Vaccine. Denver to Take Part in Trial of Inoculation That Has Its Skeptics," *Denver Post*, June 3, 1998; Maggie Fox, "AIDS Vaccine Goes into Final Trials in People," Reuters, June 3, 1998; Rick Weiss, "Large-Scale Test of AIDS Vaccine Set," *Washington Post*, June 4, 1998.

386: So even though the overall . . . Author interviews.

387: More than 95 percent . . . Author interviews.

388: These safeguards . . . VaxGen and Bangkok Vaccine Evaluation Group, "World's First Large-Scale Trial for Preventive HIV Vaccine Enrolled in Developing Country," joint press release, August 31, 2000.

388: Another volunteer . . . Kavitha Rao, "A large HIV-Vaccine Trial in Thailand Presents Ethical Dilemmas," *AsiaWeek*, May 7, 1999, online version.

390: The Gates Foundation windfall . . . By 2000, the Bill and Melinda Gates Foundation had become the world's biggest investor in vaccines for the developing world, donating $750 million to provide childhood vaccines to the poorest nations on earth. In 2001, the foundation pledged another $100 million to IAVI over five years. This will enable IAVI to move three experimental vaccines into clinical trials and to fund preclinical development for several others.

390: When the IPO was . . . Edward Iwata, "Net IPOs Ride a Bay Area Wave," *San Francisco Examiner*, July 4, 1999.

395: Even as the party goers . . . Brian Deer, "His Vaccine Could Go into Millions of People. But It Could Be One of Medicine's Greatest Mistakes," *Sunday Times* (London), October 3, 1999.

395: The editors of *Nature* . . . William E. Schmidt, "British Paper and Science Journal Clash on AIDS," *New York Times*, December 10, 1993.

GLOSSARY

adjuvant: a substance sometimes included in a vaccine to boost the immune system's response to the vaccine.

adverse event: in a clinical trial, an unwanted effect detected in participants. The term is used whether or not the effect can be attributed to the vaccine under study.

adverse reaction (side effect): in a clinical trial, an unwanted side effect caused by the study vaccine.

AIDS (acquired immunodeficiency syndrome): the late stage of HIV disease, characterized by a deterioration of the immune system and a susceptibility to a range of opportunistic infections and cancers.

AIDSVAX™: trade name for genetically engineered gp120 vaccines that originated at Genentech, then were developed by the spin-off company, VaxGen. There are two versions, a bivalent B/B being tested in the United States, and a B/E version being tried in Thailand.

allergy: immune reactions to a non-disease-causing antigen. Allergic symptoms can range from relatively mild (e.g., sneezing when exposed to pollen) to moderate (e.g., blistering rash from contact dermatitis) to severe (e.g., difficulty breathing in food or drug allergy). A life-threatening allergic reaction, called anaphylaxis, causes respiratory distress, circulatory collapse, and death if not treated promptly.

ALVAC-HIV™: a genetically engineered HIV vaccine composed of a live, weakened canarypox virus (ALVAC™), into which parts of genes for noninfectious components of HIV have been inserted. When ALVAC™ infects a human cell, the inserted HIV genes direct the cell to make HIV proteins. These proteins are presented on the cell surface, where they provoke the immune system to mount an immune response to HIV. ALVAC™ can infect but not grow in human cells, an important safety feature. (See also canarypox.)

amino acid: any of the twenty-six chemical building blocks of proteins.

anamnestic response: literally means "does not forget." Used to refer to immunologic memory, in which immune response is substantially stronger when it encounters an antigen for the second (or third, etc.) time. (See also memory cells.)

anion: an atom or molecule that is negatively charged.

antibody: a protein in blood or other body fluids that binds to specific antigens on harmful microorganisms and toxins and helps destroy them. Antibodies, also called immunoglobulins, are produced by B lymphocytes when antigens are detected. Each specific antibody binds only to the specific antigen that stimulated its production. (See also antigen; immunoglobulin; binding antibody; enhancing antibody; functional antibody; neutralizing antibody.)

antibody-mediated immunity: see humoral immunity.

antigen: any substance that stimulates the immune system to produce antibodies. Antigens are often foreign substances such as invading bacteria or viruses. (See also immunogen.)

antigen-presenting cell (APC): B cell, macrophage, dendritic cell, or other cell that ingests foreign bodies such as viruses and displays the resulting antigen fragments on its surface, where they attract and activate helper T cells that respond specifically to that antigen. (See also dendritic cell; macrophage.)

anti-inflammatory drug: a drug that suppresses inflammation (tissue damage caused by an immune response); includes aspirin, steroids, and nonsteroidal anti-inflammatory drugs (NSAIDS) such as ibuprofen.

anti-microbial drug: a drug that kills microorganisms or stops their multiplication; includes antibiotics for bacterial infections, antivirals for virus infections, and antimycotics for fungus infections.

apoptosis: cellular suicide, also known as programmed cell death. A possible mechanism used by HIV to suppress the immune system. HIV may induce apoptosis both in HIV-infected and uninfected cells of the immune system.

arm: a group of participants in a clinical trial, all of whom receive the same treatment, intervention, or placebo. The other arm(s) receive(s) a different treatment.

ARV (AIDS-related virus): the name given to the AIDS virus by Jay Levy; later designated HIV.

assay: a lab test to determine the amount of a particular substance in a mixture, such as the number of T4 cells or HIV viruses in a blood sample.

attenuated: weakened. Attenuated viruses are used as vaccines when they can stimulate a strong immune response without causing disease. Examples of attenuated virus products include the oral polio vaccine and injected vaccines for measles, mumps, and rubella.

autoimmunity: a misguided immune response directed toward the body's own cells. In HIV vaccination, autoimmunity could theoretically result from immunization.

autologous: of the same biological origin.

B lymphocyte (B cell): one of the two major classes of lymphocytes, B lymphocytes are white blood cells of the immune system that are derived from the bone marrow and spleen. B cells develop into plasma cells, which produce antibodies.

baculovirus: an insect virus used in the production of subunit vaccines. By splicing genetic material from HIV into the baculovirus genome, then combining this construct with insect cells, mass quantities of HIV protein encoded by the genetic insertion can be produced. MicroGeneSys gp160 vaccine was made in this manner. (See also expression system.)

basic science: research that focuses on how an organism or biological process works, as opposed to clinical science, which is directed toward prevention and treatment of a disease.

baseline: the time when measurements are taken just before the intervention takes place in a clinical trial. Measurements taken at later times may be compared with baseline values to assess the impact of the intervention.

binding antibody: an antibody that attaches to some part of HIV or another pathogen. Binding antibodies may or may not lead to the killing of the virus.

biomedical: the application of the natural sciences (biology, biochemistry, etc.) to the study of medicine.

biotechnology: the commercialization of molecular biology that began in the 1970s. Biotech firms use genetic engineering and similar techniques to manufacture products such as laboratory assays, therapeutic drugs, and vaccines.

blind study: a clinical trial in which participants do not know whether they are in the experimental or control arm of the study. (See also double-blind study.)

booster: a second or later vaccine dose given after the primary dose(s) to increase the immune response to the original vaccine antigen(s). The vaccine given as the booster dose may or may not be the same as the primary vaccine. (See also prime-boost.)

bDNA (branched DNA) assay: laboratory test for measuring the amount of virus in blood plasma. The test detects an amplified luminescent signal whose brightness depends on the amount of viral RNA present.

breakthrough infection: an infection, with the pathogen that a vaccine is intended to prevent, that occurs in a volunteer during the course of a vaccine trial. Such an infection is caused by exposure to the infectious agent and may occur before or after the vaccine has taken effect or all doses have been given.

canarypox: a virus that infects birds and is used as a live vector for HIV vaccines. It can carry a large quantity of foreign genes. Canarypox virus cannot grow in human cells, an important safety feature. (See also ALVAC-HIV™; vector.)

capsid: the simple protein coat of a virus. Some viruses have an additional outer layer called an envelope.

carriers: individuals who are infected with HIV but have no symptoms.

case definition: an arbitrary list of medical criteria used by epidemiologists for surveillance or reporting purposes; not necessarily the same as the clinical criteria that a physician would use to diagnose an individual patient.

CAT gene marker: used in laboratory experiments, this gene codes for chloramphenicol acetyltransferase, a substance that is easily detectable with exposure to low-level radioactivity.

cation: an atom or molecule that is positively charged.

CD: abbreviation for "cluster of differentiation," referring to cell surface molecules that are used to identify stages of maturity of immune cells, for example, CD4 T cells.

CD4 T lymphocyte: immune cell that carries a marker on its surface known as "cluster of differentiation 4" (CD4). These cells are the primary targets of HIV. Also known as helper T cells, CD4 T cells help orchestrate the immune response, including antibody responses as well as killer T cell responses. (See also T cell.)

CD8 T lymphocyte: immune cell that carries the "cluster of differentiation 8" (CD8) marker. CD8 T cells may be cytotoxic T lymphocytes or suppressor T cells. (See also cytotoxic T lymphocyte [CTL]; T cell.)

cell line: population of cells capable of dividing indefinitely in culture.

cell-mediated immunity (cellular immunity): the immune response coordinated by helper T cells and CTLs. This branch of the immune system targets cells infected with microorganisms such as viruses, fungi, and certain bacteria.

challenge: in vaccine experiments, the deliberate exposure of an immunized animal to the infectious agent. Challenge experiments are never done in human HIV vaccine research.

centrifuge (ultracentrifuge): a lab apparatus that spins at high speed and separates the components in a vial of blood (or other liquid) into different layers.

CHO (Chinese hamster ovary) cell: a cell used as a "factory" in genetic engineering to make certain subunit vaccines. CHO cells are derived from mammals and are advantageous because they add carbohydrates (a sugar coat) to the protein, much like naturally infected human cells do. (See also expression system.)

clade: also called a subtype. A group of related HIV isolates classified according to their degree of genetic similarity (such as of their envelope proteins). There are currently two groups of HIV-1 isolates, M and O. M consists of at least nine clades, A through I. Group O may consist of a similar number of clades. (See also isolate.)

clinical trial: testing a vaccine in humans. (See Phase I vaccine trial; Phase II vaccine trial; Phase III vaccine trial.)

clone: a genetic duplicate.

cohort: groups of individuals who share one or more characteristics in a research study and who are followed over time. For example, a vaccine trial might include two cohorts, a group at low risk for HIV and a group at higher risk for HIV.

complement: blood proteins that play an important role in the immune response. Generally, complement proteins amplify the effects of antibodies and inflammation.

complementary nucleotide sequence: two DNA sequences are said to be complementary if they can fit together to form a perfectly paired double helix.

control: in vaccine clinical trials, the control group is given either the standard treatment for the disease (in a therapeutic trial) or an inactive substance called a placebo (in a preventive study). The control group is compared with one or more groups of volunteers given experimental vaccines, so that vaccine effects will be more readily apparent.

core: the protein capsule surrounding a virus's DNA or RNA. In HIV, p55, the precursor molecule to the core, is broken down into the smaller molecules p24, p17, p7 and p6. HIV's core is primarily composed of p24.

correlates of immunity (correlates of protection): the immune responses that must be present to protect an individual from a certain infection. The precise correlates of immunity in HIV transmission are unknown.

culture: to grow microorganisms or cells in a specially prepared substance (the culture medium).

cytokine: a soluble, hormone-like protein produced by white blood cells that acts as a messenger between cells. Cytokines can stimulate or inhibit the growth and activity of various immune cells. Cytokines are essential for a coordinated immune response and can also be used as immunologic adjuvants. HIV replication is regulated by a delicate balance among cytokines.

cytoplasm: the contents of a cell that lie outside the nucleus but within the cell's outer membrane.

cytotoxic T lymphocyte (CTL): immune system cell that can destroy cells infected with viruses, fungi, or certain bacteria. CTLs, also known as killer T cells, carry the CD8 marker. CTLs kill virus-infected cells, whereas antibodies generally target free-floating viruses in the blood. CTL responses are a proposed but unproven correlate of HIV immunity. (See also CD8+ T lymphocyte.)

deletion: elimination of a gene either in nature or in the laboratory.

dendritic cell: immune cell with threadlike tentacles called dendrites used to enmesh antigen, which they present to T cells. Langerhans cells, found in the skin, and follicular dendritic cells, found in lymphoid tissues, are localized types of dendritic cells. (See also antigen-presenting cell.)

DNA (deoxyribonucleic acid): a chain of molecules found within the nucleus of each cell in most animals and plants. DNA carries the genetic information that cells need to reproduce and perform their functions. The DNA molecule has a double-stranded, helical shape.

DNA vaccine (nucleic acid vaccine): direct injection of a genetic material that codes for antigenic proteins, which induces human cells to produce those antigens in order to trigger an appropriate immune response.

domain: a region of a gene or gene product. A neutralizing domain is a specific site on the virus to which a neutralizing antibody is directed.

dose-ranging study: a clinical trial in which two or more doses (starting low and proceeding to higher doses) of a vaccine are tested against each other to determine which works best and has acceptable side effects.

dose-response relationship: the relationship between the size of the dose and the magnitude of the response. In vaccine research, a dose-response effect means that as the dose of the vaccine increases, so does the level of the immune response (antibodies and/or CTL activity).

double-blind study: a clinical trial in which neither the study staff nor the participants know which participants are receiving the experimental vaccine and which are receiving a placebo or another therapy. Double-blind trials are thought to produce objective results, since the outcome is not affected by the expectations of researchers or volunteers.

DSMB (Data and Safety Monitoring Board): a committee of independent clinical research experts who review data while a clinical trial is in progress. The DSMB ensures that participants are not exposed to undue risk and looks for differences between the experimental and control groups. The DSMB can break the code used to "blind" a study, so its members can tell which group received the vaccine and which group did not. The DSMB may recommend that a trial be modified or stopped if there are safety concerns or if the trial objectives have been achieved ahead of schedule.

Escherichia coli: a rod-shaped bacterium that is ubiquitous in the gut of humans and other mammals, widely used in biomedical research.

EBV (Epstein-Barr virus) cell line: a herpes virus; in vaccine research, used to make target cells for CTL assays.

efficacy: in vaccine research, the ability of a vaccine to produce a desired clinical effect, such as protection against a specific infection, at the optimal dosage and schedule in a given population. A vaccine may be tested for efficacy in Phase III trials if it appears to be safe and shows some promise in smaller Phase I and II trials.

electrophoresis: a lab technique in which an electric field is applied to a solution in order to sort proteins or DNA fragments according to size.

ELISA (enzyme-linked immunoabsorbent assay): a blood test that detects antibodies based on a reaction that leads to a detectable color change in the test tube. The HIV ELISA is commonly used as the initial screening test because it is relatively easy and inexpensive to perform. Because the HIV ELISA is designed for optimal sensitivity—that is, it detects all persons with HIV antibodies as well as some who don't have them (false positives)—a positive HIV ELISA test must be confirmed by a second, more specific test such as an HIV Western Blot.

empirical: based on experience or observational information and not necessarily on proven scientific data. In the past, vaccine trials have been performed based exclusively on empirical data and without a full understanding of the disease processes or correlates of immunity.

emulsion: a suspension of droplets of one liquid in another liquid (such as oil and water). The two liquids do not actually combine but are instead suspended within one another.

endpoint: the results of an intervention, such as vaccination, compared across study groups in a clinical trial. In early vaccine trials, common endpoints are safety and specific types and intensities of immune responses (neutralizing antibodies, CTL responses). In an efficacy trial, the endpoint might be protection against infection or protection against disease.

enhancing antibody: a type of binding antibody, detected in the test tube and formed in response to HIV infection, that may enhance the ability of HIV to produce disease. Theoretically, enhancing antibodies could attach to HIV virions and enable macrophages to engulf the viruses. However, instead of being destroyed, the engulfed virus may remain alive within the macrophage, which then can carry the virus to other parts of the body. It is currently unknown whether enhancing antibodies have any effect on the course of HIV infection. Enhancing antibodies can be thought of as the opposite of neutralizing antibodies.

enzyme: a protein produced by cells to accelerate a specific chemical reaction without itself being altered. Enzymes are generally named by adding the suffix "-ase" to the name of the substance on which the enzyme acts (for example, protease is an enzyme that acts on proteins).

env: a gene of HIV that codes for gp160, the precursor molecule that breaks down into the envelope proteins gp120 and gp41. (See also gp.)

envelope: outer surface of a virus, also called the coat. Not all viruses have an envelope. (See also virus; env.)

epidemiology: the study of the frequency and distribution of disease in human populations.

epitope: a specific site on an antigen that stimulates specific immune responses, such as the production of antibodies or activation of immune cells.

expression system: in genetic engineering, the cells into which a gene has been inserted to manufacture desired proteins. Chinese hamster ovary (CHO) cells and baculovirus/insect cells are two expression systems that are used to make recombinant HIV vaccines.

false-negative, false-positive results: erroneous results that arise from two different types of errors in a screening or diagnostic test. A test that is not sensitive enough will yield false-negative results, so that people who really have a condition or trait will escape detection. A test that is not sufficiently specific will produce false-positive results, so that people who do not have a condition or trait will be told that they do.

fatty acids: a compound with a particular chemical structure that is used as a major source of energy during metabolism and as the starting point for the synthesis of other types of lipids.

functional antibody: an antibody that binds to an antigen and has an effect that can be demonstrated in laboratory tests. For example, neutralizing antibodies are functional antibodies that inactivate HIV or prevent it from infecting other cells.

gag: a gene of HIV that codes for p55, the core protein p55 is the precursor of HIV proteins p17, p24, p7 and p6 that form HIV's capsid or core, the inner protein shell surrounding HIV's strands of RNA.

gD: a glycoprotein on the herpes virus.

gene: a region of DNA that controls a distinct hereditary characteristic, which usually corresponds to a single protein.

Genevax™: trade name for DNA vaccines designed by David Weiner at the University of Pennsylvania and licensed to Wyeth-Lederle Vaccines.

genetic code: a set of rules that governs how DNA is translated, by a series of intermediate steps, into proteins.

gene sequence: the exact string of nucleotides that makes up a gene.

genetic engineering: the laboratory technique of recombining genes to produce proteins used as reagents in experiments, or for drugs and vaccines.

genome: the complete set of genes in a cell or organism; the DNA that carries this information.

gp (glycoprotein): a protein molecule that is glycosylated, that is, coated with a carbohydrate, or sugar. The outer coat proteins of HIV are glycoproteins. The number after the gp (e.g., gp160, gp120, gp41) is the molecular weight of the glycoprotein.

gp41: glycoprotein 41. A protein imbedded in the outer envelope of HIV that anchors gp120. gp41 plays a key role in HIV's infection of CD4+ T cells by facilitating the fusion of the viral and cell membranes. Antibodies to gp41 can be detected on a screening HIV ELISA.

gp120: glycoprotein 120. One of the proteins that forms the envelope of HIV. gp120 projects from the surface of HIV and binds to the CD4 molecule on helper T cells. gp120 has been a logical target for experimental HIV vaccines because the outer envelope is the first part of the virus that encounters antibodies.

gp160: glycoprotein 160, a full-length version of HIV envelope proteins gp41 and gp120.

growth factors: an extracellular signaling molecule that stimulates cells to grow or proliferate; most growth factors have other actions as well.

half-life: the time required for half the amount of a substance to be eliminated from the body or to be converted to another substance.

helper T cell: lymphocyte bearing the CD4 marker. Helper T cells are the chief regulatory cells of the immune response. They are responsible for many immune system functions, including turning antibody production on and off, and are the main target of HIV infection. (See also CD4 T lymphocyte.)

hemophilia: a hereditary disorder in which patients bleed excessively because they lack one of several clotting factors, most commonly a substance called factor VIII. Many hemophiliacs were treated with factor VIII distilled from the blood of thousands of donors, which made them extremely vulnerable to HIV infection before it was possible to screen blood for signs of infection. Genetically engineered factor VIII is now used to treat this disease.

hepatitis B: a chronic, untreatable viral infection that gradually destroys liver function, often by causing liver cancer. Hepatitis B can be prevented by immunization.

hepatitis B surface antigen: a genetically engineered copy of this surface protrusion on the hepatitis B virus is used as the antigen in the successful vaccine against this disease.

heterologous: of a different biological origin.

HIV (human immunodeficiency virus): a human retrovirus in the lentivirus family, this RNA virus uses the enzyme reverse transcriptase to integrate its genome into human cells, where it proliferates and kills the cells. It causes progressive immune deficiency, which leads to opportunistic infections and malignancies and eventually to death.

HLA (human leukocyte antigen): two major classes of molecules on cell surfaces.

HLA class I: molecules that exist on all nucleated cells and identify the cell as "self." In addition, if the cell is infected by a virus or other microbe, the cell displays the invader's antigens in combination with the cell's HLA class I molecules. The presence of the foreign peptide antigen with the HLA class I molecule activates CD8-positive CTLs specific for that antigen.

HLA class II: molecules that are found on antigen-presenting cells such as macrophages. These cells process soluble antigens such as toxins or other proteins made by microbes and then display them on their surface as peptide antigens in combination with HLA Class II molecules. Helper T cells specific for these antigens are then able to recognize and respond to the presence of the invading microbe.

homologous: similar in appearance, structure, and usually function. For HIV, the same strain of the virus.

hormone: an extracellular chemical signal that is produced by endocrine glands and acts on target tissues located elsewhere in the body.

host: a plant or animal harboring another organism.

HTLV-III (human T cell leukemia virus III): the name given to the AIDS virus by Robert Gallo, later designated HIV.

human growth factor hormone (hGh): officially known as somatostatin, production of this hormone during childhood governs height. A genetically engineered version of hGh is used to treat hGh deficiency.

humoral immunity: immunity that results from the activity of antibodies in blood and lymphoid tissue.

hypothesis: a tentative statement or supposition, which may then be tested through research.

immortalized cells: a genetically engineered cell line that reproduces indefinitely.

immune complex: the result of a reaction between an antigen and a specific antibody. This combination of antigen bound by antibody may or may not cause adverse effects in a person.

immune deficiency: a breakdown or inability of certain parts of the immune system to function, thus making a person susceptible to diseases that they would not ordinarily develop.

immune response: the body's reaction to the invasion of foreign substances.

immunity: natural or acquired resistance provided by the immune system to a specific disease. Immunity may be partial or complete, specific or nonspecific, long-lasting or temporary.

immunization: the process of inducing immunity by administering an antigen (vaccine) to allow the immune system to prevent infection or illness when it subsequently encounters the infectious agent.

immunoassay: a lab procedure that identifies and measures a biological substance, such as an antigen.

immunogen: a substance capable of provoking an immune response. Also called an antigen.

immunocompetent: capable of developing an immune response; possessing a normal immune system.

immunogenicity: the ability of an antigen or vaccine to stimulate immune responses.

immunoglobulin: a general term for antibodies, which bind to invading organisms, leading to their destruction. There are five classes of immunoglobulins: IgA, IgG, IgM, IgD and IgE. (See also antibody.)

immunology: the branch of medicine dealing with disorders of the immune system.

immunotherapy: a treatment that stimulates or modifies the body's immune response.

incidence: the rate of occurrence of some event, such as the number of individuals who get a disease divided by a total given population per unit of time. (Contrast with prevalence.)

inclusion/exclusion criteria: the medical or social reasons that a person may or may not qualify for participation in a clinical trial. For example, some trials may exclude people with chronic liver disease or with certain drug allergies; others may include only people with a low CD4 T-cell count.

IND (investigational new drug): the status of an experimental drug after the FDA agrees that it can be tested in people.

induce: in research, to bring on an effect.

informed consent: an agreement signed by prospective volunteers for a clinical research trial that indicates their understanding of (1) why the research is being done, (2) what researchers want to accomplish, (3) what will be done during the trial and for how long, (4) what risks are involved, (5) what, if any, benefits can be expected from the trial, (6) what other interventions are available, and (7) the participant's right to leave the trial at any time.

in vitro: an artificial environment created outside a living organism (e.g., in a test tube or culture plate) used in experimental research to study a disease or biologic process.

in vivo: testing within a living organism, e.g., human or animal studies.

interferons: naturally produced glycoproteins that normally fight off viral infections.

interleukin 2 (IL2): a type of cytokine that is produced by lymphocytes and other white blood cells and acts as a cell growth factor.

IRB (Institutional Review Board): a committee of physicians, statisticians, community advocates, and others that reviews clinical-trial protocols before they can be initiated. IRBs ensure that the trial is ethical and that the rights of participants are adequately protected.

isolate: a particular strain of HIV-1 taken from a person.

Kaposi's sarcoma: cancer of the circulatory system; usually found only in people whose immune systems are compromised by diseases such as HIV.

laboratory-adapted: a strain of virus adapted to grow in immortalized cell lines instead of fresh human lymphocytes; often used in research and development of vaccines and laboratory assays.

LAI: an HIV-1 isolate used in HIV vaccine development. LAI is also referred to as IIIB or LAV. LAI belongs to clade B, the subtype to which most HIV-1 found in America and Europe belongs. (See also clade.)

LAV (lymphadenopathy associated virus): the name given to the virus that causes AIDS by Luc Montagnier; later designated HIV.

leukemia: a disease of organs that form blood cells (bone marrow, spleen, etc.) causing white blood cells to increase.

liposomes: artificially made lipids (fatty or waxy molecules) that are used to deliver drugs to a specific organ.

live-vector vaccine: a vaccine that uses a non-disease-causing organism (virus or bacterium) to transport HIV or other foreign genes into the body, thereby stimulating an effective immune response to the foreign products. This type of vaccine is important because it is particularly capable of inducing CTL activity. Examples of organisms used as live vectors in HIV vaccines are vaccinia, canarypox, and Venezuelan equine encephalitis.

lymph glands, lymph nodes: the body's system for filtering dead cells, including viruses and bacteria, from lymphocytes. The lymph system parallels major blood vessels, and nodes are especially plentiful in the neck and groin. Swollen lymph nodes in these areas often indicate chronic infection.

lymphadenopathy: chronically swollen lymph nodes.

lymphocyte: a type of white blood cell produced in the lymphoid organs that is primarily responsible for immune responses. Present in the blood, lymph, and lymphoid tissues. (See also B cell and T cell.)

lymphoid tissue: tonsils, adenoids, lymph nodes, spleen, and other tissues that act as the body's filtering system, trapping invading microorganisms and presenting them to squadrons of immune cells that congregate there.

macrophage: a large immune system cell in the tissues that devours invading pathogens and other intruders. Macrophages stimulate other immune cells by presenting them with small pieces of the invaders. Macrophages can also harbor large quantities of HIV without being killed, acting as reservoirs of the virus.

mammalian cells: cells from mammals.

marker: in immunology, an antigen that is used to identify a cell. In genetics, a gene that coincides with a specific event, such as an allergic reaction to a drug.

mean: the arithmetic average, or the sum of all the values divided by the number of values.

median: the midpoint value obtained by ranking all values from highest to lowest and choosing the value in the middle. The median divides a population into two equal halves.

medium, culture medium: in research, a specially prepared mixture for growing microorganisms or cells.

memory cell: memory cells are a subset of T cells and B cells that have been exposed to specific antigens and can then proliferate (recognize the antigen and divide) more readily when the immune system reencounters the same antigens. (See also anamnestic response.)

MHC (major histocompatibility complex): the gene cluster that controls certain aspects of the immune response. Among the products of these genes are the histocompatibility antigens, such as HLA class I antigens, which are present on every cell with a nucleus and serve as markers to distinguish self from non-self. (See also HLA.)

microbe: any microscopic living organism.

microencapsulated: surrounded by a thin layer of biodegradable substance referred to as a microsphere. A means of protecting a drug or vaccine antigen from rapid breakdown. Microencapsulation may also enhance an antigen's absorption and the immune response to that antigen.

microorganism: a microscopic organism such as bacteria, viruses, fungi, etc

mitogen: an extracellular substance, such as a growth factor or other chemical, that stimulates cell proliferation.

MN: an HIV-1 strain belonging to clade B, the clade to which most HIV-1 found in North America and Europe belong. MN is a "lab-adapted" strain that is grown in immortalized cell lines. It is used in vaccine development. (See also clade.)

molecule: two or more atoms that are bonded together.

molecular biology: study of the biochemistry of cells, especially DNA biochemistry.

monoclonal antibody: custom-made, identical antibody that recognizes only one epitope.

monocyte: a large white blood cell in the blood that ingests microbes or other cells and foreign particles. When a monocyte passes out of the bloodstream and enters tissues, it develops into a macrophage.

monovalent vaccine: a vaccine that contains only one antigen.

mucosal immunity: resistance to infection across the mucous membranes Mucosal immunity depends on immune cells and antibodies present in the linings of reproductive tract, gastrointestinal tract, and other moist surfaces of the body exposed to the outside world.

mutagenesis: deliberately introducing a mutation into genes.

mutation: a change in genetic material. Mutations can occur spontaneously (e.g., from environmental toxins). In research, mutations are often deliberately induced.

naked DNA: DNA that has been spliced into a plasmid, but is not otherwise encapsulated, which is then introduced into animals or humans as a vaccine.

nef: a virulence gene common to SIV and HIV that regulates the production of the virus in host cells. Vaccines made of SIV virions from which nef has been removed (nef-deleted) showed early promise as a vaccine in monkeys, but most of the animals later developed simian AIDS.

neutralizing antibody: an antibody that keeps a virus from infecting a cell, usually by blocking receptors on the cells or the virus.

neutralizing domain: a section of HIV (most commonly on the envelope protein gp120) that elicits antibodies with neutralizing activity. (See also V3 loop.)

NK cell (natural killer cell): a nonspecific lymphocyte. NK cells, like killer T cells, attack and kill cancer cells and cells infected by microorganisms. NK cells are "natural" killers because they do not need to recognize a specific antigen in order to attack and kill.

nucleus: within living cells, the structure where the DNA blueprint for the organism is stored within a protective membrane that walls it off from the cytoplasm.

neurology: the branch of medicine that deals with the brain and nervous system.

neuropeptide: a chemical that aids communication from one nerve cell to another.

neutralize: to make a pathogen or chemical harmless.

nucleic acid: the complex of nucleotides and linking proteins that make up DNA and RNA.

nucleocapsid: the nucleic acid core and protein coat of a virus, taken together.

open-label trial: a clinical trial in which doctors and participants know which vaccine is being administered to all participants.

opportunistic infection: illness due to an organism that usually does not cause disease in a person with a normal immune system. People with advanced HIV infection suffer opportunistic infections of the lungs, brain, eyes, and other organs.

p24: a protein in HIV's inner core. The p24 antigen test looks for the presence of this protein in a person's blood.

parenteral: administered intravenously or by injection. For example, medications or vaccines may be administered by injection into the fatty layer immediately below the skin (subcutaneous) or into the muscle (intramuscular). Medications, but not vaccines, can also be administered into a vein (intravenously).

pathogen: a microorganism that causes disease.

pathogenesis: the origin and development of a disease. More specifically, the way a microbe (bacteria, virus, etc.) causes disease in its host.

PBMC (peripheral blood mononuclear cell): cells in the bloodstream that have one round nucleus, e.g., lymphocytes and monocytes. Usually, the majority of circulating PBMCs are lymphocytes.

PCR (polymerase chain reaction): a sensitive laboratory technique used to detect and repeatedly copy small amounts of RNA or DNA. Some PCR tests can also quantify the amount of RNA or DNA. PCR is used to measure viral load in people infected with HIV.

peptide: a short compound formed by linking two or more amino acids. Proteins are made of multiple peptides.

PHA (phytohemagglutinin): a plant chemical used to stimulate the multiplication (proliferation) of T lymphocytes in laboratory tests.

Phase I vaccine trial: a closely monitored clinical trial of a vaccine conducted in a small number of healthy volunteers. A Phase I study is designed to determine the vaccine's safety in humans, its metabolism and pharmacologic actions, and side effects associated with increasing doses.

Phase II vaccine trial: a controlled clinical study of a vaccine to identify common short-term side effects and risks associated with the vaccine and to collect information on its immunogenicity. Phase II trials enroll some volunteers who have the same characteristics as persons who would be enrolled in an efficacy (Phase III) trial of a vaccine. Phase II trials enroll up to several hundred participants and have more than one arm.

Phase III vaccine trial: a large controlled study to determine the ability of a vaccine to produce a desired clinical effect, such as preventing infection or disease, at an optimally selected dose and schedule. These trials also expand on safety data collected in earlier trials, which will be needed to evaluate the overall benefit-risk relationship of the vaccine and to provide adequate basis for labeling. Phase III trials for treatments may require only several hundred volunteers, whereas efficacy trials for preventive vaccines typically involve thousands of people and last several years.

pharmacokinetics: the processes of absorption, distribution, metabolism, and excretion of a drug or vaccine.

pituitary: a gland at the base of the brain that produces several hormones, including human growth hormone.

placebo: an inactive substance administered to some study participants while others receive the agent under evaluation, to provide a basis for comparing effects.

plasmid: a ring of DNA found in the cytoplasm of bacteria, which replicates independently of the genetic material stored in the nucleus.

pol: a gene of HIV that codes for the enzymes protease, reverse transcriptase, and integrase.

polymerase: an enzyme that stitches together genetic material, either RNA or DNA, from nucleotide building blocks.

polyvalent vaccine: a vaccine that is produced from multiple viral strains or is made to induce immune responses against multiple strains.

prevalence: the number of people in a given population affected with a particular disease or condition at a given time. Prevalence can be thought of as a snapshot of all existing cases at a specified time. (Contrast with incidence.)

preventive HIV vaccine: a vaccine designed to prevent HIV infection or disease.

primary isolate: a strain of virus isolated from the blood of an infected person; grown in the laboratory in fresh human lymphocytes and handled in ways that minimize adaptations or changes.

priming: giving one vaccine first to induce certain immune responses, followed or accompanied by a second type of vaccine. The intent of priming is to induce certain immune responses that will be enhanced by the booster dose(s).

prime-boost: in HIV vaccine research, administration of one type of vaccine, such as a live-vector product, followed or accompanied by a second type, such as a recombinant subunit vaccine. The intent of this combination regimen is to induce different types of immune responses and enhance the overall immune response, a result that may not occur if only one type of vaccine is given for all doses.

propagation deficient: a virus that has been altered so that it cannot copy itself within host cells.

prophylaxis: prevention of disease.

protease inhibitor: one of a class of anti-HIV drugs designed to inhibit the enzyme protease and interfere with virus replication. Protease inhibitors prevent the cleavage of HIV precursor proteins into active proteins, a process that normally occurs when HIV replicates.

protein: compounds of amino acids that are essential to all life.

protocol: the detailed plan for a clinical trial that states the trial's rationale, purpose, vaccine dosages, routes of administration, duration, eligibility criteria, and other aspects of trial design.

pseudovirion: a virus-like particle that resembles a virus but does not contain its genetic information and cannot replicate. In some viral diseases, pseudovirions can interfere with infection by the real infectious virus.

randomized trial: a study in which participants are assigned by chance to one of two or more intervention arms or regimens. Randomization minimizes the differences among groups by equally distributing people with particular characteristics among all the trial arms.

reactogenicity: the capacity of a vaccine to produce adverse reactions.

reagent: any chemical used in a laboratory test or experiment.

receptor: a molecule on the surface of a cell that serves as a recognition or binding site for antigens, antibodies, drugs, vaccines, or other cellular or immunologic components.

recombinant DNA: a technology that involves inserting genetic material from one organism into another organism, so that the recipient will generate large quantities of the protein encoded by the inserted material.

regulatory gene: HIV genes (nef, rev, tat, vpr) that regulate viral replication in infected cells.

replicate: the process of making an exact genetic copy of an organism from DNA or RNA.

replicon: a genetically engineered form of Venezuelan equine encephalitis virus that cannot replicate itself in human cells, because essential structural genes have been removed.

restriction enzyme: an enzyme that cuts DNA at a specific site.

retrovirus: HIV and other viruses that carry their genetic material in the form of RNA, rather than DNA, and use the enzyme reverse transcriptase to transcribe it into DNA. In most animals and plants, DNA is usually made into RNA, hence "retro" is used to indicate the opposite direction.

reverse transcriptase: the enzyme produced by HIV and other retroviruses that enables them to direct a cell to synthesize DNA from their viral RNA.

RNA (ribonucleic acid): a single-stranded molecule composed of chemical building blocks, similar to DNA. The RNA segments in cells represent copies of portions of the DNA sequences in the nucleus. RNA is the sole genetic material of retroviruses.

sequencing: the process of determining the exact order of nucleic acids of a strand of DNA or RNA.

seroconversion: the development of antibodies to a particular antigen. When people develop antibodies to HIV or an experimental HIV vaccine, they "seroconvert" from antibody-negative to antibody-positive. Vaccine-induced seroconversion does not represent an infection. Instead, vaccine-induced seroconversion is an expected response to vaccination that may disappear over time.

serostatus: positive or negative results of a diagnostic test, such as an ELISA, for a specific antibody.

SF2: an HIV-1 strain used in vaccine development. SF2 belongs to clade B, the clade to which most HIV-1 strains found in North America and Europe belong. (See also clade.)

SHIV: genetically engineered hybrid virus having an HIV envelope and an SIV core.

side effect: (see adverse reaction.)

SIV (simian immunodeficiency virus): an HIV-like virus that infects and causes an AIDS-like disease in some species of monkeys.

somatostatin: (see human growth hormone.)

splicing: the process of joining two previously unrelated pieces of DNA or RNA.

staging: a way of tracking the progression of a chronic disease. Criteria for staging are based on the patient's symptoms and results of lab tests.

statistical significance: the probability that an event or difference occurred as the result of the intervention (vaccine) rather than by chance alone. This probability is determined by using statistical tests to evaluate collected data. Guidelines for defining significance are chosen before data collection begins.

supernatant: the liquid portion of a mixture after it has been separated into layers using a centrifuge.

surface antigen, surface protein: a structure on the outside of a virus. Antibodies attach to surface antigens and dispose of the virus.

sterilizing immunity: an immune response that completely prevents the establishment of an infection.

strain: one type of HIV. HIV is so heterogeneous that no two isolates have exactly the same genetic sequence. When HIV is isolated from an individual and worked on in the lab, it is given its own unique identifier, or strain name (i.e, MN, LAI).

stratification: separation of a study cohort into subgroups or strata according to specific characteristics.

subtype: also called a clade. With respect to HIV isolates, a classification scheme based on genetic differences.

subunit vaccine: a vaccine that contains only part of the virus or other microorganism. HIV subunit vaccines produced by genetic engineering are made of only one or two HIV proteins, which have been grown in expression systems.

surrogate marker: an indirect measure of disease progression. In HIV disease, the number of CD4+ T cells per cubic millimeter of blood is often used as a surrogate marker for severity of disease.

syncytia: giant cells formed by the fusion of an HIV-infected blood cell with one or more uninfected ones.

synthesize: artificially building a compound from natural elements.

T cell: white blood cell critical to the immune response. Among these are CD4 T cells and CD8 T cells. The "T" stands for the thymus, where T lymphocytes mature. (See also lymphocyte.)

T lymphocyte proliferation assay: a test used to measure how well memory T cells recall antigens or microbes, such as HIV.

therapeutic HIV vaccine: a vaccine designed to boost the immune response to HIV in a person already infected with the virus. Also referred to as an immunotherapeutic vaccine.

tissue plasminogen activator (tPA): an enzyme that dissolves blood clots.

trials: (see clinical trials.)

ultracentrifuge: (see centrifuge.)

V3 loop: a section of the HIV gp120 surface protein that appears to be important in stimulating neutralizing antibodies but which mutates so easily that antibodies against one strain's V3 loop may do little against other strains (See also neutralizing domain.)

vaccine: a preparation that stimulates an immune response that can prevent an infection or create resistance to an infection.

vaccinia: a cowpox virus, harmless to humans, used in human smallpox vaccines. Employed as a vector in HIV vaccines to transport HIV genes into the body.

vector: in vaccine research, a bacterium, virus, or plasmid that does not cause disease in humans and can be safely used to transport genes coding for antigens into the body to induce an immune response. (See also vaccinia and canarypox.)

Venezuelan equine encephalitis (VEE): a virus native to South America that can infect humans and cause fever and encephalitis. A weakened form of VEE is being tested as a live-vector vaccine against HIV and other infectious diseases. When the virus's structural genes are removed, it cannot replicate in human cells; this form is known as a VEE replicon particle.

viremia: the presence of virus in the bloodstream.

virion: a mature infectious virus particle released by an infected cell.

virulence: the ability of an organism to cause disease.

virus: a microorganism composed of a piece of genetic material—RNA or DNA—surrounded by a protein coat. To replicate, a virus must infect a cell and direct its cellular machinery to produce new viruses.

Western blot: a blood test that uses radioactive antibodies to detect specific proteins from a virus such as HIV. This test is most often used to confirm a positive ELISA.

BIBLIOGRAPHY

BOOKS

Ashe, Penelope. *Naked Came the Stranger.* New York: Lyle Stuart, 1969.

———. *Physicians Desk Reference.* 50th ed. Montvale, NJ: Medical Economics, 1996.

Alberts, Bruce, Dennis Bray, Julian Lewis, Martin Raff, Keith Roberts, and James D. Watson. *The Molecular Biology of the Cell.* 3rd ed. New York: Garland Publishing, 1994.

Baron, Samuel, ed. *Medical Microbiology.* 4th ed. Galveston: University of Texas Medical Branch at Galveston, 1996.

Benjamini, Eli, Geoffrey Sunshine, and Sidney Leskowitz. *Immunology: A Short Course.* 3rd ed. New York: Wiley-Liss, 1996.

Beyrer, Chris. *War in the Blood: Sex, Politics, and AIDS in Southeast Asia.* London and New York: Zed Books, 1998.

Burkett, Elinor. *The Gravest Show on Earth: America in the Age of AIDS.* New York: Picador USA, 1995.

Child, Julia, Louisette Bertholle, and Simone Beck. *Mastering the Art of French Cooking* Vol. 1 (updated). New York: Alfred A. Knopf, 1983.

Epstein, Steven. *Impure Science: AIDS, Activism, and the Politics of Knowledge.* Berkeley: University of California Press, 1997.

Fenner, Frank, D. A. Henderson, I. Arita, J. Jezek, and I. D. Ladnyi. *Smallpox and Its Eradication.* Geneva: World Health Organization, 1988.

Fettner, Ann Giudici. *Viruses: Agents of Change.* New York: McGraw-Hill, 1990.

Fettner, Ann Giudici, and William A. Check. *The Truth About AIDS: Evolution of an Epidemic.* Rev. ed. New York: Holt, Rinehart and Winston, 1985.

Galambos, Louis, with Jane Eliot Sewell. *Networks of Innovation: Vaccine Development at Merck, Sharp & Dohme, and Mulford, 1895–1995.* Cambridge and New York: Cambridge University Press, 1995.

Gallo, Robert. *Virus Hunting: AIDS, Cancer, and the Human Retrovirus: A Story of Scientific Discovery.* New York: Basic Books, 1991.

Garrett, Laurie. *The Coming Plague: Newly Emerging Diseases in a World out of Balance.* New York: Farrar Straus Giroux, 1994.

Grady, Christine. *The Search for an AIDS Vaccine.* Bloomington and Indianapolis: University of Indiana Press, 1995.

Hall, Stephen S. *Invisible Frontiers: The Race to Synthesize a Human Gene.* New York: Atlantic Monthly Press, 1987.

Lasky, Lawrence, ed. *Technological Advances in Virus Development: UCLA Symposia on Molecular and Cellular Biology, New Series.* New York: Alan R. Liss, 1988.

Kaufmann, Stefan H. E., ed. *Concepts in Vaccine Development.* Berlin and New York: Walter deGruyter, 1996.

Kenney, Martin. *Biotechnology: The University-Industrial Complex.* New Haven and London: Yale University Press, 1986.

Koprowski, Hilary, and Michael B.A. Oldstone, eds. *Microbe Hunters: Then and Now.* Bloomington, IL: Medi-Ed Press, 1996.

Mann, Jonathan, and Daniel Tarantola, eds. *AIDS in the World II: Global Dimensions, Social Roots, and Responses.* New York and Oxford: Oxford University Press, 1996.

Marsa, Linda. *Prescription for Profits: How the Pharmaceutical Industry Bankrolled the Unholy Marriage Between Science and Business.* New York: Scribner, 1997.

McLaughlin, Loretta. *The Pill, John Rock, and the Church: The Biography of a Revolution.* Boston: Little, Brown and Company, 1982.

Nussbaum, Bruce. *Good Intentions: How Big Business and the Medical Establishment Are Corrupting the Fight Against AIDS.* New York: Penguin, 1990.

Porter, Roy. *The Greatest Benefit to Mankind: A Medical History of Humanity.* New York and London: W. W. Norton & Company, 1997.

Powell, Michael F., and Mark J. Newman, eds. *Vaccine Design: The Subunit and Adjuvant Approach.* New York: Plenum Press, 1995.

Shilts, Randy. *And the Band Played On: Politics, People, and the AIDS Epidemic.* New York: St. Martin's Press, 1987.

———. *Conduct Unbecoming: Gays and Lesbians in the U.S. Military.* New York: St. Martin's Press, 1993.

Shorter, Edward. *The Health Century: A Companion to the PBS Television Series.* New York: Doubleday, 1987.

Starr, Douglas. *Blood: An Epic History of Medicine and Commerce.* New York: Alfred A. Knopf, 1998.

Starr, Paul. *The Social Transformation of American Medicine.* New York: Basic Books, 1982.

Teitelman, Robert. *Gene Dreams: Wall Street, Academia, and the Rise of Biotechnology.* New York: Basic Books, 1989.

SCIENTIFIC ARTICLES

Ada, G., W. Koff, and J. Petricciani. "The Next Steps in HIV Vaccine Development." *AIDS Research and Human Retroviruses* 8 (8) (1992):1317–1319.

Agosto, Moises, et al. "Letter to the Editor," *Science,* May 8, 1998 (280):803.

Alter, H. J. "Transmission of HTLV-III Infection from Human Plasma to Chimpanzees: An Animal Model for AIDS." *Science,* November 2, 1984 (226):549–552.

Angell, M. "Editorials: The Ethics of Clinical Research in the Third World." *New England Journal of Medicine,* September 18, 1997 (337):847–849.

Barre-Sinoussi, Françoise, J. C. Chermann, F. Rey et al. "Isolation of a T-Lymphotrophic Retrovirus from a Patient at Risk for Acquired Immunodeficiency Syndrome (AIDS)." *Science,* May 20, 1983 (220):868–870.

Berman, P. W., A. M. Gray, T. Wrin, J. C. Vennari, D. J. Eastman, G. R. Nakamura, D. P. Francis, G. Gorse, and D. H. Schwartz. "Genetic and Immunologic Characterization of Viruses Infecting MN-rgp120-Vaccinated Volunteers." *Journal of Infectious Diseases* 176 (August 1997):384–397.

Berman, P. W., T. J. Gregory, L. Riddle, G R. Nakamura, M. A. Champe, J. P. Porter, F. M. Wurm, R. D. Hershberg, E. K. Cobb, and J. W. Eichberg. "Protection of Chimpanzees from Infection by HIV-1 After Vaccination with Recombinant Glycoprotein But Not gp120." *Nature* 345 (1990):622–625.

Boyer, J. D., K. E. Ugen, B. Wang, M. Agadjanyan, L. Gilbert, M. L. Bagaarazzi, M. Chattercoon, P. Front, A. Javadian, W. V. Williams, Y. Refaeli, R. B. Ciccarelli, D. McCallus, L. Coney, and D. B. Weiner. "Protection of Chimpanzees from High-Dose Heterologous HIV-1 Challenge by DNA Vaccination." *Nature Medicine* 3 (May 1997):1–7.

Brundage, J. F., D. S. Burke, L. I. Gardner, J. G. McNeil, M. Goldenbaum, R. Visintine, R. R. Redfield, M. Peterson, and R. N. Miller. "Tracking the Spread of the HIV Infection Epidemic Among Young Adults in the United States: Results of the First Four Years of Screening Among Civilian Applicants for U.S. Military Service." *Journal of AIDS* 3 (1990):1168–1180.

Carney, Desmond N., and Heine H. Hansen, "Editorial: Non-Small-Cell Lung Cancer—Stalemate or Progress?" *New England Journal of Medicine,* October 26, 2000 (343):1261–1263.

Celentano, D. D., K. C. Bond, C. M. Lyles, S. Eiumtrakul, V. F.-L. Go, C. Beyrer, C. Chiangmai, K. E. Nelson, C. Khamboonruang, and D. Vaddhanaphuti. "Preventive Intervention to Reduce Sexually Transmitted Infections: A Field Trial in the Royal Thai Army." *Archives of Internal Medicine* 160 (4) (February 28, 2000):535–540.

Chakrabarti, S., M. Robert-Guroff, F. Wong-Staal, R. C. Gallo, and B. Moss. "Expression of the IITLV-III Envelope Gene by a Recombinant Vaccinia Virus." *Nature* 320 (1986):535–537.

Cohen, Stanley, A. Chang, H. Boyer, and R. Helling. "Construction of Biologically Functional Bacterial Plasmids In Vitro," *Proceedings of the National Academy of Sciences* 70 (November 1973):3240–3244.

Corey, Lawrence, A. J. Nahmias, M. E Guinan, J. K. Bendetti, C. W. Critchlow, and K. K. Holmes. "A Trial of Topical Acyclovir in Genital Herpes Simplex Infections." *New England Journal of Medicine* 306 (1982):1313–1319.

Daar, E. S., X. L. Li, T. Moudgil, and David D. Ho. "High Concentrations of Recombinant CD4 Are Required to Neutralize Primary Human Immunodeficiency Virus Type 1 Isolates." *Proceedings of the National Academy of Sciences* 87 (1990):6547.

Davis, Nancy L., et al., "Attenuation Mutations in the E2 Glycoprotein Gene of Venezuelan Equine Encephalitis Virus: Construction of Single and Multiple Mutants in a Full-Length cDNA Clone." *Virology* 183 (1991):20–31.

Davis, Nancy L., K. Brown, and Robert Johnston. "A Viral Vaccine Vector That Expresses Foreign Genes in Lymph Nodes and Protects Against Mucosal Challenge." *Journal of Virology* 70:3781–3787.

Davis, Nancy L., I. J. Caley, K. W. Brown, M. R. Betts, D. M. Irlbeck, K. M. McGrath, M. J. Connell, D. C. Montefiori, J. A. Frelinger, R. Swanstrom, P. Johnson, and R. E. Johnston. "Vaccination of Macaques Against Pathogenic SIV with VEE Virus Replicon Particles." *Journal of Virology* 74 (January 2000):371–378.

Donnelly, J. J., A. Freidman, D. Martinez, D. L. Montgomery, J. W. Shiver, S. L. Motzel, J. B. Ulmer, and M. A. Liu. "Preclinical Efficacy of a Prototype DNA Vaccine: Enhanced Protection Against Antigenic Drift in Influenza Virus." *Nature Medicine* 1 (6) (June 1995).

Editor's note, in correspondence section, *New England Journal of Medicine*, March 19, 1998 (338):841.

Emini, E. A. "Hurdles in the Path to an HIV-1 Vaccine." *Scientific American Science and Medicine*, May–June 1995:38–47.

Ferrari, G., W. Humphrey, M. J. McElrath, J.-L. Excler, A.-M. Duliege, M. L. Clements, L. C. Corey, D. P. Bolognesi, and K. J. Weinhold. "Clade B-based HIV-1 Vaccines Elicit Cross-Clade Cytotoxic T Lymphocyte Reactivities in Uninfected Volunteers." *Proceedings of the National Academy of Sciences* 94 (February 1997):1396–1401.

Fields, B. N. "AIDS: Time to Turn to Basic Science." *Nature* 369 (1994):95–96.

Gallo, Robert, P. S. Sarin, E. P Gelmann et al. "Isolation of Human T-Cell Leukemia Virus in Acquired Immune Deficiency Syndrome (AIDS)." *Science*, May 20, 1983 (220):865–867.

Graham, B. S., and P. F. Wright. "Candidate AIDS Vaccines." *New England Journal of Medicine*, November 16, 1995 (333):1331–1339.

Hanson, C. V. "Measuring Vaccine-Induced HIV Neutralization: Report of a Workshop." *AIDS Research and Human Retroviruses* 10 (6) (1994):645–648.

Hevey, M., et al. "Marburg Virus Vaccines Based upon Alphavirus Replicons Protect Guinea Pigs and Nonhuman Primates." *Virology* 251 (1998):28–37.

Hu, S.-L., S. G. Kosowski, and J. M. Dalrymple. "Expression of AIDS Virus Envelope Gene in Recombinant Vaccinia Viruses." *Nature* 320 (1986):537–540.

LaRosa, J., J. P. Dande, and K. Weinhold. "Conserved Sequence and Structural Elements in the HIV-1 Principal Neutralizing Determinant." *Science*, August 24, 1990 (249):932.

Levy, J. A., A. D. Hoffman, S. M. Kramer, J. A. Landis, and J. M. Shimabukobo "Isolation of Lymphocytopathic Retroviruses from San Francisco Patients with AIDS." *Science*, August 24, 1984 (225):840–842.

Levy, Jean-Paul. "Letter to the Editor." *Science*, May 8, 1998 (280):803.

Liljestrom, P., and H. Garoff. "A New Generation of Animal Cell Expression Vectors Based on the Semliki Forest Virus Replicon." *Bio/Technology* 9 (1991):1356–1361.

Luciw, P. A., S. J. Potter, K. Steimer, and D. Dina. "Molecular Cloning of AIDS-Associated Retrovirus." *Nature* 312 (1984):760–763.

Lurie, P., and S. M. Wolfe. "Sounding Board: Unethical Trials of Interventions to Reduce Perinatal Transmission of the Human Immunodeficiency Virus in Developing Countries." *New England Journal of Medicine*, September 18, 1997 (337):853–856.

Mascola, J. R., J. G. McNeil, and D. S. Burke. "AIDS Vaccines: Are We Ready for Human Efficacy Trials?" *Journal of the American Medical Association*, August 10, 1994 (272):488–489.

Mastro, Timothy D., and Isabelle de Vincenzi. "Probabilities of Sexual HIV-1 Transmission." *AIDS* 10 (1996):S75–S82.

Matthews, T. J. "Tenth Anniversary Perspective on AIDS: Dilemma of Neutralization Resistance of HIV-1 Field Isolates and Vaccine Development." *AIDS Research and Human Retroviruses* 10 (6) (1994):631–632.

McCutchan, F. E., P. A. Hegerich, T. P. Brenna, P. Pharnuphak, P. Singharaj, A. Jugsudee, P. W. Berman, A. M. Gray, A. K. Fowler, and D. S. Burke. "Genetic Variants of HIV-1 in Thailand." *AIDS Research and Human Retroviruses* 8 (1992):1887–1895.

McDonnell, W. M., and F. K. Askari. "Molecular Medicine: DNA Vaccines." *New England Journal of Medicine*, January 4, 1996 (334):42–45.

McElrath, M. J., R. F. Siliciano, and K. J. Weinhold. "HIV Type 1 Vaccine-Induced Cytotoxic T Cell Responses in Phase I Clinical Trials: Detection, Characterization, and Quantification." *AIDS Research and Human Retroviruses* 13 (3) (1997):211–216.

McNeil, J. G., J. F. Brundage, Z. F. Wann, D. S. Burke, R. N. Miller, and the Walter Reed Retrovirus Research Group. "Direct Measurement of Human Immunodeficiency Virus Seroconversions in a Serially Tested Population of Young Adults in the United States Army, October 1985 to October 1987." *New England Journal of Medicine*, June 15, 1989 (320):1581–1585.

Murthy, K. K., E. K. Cobb, S. R. Rouse, H. M. McClure, J. S. Payne, M. T. Salas, and G. R. Michalek. "Active and Passive Immunization Against HIV Type A Infection in Chimpanzees." *AIDS Research and Human Retroviruses* 14 (S3) (1998):S271–276.

Panicali, D., S. W. Davis, R. L. Weinberg, and E. Paoletti. "Construction of Live Vaccines by Using Genetically Engineered Poxviruses: Biological Activity of Recombinant Vaccinia Virus Expressing Influenza Virus Hemagglutinin. *Proceedings of the National Academy of Sciences* 80 (1983):5364–5368.

Panicali, D., S. W. Davis, S. R. Mercer, and E. Paoletti. "Two Major DNA Variants Present in Serially Propagated Stocks of the WR Strain of Vaccinia Virus." *Journal of Virology* 42 (1981):734–741.

Panicali, D., and E. Paoletti. "Construction of Poxviruses as Cloning Vectors: Insertion of the Thymidine Kinase Gene from Herpes Simplex Virus into the DNA of Infectious Vaccinia Virus." *Proceedings of the National Academy of Sciences* 79 (1982):4927–4931.

Paoletti, E., B. R. Pipinskas, C. Adamsonoff, S. Mercer, and D. Panicali. "Construction of Live Vaccines Using Genetically Engineered Poxviruses: Biological Activity of Vaccinia Virus Recombinants Expressing the Hepatitis B Virus Surface Antigen and the Herpes Simplex Virus Glycoprotein E." *Proceedings of the National Academy of Sciences* 81 (1984):193–197.

Perkus, Marion E., A. Piccini, B. R. Lipinskas, and E. Paoletti. "Recombinant Vaccinia Virus: Immunization Against Multiple Pathogens." *Science,* September 6, 1985 (229):981–984.

Phanuphak, Praphan. "Occasional Notes: Ethical issues in Studies in Thailand of the Vertical Transmission of HIV." *New England Journal of Medicine,* March 19, 1998 (338):834.

Pushko, P., et al. "Replicon-Helper Systems from Attenuated Heterologous Pathogens In Vivo." *Virology* 239 (1997):389–401.

Redfield, R. R., D. C. Wright, and E. C. Tramont. "The Walter Reed Staging Classification for HTLV-III, LAV Infection." *New England Journal of Medicine* 314 (1986):131–132.

Richmond, Douglas D. "HIV Therapeutics." *Science,* June 28, 1996 (272):1887.

Schultz, A. M., and Shiu-Lok Hu. "Primate Models for HIV Vaccines." *AIDS* 7 (S1) (1993):S161–S170.

Tang, D., M. DeVit, and S. A. Johnston. "Genetic Immunization Is a Simple Method for Eliciting an Immune Response." *Nature* 356 (1992):152–154.

Ulmer, J. B., J. J. Donnelly, S. E. Parker, G. H. Rhodes, P. L Felgner, V. J. Swarkl, S. H. Gromkowski, R. R. Deck, C. M. DeWitt, A. Friedman, L. A. Hawe, K. R. Leander, D. Martinez, H. C. Perry, J. W. Shiver, D L. Montgomery, and M. A. Liu. "Heterologous Protective Immunity to Influenza A by Inramuscular Injection of DNA Encoding a Conserved Viral Protein." *Science,* March 19, 1993 (259):1745–1749.

Valenzuela, P., et al. "Synthesis and Assembly of Hepatitis B Virus Surface Antigen Particles in Yeast." *Nature* 298 (1982):347–350.

Various authors. "Correspondence: Ethics of Placebo-Controlled Trials of Zidovudine to Prevent the Perinatal Transmission of HIV in the Third World." *New England Journal of Medicine,* March 19, 1998 (338):836–844.

Varmus, H., and D. Satcher. "Sounding Board: Ethical Complexities of Conducting Research in Developing Countries." *New England Journal of Medicine,* October 2, 1997 (337):1003–1005.

Wang, B., D. B. Weiner et al. "Gene Inoculation Generates Immune Responses Against Human Immunodeficiency Virus Type 1." *Proceedings of the National Academy of Sciences* 90 (1993):4156–4160.

Weniger, B. G., K. Limpakarnjanarat, K. Ungchusak et al. "The Epidemiology of HIV Infection and AIDS in Thailand." *AIDS* 5 (1991):S71–S85.

Wolff, J. A., R. W. Malone, P. Williams, W. Chong, G. Acsadi, A. Jani, and P. L. Felgner. "Direct Gene Transfer into Mouse Muscle In Vivo." *Science,* March 23, 1990 (247):1465–1468.

Wong-Staal, F., and R. C. Gallo. "The Family of Human T-Lymphotrophic Leukemia Viruses: HTLV-I as the Cause of Adult T Cell Leukemia and HTLV-III as the Cause of Acquired Immunodeficiency Syndrome." *Blood* 65 (February 1985):253–263.

OTHER DOCUMENTS

AFRIMS-RIHES Vaccine Evaluation Group (ARVEG). "ARVEG V6P17 Protocol: Recruitment and Safety Data," n.d., probably late 1996–early 1997.

"AIDS Research: Which Institutions Are Most Productive and Influential?" *Scientist*, October 18, 1993 (7):14.

AIDS Vaccine Advocacy Coalition. *8 Years and Counting: What Will Speed Development of an AIDS Vaccine?* Washington, DC: AVAC, May 1999.

———. *9 Years and Counting: Will We Have an AIDS Vaccine by 2007?* San Francisco: AVAC, May 1998.

Allison, Malorye. "AIDS Therapy: Combating HIV in the Nineties." *Harvard Health Letter*, September 1991.

Altman, Lawrence K. "AIDS Experts Leave Journal After Studies Are Criticized." *New York Times*, October 15, 1997.

———. "AIDS Now Seen as a Worldwide Health Problem." *New York Times*, November 29, 1983.

———. "The Doctor's World: A Setback in Hunt for AIDS Vaccine." *New York Times*, June 28, 1994.

———. "The Doctor's World: After setback, first AIDS vaccine trials are planned. Even a weak vaccine would help slow the epidemic," *New York Times*, November 29, 1994.

———. "The Doctor's World: Combination Strategy Reinvigorates Search for AIDS Vaccine." *New York Times*, February 26, 1996.

———. "The Doctor's World: Discussing Possible AIDS Cure Raises Hope, Anger and Question: What Exactly Is Meant by 'Cure'?" *New York Times*, July 16, 1996.

———. "FDA Authorizes First Full Testing for HIV Vaccine. Results Due in 4 Years. Experiment Will Be Conducted on Volunteers in Thailand and in North America." *New York Times*, June 4, 1998.

———. "Panel Rejects Wider Testing to Develop AIDS Vaccine." *New York Times*, June 18, 1994.

———. "U.N. Reports 3 Million New HIV Cases Worldwide for '96." *New York Times*, November 27, 1996.

———. "Vaccine Protects Two Chimps from AIDS." *New York Times*, April 30, 1997.

"American Home Products Buys Biotechnology Concern." Bloomberg News, *New York Times*, May 12, 1998.

"Apollon, Inc. Is Another Early-Stage Biotech Company Jumping on the IPO Bandwagon . . . " *Genetic Engineering News*, November 1, 1997:25.

"Apollon Will Offer 2.5 Mil Shares, with Proceeds Being Used for Research and Development." *Going Public: The IPO Reporter*, November 24, 1997 (21):10.

Armstrong, Larry. "Besting AIDS and the Drug Giants." *Business Week*, June 9, 1997.

Arnold, David. "Another Look at History Spurs Drive to Rename Amherst." *Boston Globe*, March 6, 2000.

"Axelrod Stricken While in Washington." United Press International, February 26, 1991.

Bain, Lisa. "Therapeutic AIDS Vaccine Clinical Trial Begins at Penn." Press release from University of Pennsylvania Medical Center, June 16, 1995.

Baltimore, David. "Fighting with HIV While It Fights Back." Presentation at National Cooperative Vaccine Development Groups, May 4, 1997. Author's transcript.

———. Interview with Christopher Lydon on *The Connection.* National Public Radio, January 22, 1997. Author's transcript.

Bernstein, Karen. "1995 Was a Very Fine Year: Performance Pays Off." *BioCentury,* January 2, 1996.

Bhatiasevi, Aphaluck. "Researcher Warns over Vaccine Trials." *Bangkok Post,* May 17, 1997.

Bloom, Barry R., and José Esparza. Letter to Professor Natth Bhamarapravati with attachments (UNAIDS panel's review of gp120), dated July 28, 1997.

Boffey, Philip M. "Campaign to Find Drugs for Fighting AIDS Is Intensified." *New York Times,* February 14, 1988.

Borman, Stu. "Criteria May Speed AIDS Vaccine Development." *Chemical and Engineering News,* February 19, 1996:9.

Bramarapravati, Natth. Letter to José Esparza, confirming receipt of gp120 panel review, dated July 31, 1997.

"Bristol-Myers and Genetic Systems Announce Merger Transaction." PR Newswire, New York, October 23, 1985.

Brown, David. "Pentagon May Hold Up AIDS Study Funds; Breast Cancer Research." *Washington Post,* February 10, 1995.

Brown, David, and Benjamin Weiser. "HIV Infections Cast Pall over Expanding Vaccine Experiments." *Washington Post,* May 30, 1994.

Brown, Phyllida. "Protein Therapy 'Stimulates Antibodies.'" *New Scientist,* August 1, 1992:8.

———. "Sex and Drugs Spread Different Types of HIV." *New Scientist,* July 25, 1992:6.

Burke, Donald S. "Uncertainties and Risks in HIV Vaccine R&D: The Case for 'Thoughtful Empiricism.'" Lecture at WHO Consultative Meeting on Scientific and Public Health Rationale for HIV Vaccine Efficacy Trials, Geneva, October 13–14, 1994.

Caldwell, Mark, "The Dream Vaccine." *Discover* (September 1997):86.

Centers for Disease Control. "AIDS Weekly Surveillance Report—United States." December 28, 1987.

———. "HIV/AIDS Surveillance Report." January 1989.

———. "HIV/AIDS Surveillance Report. US. HIV and AIDS Cases Reported Through December 1993." Year-end edition, vol. 5, no. 4, released March 1994.

———. "Kaposi's Sarcoma and *Pneumocystis* Pneumonia Among Homosexual Men—New York and California." *Morbidity and Mortality Weekly Report,* July 3, 1981 (30):305–308.

———. "*Pneumocystis* Pneumonia—Los Angeles." *Morbidity and Mortality Weekly Report,* June 5, 1981 (30):250–252.

Chase, Marilyn. "Demand for MS Drug May Help Chiron Corp. Emerge from the Pack." *Wall Street Journal,* September 1, 1993.

Chiron Corporation. Annual Report, 1994. Emeryville, February 1995.

————. "Chiron Announces Plans to Close St. Louis, Missouri, Manufacturing Site." Press release, March 5, 1998.

————. "Chiron Completes Acquisition of Vaccines Business from Hoechst AG." Press release, April 1, 1998.

————. "A Subunit Approach to Vaccination Against HIV." RFP #90-015, Department of Health Services, submitted January 31, 1990.

Chiron Corp. v. Abbott Laboratories (22300/4), U.S. District of California/Northern District. Deposition of Paul Luciw, taken in January and May 1995.

"Chiron Stock Falls as Tender Offer Is Completed." Reuters, *New York Times*, January 5, 1995.

Clements, Mary Lou. "Historical Perspectives on Vaccine Development." Notes for presentation at meeting of the Vaccine Working Group, April 21–22, 1994.

Clinton, William J. "Commencement Address at Morgan State University." Office of the press secretary, the White House, May 18, 1997.

Cohen, Jon. "Army Investigates Researcher's Report of Clinical Trial Data." *Science*, November 6, 1992 (258):883.

————. "Congress Plays Doctor; How Come Capitol Hill Is Choosing a New AIDS Vaccine?" *Washington Post, Outlook*, November 1, 1992.

————. "The HIV Vaccine Paradox." *Science*, May 20, 1994 (264):1072.

————. "Looking for Lin HIV's Battle with Immune System." *Science*, May 23, 1997 (276):1196–1197.

————. "New AIDS Chief Takes Charge." *Science*, March 11, 1994 (263):1364–1366.

————. "NIH Panel OKs Vaccine Test—in a New Form." *Science*, December 4, 1992 (258):1569.

————. "Trials Set in High-Risk Populations" *Science*, December 11, 1992 (258):1729.

————. "Will Media Reports KO Upcoming Real-Life Trials?" *Science*, June 17, 1994 (264):1660.

Collins, Huntly. "Bill Gates Donates $25 Million for AIDS." *Philadelphia Inquirer*, May 4, 1999.

————. "Trials of AIDS Vaccine Get Started in Phila. It's the First Vaccine to Undergo Large-Scale Testing. Researchers Don't Give It Much Chance." *Philadelphia Inquirer*, June 24, 1998.

Crewdson, John. "The Great AIDS Quest." *Chicago Tribune*, November 19, 1989 (special section).

————. "New Doubts on AIDS Vaccine; 5 Study Volunteers Infected; U.S. Debates Future of Trials." *Chicago Tribune*, May 29, 1994.

Cross, Jeannie H., "Audit Blasts Health Officials for Conflicts of Interest, Cheating State." United Press International, December 27, 1989.

D'Adesky, Anne-Christine. "The AIDS Dream Team." *Out* (February 1997):72.

————. "Dr. Baltimore's Vaccine Dreams." *Out* (April 1997):33.

DAIDS. AVEG. "Outline of Protocol 202." N.d.

————. "AVEG Protocol Activity Overview Chart." April 1997.

———. "Guidelines of Clinical and Research Data Which Will Facilitate the Decision-Making Process for Entry of Candidate Vaccines into Pivotal Phase III Efficacy Trials." Draft, April 28, 1993, and finished document, September 1993.

———. "Guidelines for Entry of HIV Vaccines into Efficacy Trials in Uninfected Volunteers." Draft B, February 15, 1993.

———. "A Phase III Trial to Evaluate the Efficacy of Candidate HIV Vaccine(s), Clinical Trial Sponsored by the Vaccine Trials and Epidemiology Branch, DAIDS, NIAID, NIH, Bethesda, MD." Draft April 1, 1993.

———. "Shell Protocol. A Phase III Trial to Evaluate the Efficacy of Candidate HIV Vaccine(s)." Draft, April 28, 1993.

———. "Table 1: AIDS Vaccine Candidates Studied by the AVEG." May 1997.

———.Draft, October 19, 1993, and draft, October 25, 1993.

———. "Trial Design Team." May 3, 1994.

"DAIDS Vaccine Briefing." Minutes of a meeting on March 23, 1993.

Deer, Brian. "His Vaccine Could Go into Millions of People. But It Could Be One of Medicine's Greatest Mistakes." *Sunday Times* (London), October 3, 1999.

DeNoon, Daniel J. "Merck Pledges Aggressive Development of HIV DNA vaccine." *Vaccine Weekly,* June 23, 1997.

Douglas, R. Gordon. "May 21, 1997, Remarks of R. Gordon Douglas, MD, President, Merck Vaccines, Merck & Co., Inc., Congressional Task Force on International HIV/AIDS, Briefing on AIDS Vaccines." Merck Public Affairs.

Eaton, Leslie, "Desperate in 1995, a Small City's Fortunes Rebound Sharply." *New York Times,* August 28, 2000.

"Editorial: A Vaccine for AIDS—New Goal for Science." *San Francisco Chronicle,* May 20, 1997.

Emmes Corporation. "Redline Version, Proposed Protocol 016A Consent Form." May 20, 1994.

Fast, Patricia, "Clinical Research Update." Handout for June 17, 1994, ARAC meeting.

———. "Memo to Interested Individuals, on AIDS Vaccine Trial News." June 2, 1994.

———. NIH letter to principal investigators, June 1, 1994.

———. "Note to Jack Killen." N.d., probably March–April 1995.

Fast, Patricia, and William Snow. "HIV Vaccine Development—an Overview." Essay posted on the American Medical Association Rx Treatment Center web site, March 25, 1997.

Fauci, Anthony S. "The AIDS Paradigm: Scientific and Policy Lessons for the 21st Century." Lecture at Annual Meeting of the Institute of Human Virology, Baltimore, August 30, 1999, author's transcription.

———. "Introductory Remarks for NIH National Collaborative Vaccine Development Group Meeting." May 4, 1997, Bethesda, MD. Author's transcript.

———. Text of opening statement for June 17, 1994, ARAC meeting, plus copies of slides accompanying presentation.

Feiffer, Jules. Untitled cartoon. Universal Press Syndicate, 1985.

Felgner, Philip L. "Nonviral Strategies for Gene Therapy." *Scientific American,* June 1997.

Fettner, Ann Giudici, with Pat Thomas. "Big Doings in Hotlanta." *New York Native*, April 1985.

Fisher, Lawrence M. "Genentech: Survivor Strutting Its Stuff." *New York Times*, October 1, 2000.

Foster, Sam. "Apollon Inc." *Venture Capital Journal*, February 1, 1998.

"$4.2 Million for Apollon AIDS Vaccine." SCRIP No. 1967 (October 18, 1994):16.

Fox, Maggie. "AIDS Vaccine Goes into Final Trials in People." Reuters, June 3, 1998.

Francis, Don. Cover letter to L. Barker, Clinical Research Program, DAIDS, May 20, 1994. Enclosure: "Design Proposal for a Large Simple Efficacy Trial of HIV Preventative Vaccines." Genentech, Inc., May 19, 1994.

Fried, Stephen. "Cocktail Hour." *Washington Post Magazine*, May 18, 1997.

Genentech Annual Report, 1996. On-line version. Chart showing revenues for 1994, 1995, 1996.

Gershon, Diane. "Chiron Buys Hoechst Vaccine Interest." *Nature Medicine* 2 (April 1996):370.

———. "Genentech Sheds gp120 Vaccine." *Nature Medicine* 2 (April 1996):370.

Gladwell, Malcolm. "A Divergent Strategy in the War on AIDS: Vaccines Can Help the Body Win, Some Say." *Washington Post*, July 20, 1992.

Gold, David, and Sam Averett. "HIV DNA Vaccines Move Slowly into Clinical Trials." *IAVI Report* (3) (July–September 1998):1.

Gorman, Christine, et al. "Man of the Year" package. *Time*, December 30, 1996–January 6, 1997, 52–87.

Green, Jesse. "Who Put the Lid on gp120?" *New York Times Magazine*, March 26, 1995.

Hamilton, Joan O'C. "Jealousy, Money, Power: A Biotech Marriage Breaks Up." *Business Week*, July 21, 1986.

Heberlein, Greg. "Biotech's New ICOS Starts Big." *Seattle Times*, July 3, 1990.

Hoff, Rod. "HIV Vaccine Trial Design." Handout for June 17, 1994, meeting of ARAC and NIAID Council.

"Hundreds at AIDS Talks Protest Reagan Policy." *Boston Globe*, June 6, 1987.

"In Memoriam: Bernard Fields: Scientist, Mentor, Visionary." *Focus: News from Harvard Medical, Dental and Public Health Schools*. February 3, 1995, 1.

"Industry News/Joint Venture Research Agreement Signed to Collaborate in Vaccine Field. ANRS, Pasteur Mérieux and Connaught Extend HIV Vaccine Collaboration for 1995 and 1996." *Vaccine Weekly*, April 17, 1995.

"An Interview with Margaret Liu." *IAVI Report* (3) (July–September 1998):1.

"Investors Sought for AIDS Vaccine Trials." *Science*, March 1, 1996 (271):1237.

"Is Chiron on the Verge of a Biotech Breakthrough?" *Business Week*, June 4, 1990.

Iwata, Edward. "Net IPOs Ride a Bay Area Wave." *San Francisco Examiner*, July 4, 1999.

Johnson, Hillary J. "Dr. David Ho and the Lazarus Equation." *Rolling Stone*, March 6, 1997.

Johnston, Peggy. "Note to Tony Fauci, Through Acting Director, DAIDS." October 18, 1993.

"Kathelyn Sue Steimer, 48, AIDS Researcher." *New York Times*, November 24, 1996.

"Key Lobbyist Wins AIDS Vaccine Trials." Associated Press, *New York Times,* October 20, 1992.

Killen, Jack. Handouts on restructuring of clinical trials networks, distributed at AIDS Research Advisory Committee meeting, June 2, 1998, Bethesda, MD.

King, Ralph T. "FDA Allows Large-Scale Trial of AIDS Vaccine." *Wall Street Journal,* June 3, 1998.

Kitayaporn, Dwip. Personal communication on the text of the consent form for Phase III VaxGen trial in Thailand. March 2, 1999.

Knox, Richard A., "Researcher Urges Early Use of Imperfect AIDS Vaccines." *Boston Globe,* July 22, 1992.

———. "Scientists Encouraged by Test of AIDS Vaccine in Chimps." *Boston Globe,* April 30, 1997.

———. "Vaccine Seen Promising in Early Stages of AIDS." *Boston Globe,* October 17, 1989.

Kolata, Gina. "Maker of an AIDS Vaccine Says Test Found No Benefit." *New York Times,* April 19, 1996.

———. "Recent Setbacks Stirring Doubts About Search for AIDS Vaccine," third of four articles in series "AIDS: Confronting the Epidemic." *New York Times,* February 16, 1988.

———. "Saying Strategy to Find Cure for AIDS Has Gone Awry, Researchers Seek Redirection." *New York Times,* May 12, 1994.

Kunanusont, Chaiyos, and Vipa Thiamchai. "Lessons from HIV Vaccine Development in Thailand." Handout prepared for Session V of workshop, "HIV Vaccines for Developing Countries: Prioritizing Vaccine Candidates for Human Trials," sponsored by the Harvard AIDS Institute, Dedham, MA, October 4–7, 1999.

Leary, Warren. "Nobel Laureate to Head Panel Pushing for AIDS Vaccine." *New York Times,* December 13, 1996.

Leder, Phillip, and Patricia Thomas. "Making Drugs from DNA." *Harvard Health Letter,* Special Supplement, July 1994.

Levine Committee. "NIH AIDS Research Program Evaluation. Vaccine Research and Development Area Review Panel, Findings and Recommendations." NIH, March 13, 1996.

———. "Report of the NIH AIDS Research Program Evaluation Working Group of the Office of AIDS Research Advisory Council." NIH, March 13, 1996.

Lewthwaite, Gilbert A. "Clinton Moves to Save Research Projects." *Baltimore Sun,* February 11, 1995.

———. "Dozens of 'Nondefense' Pentagon Programs Fall Under Scrutiny." *Baltimore Sun,* February 3, 1995.

Maccoby, Michael. "Narcissistic Leaders: The Incredible Pros, the Inevitable Cons." *Harvard Business Review,* January–February 2000.

MacIlwain, Colin. "MicroGeneSys Drops Out of NIH Trial for AIDS Vaccine." *Nature,* March 25, 1993 (362):277.

Matthews, Jessica. "Pork-Barrel Research." Editorial, *Washington Post,* November 2, 1992.

Maugh, Thomas H., Marlene Cimons, and John-Thor Dahlburg. "Can Clinton Kick Quest for AIDS Vaccine into Gear?" *Los Angeles Times,* May 25, 1997.

McFadden, Robert D. "David Axelrod, Health Chief Under Cuomo, Is Dead at 59." *New York Times,* July 5, 1994.

McKenna, M.A.J. "AIDS Scientists Regroup." *Atlanta Journal and Constitution,* February 1, 1998.

McNeil, John, "Proposal for *Your Organization*—Military Medical Consortium for Applied Retroviral Research Cooperative Research, Development, Testing and Evaluation of HIV-1 Prophylactic Vaccines: Thailand." Draft of a letter, June 1993.

Meier, Barry. "Political Battle over an AIDS Drug." *New York Times,* November 2, 1993.

———. "Scientists Assail Congress on Bill for Money to Test an AIDS Drug." *New York Times,* October 26, 1992.

Merck. News release. "Fact Sheet" (on the West Point site). October 1, 1997.

Merck & Co. "Annual Report 1996."

"Mérieux, State of NY Fund Virogenetics to Develop Poly-Vaccines." *Biotechnology Newswatch,* March 3, 1986

Milburn, Karen. "Management Shakeup at Biotech Star ICOS." *Seattle Times,* September 28, 1991.

Ministry of Public Health, Thailand. Agenda for Thai HIV Vaccine Scientific Subcommittee meeting, February 11–13, 1998, Siam City Hotel, fax from Dr. Praphan Pranuphak, dated January 19, 1998.

"MIT Laureate to Head AIDS Vaccine Search." Reuters, *Boston Globe,* December 13, 1996.

Mitchell, Alison. "Clinton Calls for AIDS Vaccine as Goal." *New York Times,* May 19, 1997.

Moses, Phyllis. "Vaccinia Virus: Reinventing the Wheel." *BioScience* 36 (3) (March 1986):148–150.

"New York State Weighs Venture to Market Vaccine." *New York Times,* October 30, 1983.

NIAID. "HIV Infection in Vaccine Trial Volunteers." Press release, dated June 6, 1994.

———. Official transcript of joint meeting of the AIDS Subcommittee of the National Advisory Allergy and Infectious Diseases Council and the AIDS Research Advisory Committee, June 17, 1994. Obtained May 1997.

———. Official seating chart for joint meeting of the AIDS Subcommittee of the National Advisory Allergy and Infectious Diseases Council and the AIDS Research Advisory Committee, June 17, 1994.

———. Press release. "NIAID Collaborates with VaxGen on Vaccine studies," August 18, 1998.

———. "Scientific Review Supports Expanded Clinical Studies of Two Candidate HIV Vaccines." Press release, dated April 29, 1994.

NIAID, DAIDS, HIV Vaccine Working Group, April 21–22, 1994. Draft agenda, April 18, 1994.

———. Meeting summary (draft), May 1994.

———. List of participants.

NIH. "NIH Plan to Implement Recommendations of the NIH AIDS Research Program Evaluation Task Force." August 1997.

NIH Office of AIDS Research. NIH Total AIDS Dollars and Expenditures for Vaccine Development and Vaccine Clinical Trials, FY 1989–98, personal communication from Stan Katzman, received 13 September 1999.

"N.Y. State Touts Vaccines for Herpes, Hepatitis, Flu, All Still on Drawing Board." *Biotechnology Newswatch*, November 7, 1983.

Panetta, Leon. Letter to William J. Perry, February 10, 1995. US Newswire.

"Pasteur Mérieux-Connaught Signs a Research Agreement with the ANRS." Canada NewsWire, April 6, 1995.

Petit, Charles. "AIDS Experts Dubious About 10-Year Target." *San Francisco Chronicle*, May 20, 1997.

"Price Waterhouse LLP Venture Capital Survey, Second Quarter 1996." Published August 19, 1996, *Mercury Center-San Jose Mercury News*.

Priest, Dana. "'Non-Defense' Projects Targeted; Pentagon Supports Some, Not All, Against GOP Attack." *Washington Post*, February 10, 1995.

Ranii, David. "Company Sets Sights on Vaccines." *Raleigh News and Observer*, January 22, 1998.

Rao, Kavitha. "A Large HIV-Vaccine Trial in Thailand Presents Ethical Dilemmas." *Asia-Week*, May 7, 1999.

Richardson, Sarah. "Crushing HIV." *Discover*, January 27, 1997.

Ross, Sonya. "Clinton Targets an AIDS Vaccine Date." *Boston Globe*, May 19, 1997.

Saba, Joseph, and Arthur Ammann. "A Cultural Divide on AIDS Research: American Values, African Realities." *New York Times*, September 20, 1997.

Saltus, Richard. "MIT Laureate to Lead Caltech." *Boston Globe*, May 14, 1997.

Sanford, David. "Back to a Future: One Man's AIDS Tale Shows How Quickly Epidemic Has Turned." *Wall Street Journal*, November 8, 1996.

Saxon, Wolfgang. "Mary Lou Clements-Mann, 51, an Expert on AIDS Vaccines. *New York Times*, September 4, 1998.

Schmeck, Harold M. "AIDS Researchers Begin Testing New Version of Smallpox Vaccine." *New York Times*, April 10, 1986.

Schmidt, William E. "British Paper and Science Journal Clash on AIDS." *New York Times*, December 10, 1993.

Schrader, Ann. "Major Test Next for HIV Vaccine. Denver to Take Part in Trial of Inoculation That Has Its Skeptics." *Denver Post*, June 3, 1998.

Schultz, Alan M. "Preclinical Research Update." Presented at the June 17, 1994, ARAC meeting.

Schwartz, John, "Pentagon Drops Plan to Test an AIDS Vaccine; Health Officials Had Opposed Single-Drug Trial." *Washington Post*, January 23, 1994.

Seacrist, Lisa. "A Dose of DNA to Fight Influenza Virus." *Science News*, June 3, 1995:343.

Sheon, Amy. "Vaccine Feasibility Research." Presented at the June 17, 1994, ARAC meeting.

"Smallpox Vaccine Assigned New Job." *Science News,* November 5, 1982.

Smith, Paul. "Army, Navy Differ in Policies on Homosexual AIDS Patients." *Army Times,* August 26, 1985.

———. "On-Base Blood Banks to Tell Military If AIDS Virus Found." *Army Times,* August 26, 1985.

Snow, Bill. "In Memory" (AVAC response to the death of Mary Lou Clements-Mann). September 15, 1998, Washington, DC.

Squires, Sally. "Army to Test AIDS Drug Despite Objections; NIH and FDA Urged That Clinical Trial Include Other Therapeutic Vaccines." *Washington Post,* April 7, 1993.

———. "Bowing to Pressure, Defense Dept. Agrees to Drop AIDS Vaccine Test." *Washington Post,* April 15, 1993.

Stephenson, Joan, "Fighting Infectious Disease Threats Via Research: A Talk with Anthony S. Fauci." *Journal of the American Medical Association,* January 17, 1996 (275):173–174.

Sternberg, Steve. "A Shot in the Dark: Prototypes Attack Virus on All Fronts." *USA Today,* May 22, 1997.

Stolberg, Sheryl Gay. "U.S. AIDS Research in Poor Nations Raises an Outcry. Some Call It Unethical. Comparisons with a Syphilis Study Arise Because Some Do Not Get Therapy." *New York Times,* September 18, 1997.

Stone, Richard. "DOD to Single Out MicroGeneSys Vaccine." *Science,* April 2, 1993.

Strow, David. "AlphaVax Touts New Model for Biotech Firms." *Triangle Business Journal,* February 27, 1998:5.

Sullivan, Andrew. "When Plagues End: Notes on the Twilight of an Epidemic." *New York Times Magazine,* November 10, 1996.

Sullivan, Ronald, "Researchers Are Hailed as New Genetics Breed." *New York Times,* October 19, 1983.

"Syntex: Bristol-Myers Joins Syntex and Genetic Systems in Oncogen Joint Venture." *Business Wire,* February 7, 1985.

Taubes, Gary. "Busting the Fraud-Busters." *Discover* (January 1997):76.

———. "Immunology: Salvation in a Snippet of DNA?" *Science,* December 5, 1997.

Thaitawat, Nusara. "On the Right Track. VaxGen Inc's HIV Vaccine Trial Launched in Bangkok Last Month Was a Breakthrough in the Battle Against AIDS." *Medicine* (Thailand), April 1999.

Thomas, Patricia. "The Montreal Conference: Warnings of Things to Come." *Medical World News,* July 24, 1989:40–49.

———. "Top Ten Medical Advances of 1995." *Harvard Health Letter* (March 1996):1.

Thongchoroen, Prasert, MD. Letter from the THAIVEG Consortium to Dr. Anthony Fauci, NIAID. June 1994.

Travis, John. "DNA Vaccine Set to Tackle HIV Infection." *Science News,* February 17, 1996:100.

"Triple-Valent Vaccine Spliced Against Herpes, Influenza, Hepatitis." *Biotechnology Newswatch,* September 16, 1985.

United States Army Medical Research and Materiel Command. Walter Reed Army Institute of Research. *Entering a 2nd Century of Research for the Soldier.* 1997. Booklet.

United States Military HIV Research Program. *Leading the Battle Against HIV.* N.d. Booklet.

Various authors. Special edition of *Science Times* devoted to sequencing of the human genome. *New York Times,* June 27, 2000.

VaxGen and Bangkok Vaccine Evaluation Group. "World's First Large-Scale Trial for Preventive HIV Vaccine Enrolled in Developing Country." Press release, August 31, 2000.

"VaxGen Vaccine Trial Gets $8 Million in U.S. Government Funding." Bloomberg News Service, October 19, 1999.

"VaxGen, Inc. Announces Initial Public Offering of 3,100,000 Shares of Common Stock." Business Wire, June 30, 1999.

Wallis, Claudia. "Brave New Vaccines: A New Gene-Spliced Injection Promises a Cheap, Effective Way to Combat Herpes, Hepatitis and the Flu." *Health* (March 1984).

Weiss, Rick, "AIDS Prevention as Global Mission: Vaccine Hunter Mixes Science, Diplomacy." *Washington Post,* August 19, 1999.

———. "Large-Scale Test of AIDS Vaccine Set." *Washington Post,* June 4, 1998.

Weiner, D. B., and R. C. Kennedy. "Genetic Vaccines." *Scientific American* (July 1999).

Weniger, Bruce G., and Max Essex. "Clearing the Way for an AIDS Vaccine." *New York Times,* January 4, 1997.

WHO Global Programme on AIDS. "Expert Group Concludes Vaccine Trials Can Go Forward." Note to correspondents, October 14, 1994.

———. List of participants. Meeting on scientific and public health rationale for HIV vaccine efficacy trials, Geneva, October 13–14, 1994.

Wolinsky, Steven M., and David D. Ho. Letter to Dr. Praphan Phanuphak, dated April 4, 1997, with transmittal memo from Phanuphak to Dr. Kachit Choopanya, deputy governor of Bangkok, dated April 18, 1997.

Wyeth-Ayerst Laboratories. "Wyeth-Lederle Acquires Apollon, Inc.—Gains Access to Biotechnology Tools for Expansion of Vaccine Research Opportunities." Press release, dated May 11, 1998.

INDEX

PUBLICAFFAIRS is a new nonfiction publishing house and a tribute to the standards, values, and flair of three persons who have served as mentors to countless reporters, writers, editors, and book people of all kinds, including me.

I. F. STONE, proprietor of *I. F. Stone's Weekly*, combined a commitment to the First Amendment with entrepreneurial zeal and reporting skill and became one of the great independent journalists in American history. At the age of eighty, Izzy published *The Trial of Socrates*, which was a national bestseller. He wrote the book after he taught himself ancient Greek.

BENJAMIN C. BRADLEE was for nearly thirty years the charismatic editorial leader of *The Washington Post*. It was Ben who gave the *Post* the range and courage to pursue such historic issues as Watergate. He supported his reporters with a tenacity that made them fearless, and it is no accident that so many became authors of influential, best-selling books.

ROBERT L. BERNSTEIN, the chief executive of Random House for more than a quarter century, guided one of the nation's premier publishing houses. Bob was personally responsible for many books of political dissent and argument that challenged tyranny around the globe. He is also the founder and was the longtime chair of Human Rights Watch, one of the most respected human rights organizations in the world.

. . .

For fifty years, the banner of Public Affairs Press was carried by its owner Morris B. Schnapper, who published Gandhi, Nasser, Toynbee, Truman, and about 1,500 other authors. In 1983 Schnapper was described by *The Washington Post* as "a redoubtable gadfly." His legacy will endure in the books to come.

Peter Osnos, *Publisher*